THE ARTERIAL SYSTEM IN HYPERTENSION

Developments in Cardiovascular Medicine

VOLUME 144

The titles published in this series are listed at the end of this volume.

The Arterial System in Hypertension

edited by

Michel E. Safar
Professor of Therapeutics, Broussais-Hôtel Dieu, Paris, France

and

Michael F. O'Rourke
Professor of Medicine, University of New South Wales, St. Vincent's Hospital, Sydney, Australia

Springer-Science+Business Media, B.V.

Library of Congress Cataloging-in-Publication Data

The Arterial system in hypertension / edited by Michel E. Safar and
  Michael F. O'Rourke.
       p.   cm. -- (Developments in cardiovascular medicine ; v. 144)
    Includes index.
    ISBN 978-0-7923-2343-3   ISBN 978-94-011-0900-0 (eBook)
    DOI 10.1007/978-94-011-0900-0
    1. Hypertension--Pathophysiology. 2. Arteries--Pathophysiology.
  I. Safar, Michel. II. O'Rourke, Michael F. III. Series.
    [DNLM: 1. Hypertension--physiopathology. 2. Arteries-
  -physiopathology.   W1 DE997VME v.144 1994 / WG 340 A785 1994]
  RC685.H8A744   1994
  616.1'3207--dc20
  DNLM/DLC
  for Library of Congress   93-1730

ISBN 978-0-7923-2343-3

Table of contents

List of contributors

ATHANASE BENETOS
Department of Internal Medicine 1, Hôpital Broussais, 96, Rue Didot,
F-75674 Paris Cedex 14, France
Chapter 12 co-author: Michel E. Safar

COLIN L. BERRY
Department of Morbid Anatomy, The London Hospital, The London Hospital Medical College, London E1 1BB, U.K.
Chapter 4 co-author: Jorge A. Sosa-Melgarejo

RENÉ GOURGON
Department of Cardiology, Hôpital Beaujon, 100, Bd. du Gal-Leclerc,
F-92118 Clichy Cedex, France
Chapter 10 co-author: Alain Cohen-Solal

ARNOLD P.G. HOEKS
Department of Biophysics, University of Limburg, P.O. Box 616, 6200 MD
Maastaricht, The Netherlands
Chapter 8

RICKY D. LATHAM
Director Laboratory for Aerospace, Cardiovascular Research (CACR),
Armstron Laboratory (AFMC), Building 125, Room B59A, Brooks AFB,
TX 78235–5301, U.S.A.
Chapter 3 co-authors: David M. Slife

STÉPHANE LAURENT
Department of Pharmacology, Hôpital Broussais, 96, Rue Didot, F-75674
Paris Cedex 14, France
Chapter 1

BERNARD I. LÉVY
INSERM Unit 141, Hôpital Lariboisière, Cardiovascular Dynamics, 41 Bd de la Chapelle, F-75010 Paris Cedex 10, France
Chapter 5 co-author: Marie Christine Mourlon-Le Grand

GÉRARD M. LONDON
Chief Nephrology Division, Hôpital Manhes, 8, Grande Rue, F-91700 Fleury-Mérogis, France
Chapter 11 co-author: Michel E. Safar
Chapter 13 co-author: Bernard I. Lévy
Chapter 14 co-author: Toshio Yaginuma

WILLIAM McFATE SMITH
Senior Research Physician, SRI, International, 333 Ravenswood Avenue, Menlo Park, CA 94025, U.S.A.
Chapter 7

JEAN-BAPTISTE MICHEL
Reaearch Director, National Institute of Health and Medical Research, Unit 367, INSERM, 17, Rue du Fer à Moulin, F-75005 Paris, France
Chapter 6 co-author: Jean-François Arnal

MICHAEL F. O'ROURKE
University of New South Wales, Medical Professiorial Unit, St. Vincent's Hospital, Victoria Street, Darlinghurst, NSW 2010, Australia
Chapter 2

MICHEL E. SAFAR
Department of Internal Medicine, Hôpital Broussais, The Hypertension Research Center and INSERM U 337, 96, Rue Didot, F-75674 Paris, Cedex 14, France
Chapter 9

Introduction

MICHEL E. SAFAR and MICHAEL F. O'ROURKE

One of the principal problems of hypertension is the precise definition of blood pressure as a cardiovascular risk factor. Clinicians indicate peak systolic pressure and end diastolic pressure in the brachial artery as the principal criteria for blood pressure measurement. Consequently, these values are used as indicators for clinical management and therapeutic adjustment. This methodology, based on indirect blood pressure measurements at the site of the brachial artery relates only to the highest and lowest pressure in that vessel, and does not give any information of the blood pressure curve itself; this carries more information than peak systolic pressure and end diastolic pressure.

As a first step in better analysis of the blood pressure curve, research workers in experimental hypertension defined in addition to peak systolic pressure and end diastolic, another blood pressure value, mean arterial pressure, i.e. the average pressure throughout the cardiac cycle, and about which pressure fluctuates. This is the pressure recorded by Hales [1] and by Poiseuille [2] in their pioneering studies. By application of Poiseuille's Law, this definition of mean arterial pressure led to the concept that increased mean arterial pressure (and therefore hypertension) was related, at any given value of cardiac output, to an increase in vascular resistance, i.e. to a reduction in the caliber of the small arteries. Although universally admitted, this definition of hypertension completely neglected the principal characteristic of the blood pressure curve in living animals and humans, i.e. the presence of cyclic changes and hence of pulsatility of blood pressure. However, if the goal of research in hypertension is to characterize elevated blood pressure as a mechanical factor related to cardiovascular risk through alterations of the arterial wall, then the totality of the blood pressure curve should be analyzed in detail. Both steady and pulsatile phenomena need to be considered.

For a long time, studies of pulsatile arterial hemodynamics have shown that the blood pressure curve should be divided into two components [3]: a steady component, mean arterial pressure, and a pulsatile component, pulse pressure. Whereas the former is relatively simple to define and remains

M. E. Safar and M. F. O'Rourke (eds.), The arterial system in hypertension. pp. 1–3.

almost constant along the tree, the latter is much more complex. Indeed, pulse pressure is due to the summation of a forward pressure wave coming from the heart, and a backward reflected wave returning from the resistant arterioles. As a consequence, pulse pressure tends to increase markedly from the central to peripheral arteries with systolic pressure increasing significantly, and diastolic pressure decreasing to a lesser degree. Thus, pulse pressure differs along the arterial tree and the factors which determine pulse pressure may influence the definition of hypertension itself. Since at any given value of ventricular ejection, pulse pressure is influenced by arterial stiffness and the timing of reflected waves, then the large arteries themselves must be considered as involved in the definition of the hypertensive vascular disease.

Since in past years large arteries were neglected in the hemodynamic definition of hypertension, several aspects of pathophysiology of the disease were largely dismissed. There are several examples of this assumption. Firstly, for evident methodological reasons, pathophysiological aspects of hypertensive vascular disease were principally studied at the site of the large arteries in the upper limb – principally the brachial. Nevertheless the deduced pathophysiological mechanisms were frequently applied to the resistant arterioles and integrated as playing a role in the disturbance of the blood pressure regulation observed in hypertension. Brachial artery diastolic pressure was often equated with peripheral resistance and systolic pressure was overlooked. This approach is particularly confusing since the buffering function of large arteries is related to pulse pressure regulation, whereas the resistant function of arterioles is related to mean arterial pressure regulation. Secondly, with the development of cellular biology, a multitude of vaso-active factors were discovered in recent decades, and then applied to the study of the mechanisms of hypertension. Several of them were described as acting on the cardiovascular system independently of blood pressure changes. Principally, growth factors were studied as acting on the trophicity of the heart vessels (cardiac and vascular hypertrophy) even in the absence of significant changes in mechanical forces. Further, these 'mechanical forces' were exclusively analyzed in terms of the level of brachial systolic and diastolic blood pressure, and the concept of tensile or shear forces (either steady or pulsatile) acting on the arterial or the arteriolar wall were usually not taken into account in the various pathophysiological analyses of the literature. Finally, the abnormalities of the structure and the function of the cardiovascular system were analyzed very differently by specialists in clinical and in experimental hypertension. Whereas in experimental hypertension the structure and function of the arterial system were studied in terms of adaptive mechanisms and conceived as the cause or consequence of the elevated blood pressure, clinicians investigated the cardiovascular system and mostly the arterial system as the principal site of the complications of the disease. Nevertheless, most of these discrepancies are easily resolved when two evident characteristics of hypertension are admitted: (1) large arteries define the exact site in which blood pressure is measured, and (2) large arteries participate largely to the definition of hypertensive vascular disease.

It is important to emphasize that the investigation of large arteries in hypertension not only affects the pathophysiology of the disease, but also has important consequences for the clinical management and the drug treatment of hypertensive subjects. In the various published therapeutic trials of hypertensive agents, the diagnosis of the disease was principally based on the level of diastolic blood pressure. This criterion was applied not only at the entry of these trials but also as a guide of therapeutic effectiveness. Thus, following treatment a large proportion of subjects with controlled diastolic blood pressure but uncontrolled systolic blood pressure were considered 'well controlled' hypertensive subjects. Thus, the point that these subjects had increased pulse pressure with possible adverse consequences on the arterial wall was not taken into account. For that reason the principal result of therapeutic trials, i.e. the reduction in incidence of strokes but with no substantial change in the incidence of ischemic coronary complications, could be due to selection bias. Indeed, the observation of controlled diastolic blood pressure but uncontrolled systolic blood pressure in treated hypertensive subjects means that a significant disturbance of the arterial wall still remains in treated hypertensive subjects and probably involves both increased arterial stiffness and increased wave reflection.

The purpose of this book is threefold: (1) to analyze the physiological connections between the function of large arteries and the blood pressure regulation, (2) to investigate the peculiarities of the arterial system in hypertension, taking into account principally those of human hypertension, and (3) to apply the described pathophysiological mechanisms to the study of the response of the arterial system to anti-hypertensive drug therapy.

References

1. Hales S. Statical essays including haemastatics. London: Wilson & Nichol, 1733.
2. Poiseuille E. Recherches sur la coeur aortique. Arch Gen Med 1828; 18: 550–54.
3. McDonald DA. Blood flow in arteries. London: Arnold, 1960: 17–54, 118–145, 238–282, 351–419.

1. Mechanical stress of the arterial wall and hypertension

STÉPHANE LAURENT

Introduction

The effects of mechanical stress on the arterial wall have extensively been described during the past decades and have been applied to the understanding of hypertension. However, in these studies, mechanical stress is most often referred to as steady stress and little work examined the effects of pulsatile stress or considered the variability of mechanical stress.

Investigators in the field of hypertension have focused primarily on the role played by mean arterial pressure in alterations of vascular structure during chronic hypertension. Arterial pressure has been assumed to play per se a determinant role in alterations of vascular structure, among a variety of determinants including neural factors, humoral agents and genetic factors. However the evidence has not been entirely convincing, since the degree of reversal of media hypertrophy, during chronic treatment of hypertension, has not matched often the degree of reduction in mean arterial pressure. Some epidemiological [1] and experimental [2, 3] studies have raised the possibility that pulse pressure may be a determinant of vascular structure. In addition, 24 hours variability has been reported to be more closely related to the severity of target-organ damage than casual blood pressure in hypertensives [4]. These data suggest that, when evaluating the effects of mechanical stress on the arterial wall, it is necessary not only to take into account steady (i.e. mean) parameters but also to consider pulsatile parameters and the variability of steady and pulsatile parameters. For instance, circumferential stress is usually calculated from mean arterial pressure, mean arterial diameter and mean wall thickness. Progress should be made in the understanding of vascular structural changes related to hypertension by taking into account not only steady parameters but also the amplitude of cyclic changes in pressure, diameter and thickness, the duration of the steady and pulsatile stress exerted on the arterial wall [5] and the variability of these stresses. Further work is needed in order to determine how each of these parameters can contribute to the fatiguing effect of arterial pressure on the arterial wall, leading to arterial degeneration.

M. E. Safar and M. F. O'Rourke (eds.). The arterial system in hypertension. pp. 5–26.
© 1993 *Kluwer Academic Publishers. Printed in the Netherlands.*

The purpose of this chapter is to briefly describe the different varieties of wall stress and to review the experimental and clinical evidences that wall stress abnormalities, observed during hypertension, determine functional and structural changes of large and small arteries.

Varieties of wall stress

Stress is the intensity of force (F) acting across a given plane in a body and, if it is evenly distributed over the area A, the stress is F/A. The units of stress are thus force per unit area [6]. The stress on a point in a plane may be resolved into those normal to the axis (tensile or compressive) and tangential to the axis (shearing stress).

Tensile and compressive stresses

Pressurizing a vessel distends the wall in the circumferential and longitudinal directions and simultaneously narrows the wall thickness. The circumferential and longitudinal stresses are tensile and the radial stress which narrows the wall thickness is compressive.

Circumferential stress
Circumferential stress is comparable to the wall tension (force) given by the law of Laplace but accounts for the finite wall thickness of arteries. Indeed the law of Laplace states that the tension (T, force per unit length) in the wall of a very thin cylindrical shell is related to transmural pressure (PT) and radius (r): $T = PT \times r$. The circumferential stress on the wall depends on the wall thickness, however.

The circumferential distending force ($F_{\theta D}$) for a thin-wall vessel (Figure 1) is the product of the transmural pressure and the area over which that distending transmural pressure is exerted, or

$$F_{\theta D} = PT \times di \times l \tag{1}$$

where PT is transmural pressure, di is internal diameter and l is vessel length. Deformation of an elastic or viscoelastic material elicits a retractive force ($F_{\theta D}$) which is the product of the wall stress in the circumferential direction and the area over which that stress is exerted, or

$$F_{\theta D} = \sigma\theta \times h \times l \tag{2}$$

where $\sigma\theta$ is circumferential stress exerted by the tissue and h is wall thickness. Because distending and retracting forces are equal ($F_{\tau D} = F_{\tau R}$) at equilibrium, Equations 1 and 2 may be set equal and solved algebraically for $\sigma\theta$. The mean $\sigma\theta$ is then

$$\sigma\theta = PT \times ri/h \tag{3}$$

where ri is internal radius.

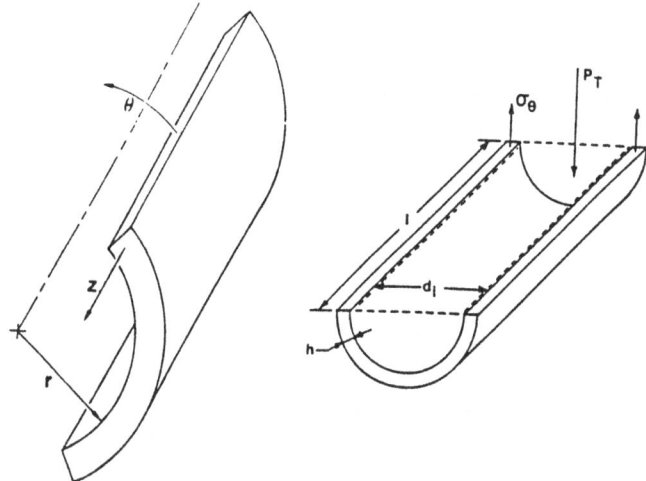

Figure 1. Diagram of arterial segment illustrating circumferential (π), longitudinal (z) and radial (r) directions. PT, transmural pressure; $\sigma\pi$, circumferential stress; *l* vessel length; *h*, wall thickness; *di*, internal diameter. From Dobrin [24].

Circumferential stress may be used to compute strain-stress relations and incremental elastic moduli in order to assess the elastic properties of the arteries. This has mainly been done in vitro, with steady increases in distending pressure [7, 8] Provided arterial wall motion is detected during each cardiac cycle, the in vivo strain-stress relation of the artery may be computed. In vivo arterial wall motion occurs predominantly in the circumferential direction; much smaller changes occur in the longitudinal direction. The shape of the diameter oscillations closely resembles the form of the pressure pulse (Figure 2). Extrathoracic systemic arteries change 8–10% in diameter with each cardiac cycle, whereas the diameter of the intrathoracic arteries changes 8–18% with each cardiac cycle [9–11]. The circumferential strain ($\epsilon\theta$) is

$$\epsilon\theta = \frac{d - do}{do} \tag{4}$$

where *d* is the observed diameter and *do* is the original diameter. Variously *do* has been defined either as the diameter of the retracted, totally unloaded vessel [8], as diameter at low or 0 mmHg pressure [7, 12], or as unstressed diameter [13, 14]. For materials having linear strain-stress relations, the ratio of stress to strain may be used to compute the Young's modulus of elasticity, the stretching force per unit cross-sectional area required to elongate a strip of a vessel wall by 100%. However, for materials with non-linear strain-stress relations, the slope of the strain-stress curve may be used to compute

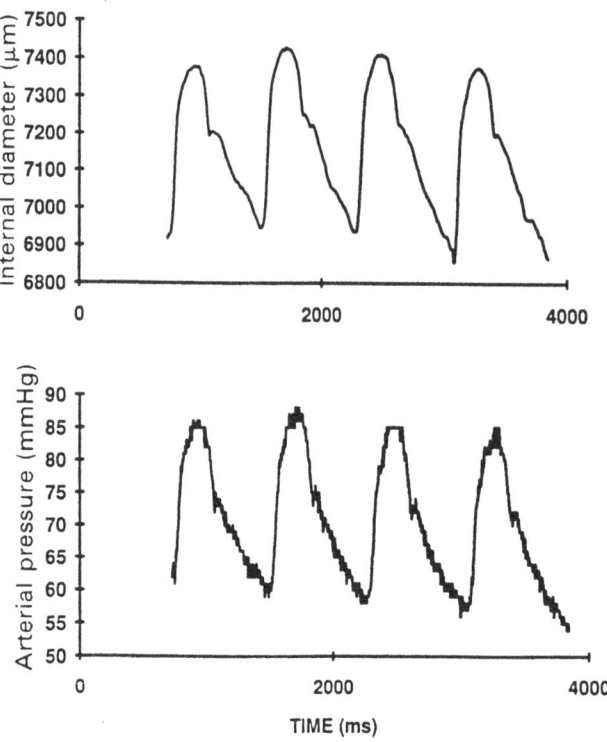

Figure 2. Simultaneous pressure (P) and diameter (D) recordings of common carotid arteries, in a 44-year-old male subject. Diameter was measured non invasively with an ultrasonic echotracking system [15] at the site of the right common carotid artery [15] and pulse pressure was measured at the site of the left common carotid artery with applanation tonometry [17].

an incremental elastic modulus, defined, for a cylindrical vessel with wall stiffnesses that are equal in all directions, as:

$$E \text{ inc} = \Delta\epsilon\theta \times 0.75/\Delta\epsilon\theta \tag{5}$$

In in vitro preparations, the stress-strain relationship is determined using the distending pressure and, at each level of distending pressure, the internal radius of the vessel and the wall thickness. Stress is calculated following Equation 3 and strain, the fractional increase in circumferential length, following Equation 4 [8].

In humans, the stiffness of vascular walls can be estimated using a non invasive approach of the pressure-diameter curve within the systolic-diastolic range. Systolic-diastolic changes in internal diameter of large arteries like the common carotid artery, the common femoral artery, the brachial artery or the radial artery, can be recorded with high resolution echotracking system [15, 16] and systolic-diastolic changes in blood pressure can be estimated using applanation tonometry [17] or photoplethysmography [16]. Mean wall thickness can now be measured at the site of the common carotid artery [18] and of the radial artery [19] and systolic-diastolic changes in wall thickness can be measured at the site of the radial artery [19]. However these clinical approaches obviously cannot determine unstressed diameter and therefore the mechanical properties of the arterial wall under fully relaxed conditions.

Longitudinal stress
Deformation in the longitudinal direction can be computed as:

$$F_{ZD} = PT \times \pi r i^2 \tag{6}$$

where F_{ZD} is the longitudinal distending force, PT is transmural pressure and *ri* is internal radius. Deformation in the longitudinal direction elicits a retractive force by the tissue, F_{ZR}, which is

$$F_Z0R = \sigma Z \times (\pi re^2 - \pi ri^2) \tag{7}$$

where σZ is longitudinal wall stress exerted by the tissue and *re* is external radius. Because distending and retractive forces are equal ($F_{ZD} = F_{ZR}$) at equilibrium, Equations 6 and 7 may be set equal and solved algebraically for σZ. The mean longitudinal stress caused by pressure so obtained is

$$\sigma Z = \frac{PT \times ri^2}{re^2 - ri^2} \tag{8}$$

By factoring the denominator, it may be shown that the longitudinal stress due to pressure (σZ) is approximately one-half the circumferential stress.

The arterial changes in length are very small in amplitude, in vivo, as reported by Lawton [20] and Patel & Fry [21]. Indeed, during each cardiac cycle the descending thoracic aorta lengthens about 1%, whereas the abdominal aorta shortens by about the same amount. The changes (5 to 11%) in length of the ascending aorta and pulmonary artery [22], which are more important, may results from gross motion of the heart. In addition, arteries are extended by a longitudinal traction force,due to the fixation of arterial side branches and the presence of periadventitial connective tissues. From experiments done with pressurized carotid arteries held at in situ length, Dobrin & Doyle [23] suggests that this interaction between pressure stress and traction stress keeps the length of arteries nearly constant.

Radial stress
Radial stress (σr) is oriented directly outward and equals transmural pressure at the intimal surface and is zero at the adventitial margin. The mean stress at midwall thickness is approximately one-half that at the intima, i.e. half the transmural pressure [24]. Therefore, it is much smaller in magnitude than circumferential or longitudinal stresses, since the latter are the products of PT and *ri/h*, which are at physiological pressures 8:1 or even 10:1. Because of its small value, σr is frequently neglected in multidirectional computations.

Components of the arterial wall bearing stress

The mechanical characteristics of relaxed vessels have been attributed to the properties of the fibrous connective tissues in the wall, specifically to those of elastin and collagen. Elastin and collagen are fibrous in nature, although elastin tends to occur in more or less continuous sheets [25]. Elastin is capable of extending more than 100% [26]. The elastic modulus of elastin, a measure of stiffness, gradually rise from very low values to about $4\ 0 \times 10^6$ dyn/cm^2 in the fully stretched state [27]. By contrast collagen is much stiffer. When the slack in the constituent fibers has been taken up, collagen can be stretched only 3–4% exhibiting an elastic modulus of 0.3–2.5×10^{10} dyn/cm^2 [24, 27]. Collagen and elastin are complexed with an amorphous substance formed of mucoprotein. This substance is not itself elastic but contributes to the elastic properties of the artery. Another constituent of the arterial wall is smooth muscle which is involved in the production of extracellular matrix, including collagen and elastin. Smooth muscle, while contributing to the tension in the wall, cannot properly be regarded as a true elastic material [28].

The structure of the arterial wall is detailed in Chapter 4, as well as the relative amounts of the various components, and their variations with age and hypertension.

Dobrin & Canfield [24], from enzymatic-degradation studies in dog carotid arteries, delineated the contributions of elastin and collagen to three-dimensional elastic properties of arteries. They suggested that elastin bears a constant portion of longitudinal stress at all vessel lengths within the physiological range, a gradually increasing portion of circumferential stress with vessel distension and a gradually increasing portion of radial stress with progressive compression of the wall. Collagen bears little longitudinal or radial stress with physiological levels of deformation but does bear a gradually increasing portion of circumferential stress with vessel distension beginning at about 60 mmHg.

The circumferential stress given by Equation 3 is the mean circumferential stress. However this stress is not uniformly distributed across the arterial wall. It has been shown by several investigators that the point stress is high at the lumen and declines curvilinearly across the wall thickness [29, 30]. This distribution closely resembles the density of the elastic lamellae at different points across the wall; elastic lamellae are close together near the lumen and are more widely spaced near the adventitia [29]. Dobrin [24] suggests that an adaptive relationship may exist between morphology and mechanical load at different locations across the wall. Wolinsky & Glagov [31] previously proposed a similar argument as they noted a virtually constant relationship between the total number of elastic lamellae in the aortic wall and the mean wall tension for a wide variety of mammalian species. Another observation is that the circumferential stress is greater on the inner radius of the aortic arch than on the outer radius; this corresponds with greater wall thickness on the inner curve.

Recent works have drawn attention to the possible involvement of the integrin-type fibronectin receptors of the rat arterial smooth muscle cell in the interconversion between contractile and synthetic phenotypes [32] and in the linkage between the extracellular matrix and smooth muscle cells [33]. The integrin family of protein has been shown to be involved in the adhesion of fibronectin to smooth muscle cells [34] and could participate to the adhesion of smooth muscle cells to collagen and elastin fibers [33]. Further studies are needed in order to determine whether the integrin-fibronectin complex may influence the elastic modulus of the arterial wall through an increase in the mass of its different constituents or through their reorganization inside the arterial wall.

Shearing stress

Another aspect of longitudinal vessel mechanics is the hemodynamically generated shear stress at the intima. Most of the work on this subject has been done in cylindrical tubes, a situation which is analogous to that of flow in blood vessels [35, 36]. Blood, like others fluids, can move in layers, or *laminae* of different velocity. The middle of the stream tends to move more rapidly than the blood adjacent to it, which in turn slides past the relatively slow-moving blood nearer the banks. The energy required to move one lamina over another lamina over another is greater for some liquids than for others. This property of a fluid is called its viscosity. Its physical definition is usually illustrated by two hypothetical fluid laminae of thickness dx, in contact over an area A, moving at velocities that differ by dv. The stress (τ) or force per unit area (F/A), required to produce that differential movement is directly proportional to the velocity gradient, or rate of shear (γ), between the layers, and the viscosity of the fluid is the proportionality constant, μ:

$$\tau = \mu \, dv/dx \qquad\qquad (9)$$

Stress is not related to absolute velocity but to the relative velocity of different laminae. Water and other liquids that behave in this way are called Newtonian fluids; their viscosity is not influenced by absolute velocity. The viscosity of non-Newtonian liquids is said to be anomalous because it changes with the forward velocity and shear rates in the stream [6, 37]. Shear rate is among the factors that determine whether fluid laminae move smoothly or irregularly. It is highest near the vessel wall, where it averages about 50/sec in the human aorta and 150/sec in the femoral artery. Steady wall shear stress (τ) may also be calculated according to the formula

$$\tau = \mu Q/\pi r^3 \qquad\qquad (10)$$

where Q is the total blood flow, r the internal radius and μ the viscosity.

Shear stress may stimulate release of endothelium-derived relaxing factor (EDRF) through a mechanism which is sensitive to velocity and viscosity and may involve K + fluxes in association with membrane hyperpolarization

[38–42]. Shear stress may also release prostaglandins [43] from endothelium or directly influence the vascular smooth muscle tone [44, 45].

Steady versus pulsatile stress

The pressure waves and the blood flow velocity waves may be described in terms of mean and pulsatile components. Mean arterial pressure is defined as the average blood pressure in the aorta and its major branches during a given cardiac cycle. It is obtained from an arterial pressure tracing, by measuring the area under the curve and dividing this area by the time interval involved [46]. Pulsatile pressure (or pulse pressure) is the difference between systolic and diastolic values. As pulsations move on through the vascular system, the properties of the arterial tree transform the shape and timing of the waves (see following chapters).

Similarly, the velocity profile oscillates with pulsatile flow in smaller arteries, becoming parabolic when flow is near its peak and less so during the diastolic period, when velocity near the wall may even reverse its direction briefly. The non-dimensional parameter α was used by Womersley [47] to characterize the motion of a viscous liquid and its value is related to the velocity profile:

$$\alpha = R(\varpi/\nu)^{1/2} \tag{11}$$

where R is the cross-section of the vessel, $\varpi = 2\pi f$ the angular frequency in radians per second of the oscillatory pressure gradient (with f the frequency in hertz) and ν the kinematic viscosity ($\nu = \mu/\rho$ where μ is the Newtonian coefficient of viscosity and ρ the density of the liquid). As the frequency of the oscillatory motion increases, α increases and the velocity profile becomes very flattened. An increase of diameter without a change of frequency will also cause an increase in α and produce a similar alteration in the profile. The liquid in the central portion of the tube is virtually unsheared and the significant velocity gradients are only found in the layers near the wall [5, 48].

Tensile and shear stresses may be calculated from the mean values of blood pressure and blood flow velocity, in Equations 3 and 10 and represent mean or 'steady' stresses. 'Pulsatile' tensile and shear stresses may be calculated from pulse pressure and pulsatile blood flow velocity. The predominant role of pulsatile stress over steady stress in alterations of vascular structure will be discussed later.

Glagov and co-workers [49], in order to correlate the excursion of shear stress over the cardiac cycle with lesion thickness, calculated pulse shear stress, defined as maximum-minimum shear stress. In addition, in order to account for the cyclic departure of the wall shear stress vector from its predominant axial alignment, they calculated an oscillatory shear index. This index represents a measure of the shear stress acting on the luminal surface due to either 'cross-flow' or reverse flow velocity components occurring during pulsatile flow.

Shear stress has often been investigated in vitro in models having rigid walls. However, the diameter of large arteries can vary by ±5 to 10% [10, 11] over the cardiac cycle and it is important to consider the effect of radial wall pulsation on this hemodynamic phenomenon. The influence of radial wall motion of the arterial wall on the shear stress that flowing blood impose on the wall has been studied by Klanchar et al. [50] who observed peak wall shear rate elevation by as much as a factor of five and the onset on strong wall shear reversal associated with a change in pressure-flow phase angle of only 20°. Alterations in phase angle of this magnitude are associated with hypertension and may be induced by vasoactive agents.

O'Rourke & Nichols [5], on the basis of engineering principles [51, 52] suggest that arterial degeneration is not caused by continually applied stresses, but is due to the fatiguing effects of cyclic stress which cause fracture of the load-bearing elastin fibers. Such fracture could lead to progressive dilation of the vessel, to transfer of stress from elastin to collagen fibers and to attempts at remodeling by the cellular elements of the wall. Indeed Prokop and co-workers [52] demonstrated, in a model of aorta, that pulsatile flow produced rapid dissection with a maximum systolic pressure of 120 mmHg while steady flow produced no dissection with pressure up to 400 mmHg. The determinant factor was the maximum rate of rise of pressure (dp/dt_{max}) in the fluid and not shear stress.

Variability of stress

If the effects of steady tensile stress on the arterial wall have been extensively described and if those of pulsatile stress have been studied by a few investigators, the effects of an excessive lability of tensile stress on the arterial wall remain purely speculative.

The blood pressure signal can be described not only as a function of time, i.e. as a steady mean arterial pressure with a pulsatile component, but also as the sum of elementary oscillatory components, defined by their frequency and their amplitude. In addition to cardiac cycle, two main rhythmic events affect the circulation: respiration and vasomotion. The respiratory activity has long been known to be accompanied by arterial pressure and heart period fluctuations, whereas the finding of slow arterial pressure oscillations (also referred to as Mayer waves), having a period of approximately 10 seconds has been more elusive [53, 54]. On the other hand, rhythmic discharges in phase with respiration have been described in the sympathetic and vagal outflows; similarly, a slower rhythm in phase with vasomotor waves has been found in the sympathetic and vagal efferent discharge [55].

In the same way than the variability of blood pressure has been analysed, the variability of tensile stress, which takes into account distending blood pressure, may be described. However, the variability of tensile stress necessitates, to be evaluated, that other factors than the variability of blood pressure should be taken into account. For example, a valid analysis of the variability of circumferential stress would require one to know the time-dependent changes of blood pressure, inernal arterial diameter and wall thickness over long periods of time. For methodological reasons, this has not been done until now. This is now possible with recently developed echotracking systems able to continuously and simultaneously record the blood pressure signal and the arterial wall signal [16]. More simply, the variability of blood pressure should probably be taken into account when dealing with the fatiguing effects of non steady stresses on the wall material. It remains, however, to be determined whether elastic properties of large arteries are influenced by an excessive lability of blood pressure and therefore by an excessive lability of tensile stress or by pulsatile stress or both. What is suggested for large arteries appears to be even more complex for arterioles, since arteriolar vasomotion could determine the low frequency component of blood pressure which in turn could determine the function and the structure of the arteriolar wall. However, the blood pressure signal which is analysed for the definition of high-and low-frequency spectral components is recorded in conduit arteries and is likely different in resistive arteries.

Shear stress and flow-dependent vasodilation

A large number of studies suggest that flow-dependent vasodilation mechanisms include shear stress. Although the mechanism coupling the increase in blood flow to the enhanced formation and release of endothelial autacoids is not yet established, it is generally assumed that the increase in fluid shear stress at the luminal surface of the endothelium is the proper stimulus for the flow-induced endothelium-dependent dilation. Substances released by vessel wall components in response to shear stress may differ, depending on the vascular preparation.

Shear stress stimulate the release of an endothelium-derived relaxing factor (EDRF) [56, 57] through a mechanism which is sensitive to velocity and viscosity and may involve K^+ fluxes in association with membrane hyperpolarization [38–42]. EDRF is now thought to be nitric oxide (NO) derived from L-arginine through the action of NO-synthetase which is inhibited by substituted L-arginine analoguee [58]. EDRF production is greater with pulsatile than steady flow [41, 42] and is frequency-related, peak release from donor rat, rabbit and pig arteries occurring at pulse frequencies of 4–6 Hz [59]. EDRF release is also modulated by transmural pressure [60] and, in experiments employing pulsatile flow is inversely related to the pulse pressure amplitude [61].

In arterioles of rat cremaster muscle, the endothelial factors involved in the mediation of the shear-stress-induced vasodilation have been demonstrated to be prostaglandins [43].

In addition, shearing stress can directly influence the vascular smooth muscle tone [62, 63], independently of the endothelium. Indeed, in rabbit ear and cerebral arteries, Bevan and co-workers [44] suggest another mechanism of relaxation to flow which involves stimulation of soluble guanylate cyclase by a smooth muscle derived relaxing factor that does appear to have L-arginine as a precursor molecule.

Flow-dependent vasodilation has been reported in man, at the site of the brachial [64] and the femoral [65] arteries, following the large increase in blood flow velocity which occurs at the site of these arteries during reactive hyperemia.

Tensile stress could interact with shear stress. Indeed Bevan & Joyce [45] showed, in isolated small rabbit ear arteries, that the magnitude of flow-induced relaxation can be correlated positively and the flow-induced constriction correlated negatively with the level of wall tone determined by norepinephrine. Busse and co-workers [66] demonstrated, in rabbit femoral arteries an increase in shear stress-dependent NO release during vasoconstriction. Whether this modulation is due to non specific mechanical factors like the level of circumferential stress or to specific agents like norepinephrine remains to be demonstrated.

Consequences for the understanding of hypertension

Tensile and shear stresses can modulate the function and the structure of large and small arteries, both acutely and chronically.

Acute arterial changes due to an increase in tensile stress

Tensile stresses, like circumferential stress, acutely modulate the geometry and the function of arteries, through the distending pressure. For instance, an increase in circumferential stress in response to an increase in distending pressure dilates large arteries and, due to the non linearity of the pressure-diameter relationship, decreases their distensibility. At the arteriolar site, an increase in circumferential stress determines geometrical changes in the opposite direction, through the myogenic response [67, 6]. Muscular medium sized arteries may have an intermediate pattern, due to their large content of smooth muscle. In humans, muscular medium-sized arteries, like the brachial and the radial artery, are indeed reactive to different stimuli, independently of distending blood pressure. They may dilate in response to an increase in flow [64] or to the activation of cardiopulmonary baroreflex [69] and constrict in response to norepinephrine [70] or mental and cold stresses [71].

Chronic arterial changes due to an increase in tensile stress

Tensile stress is a strong determinant of the vascular structure, among other factors including sympathetic activity [72] and humoral factors like angiotensin II [73]. The chronic increase in blood pressure and therefore in steady tensile stress, as occurs during hypertension, has extensively been reported to induce vascular hypertrophy [74] associated with an increase in the thickness of the smooth muscle layer [75] and a decrease in lumen diameter of resistance vessels, resulting in an increase of media/lumen ratio [76], and thus increased in minimal resistance [77]. According to equation 3 (σ = PT $\times$ l/h), the hypertrophy of the arterial wall compensate for the increase in blood pressure and makes it possible to maintain a normal level of circumferential stress. Arterial pressure is only one of the determinants of vascular hypertrophy in chronic hypertension, which include also neural stimuli, humoral factors and genetic factors. The ratio of vessel media thickness to lumen diameter has been reported to increase with intravascular pressure, not only in large arteries [78, 79] but also in peripheral arterioles [80] including coronary resistance vessels [81]. Although these experimental data have been confirmed, in humans, by some studies in isolated subcutaneous resistance vessels [82], in isolated intramyocardial arterioles [83] and in isolated medium sized arteries [84], very few data concern large arteries in vivo:: circumferential stress has recently been shown to be maintained constant by arterial wall hypertrophy in hypertensives, at the site of the radial artery [65]; an increased intima+media thickness has been measured non-invasively at the site of the common carotid arteries of hypertensives [18]. From the point of view of proximal large arteries, hypertension is often looked upon as an accelerated form of aging, with a progressive increase in arterial stiffness [5]. If hypertension-induced decrease in arterial distensibility has consistently been reported for proximal large arteries, like the aorta [85] and the common carotid artery [11] in man, by contrast (a) the distensibility of arterial wall material is increased in small arteries from SHR [86], including cerebral small arteries [87], and (b) isobaric distensibility of a distal medium-sized artery, the radial artery, is increased in hypertensives [88]. As has been emphasized by Baumbach et al. [87], this reduction in elastic modulus of the materials constituting the vascular wall would be a means by which the vasculature can functionally maintain its distensibility characteristics despite the relatively increased wall thickness required by the increased intravascular pressure.

Dilation of large arteries with age has been extensively described [5, 90]. O'Rourke and co-workers suggested [5] that enlargement of arterial diameter with aging could be due to the fracture of load-bearing elastin fibers in response to the fatiguing effect of tensile stress. Arterial dilation occurs in proximal arteries, such as the common carotid artery and the thoracic and abdominal aorta, where it is accelerated by hypertension, but does not occur in peripheral muscular arteries like the common femoral, the brachial and the radial arteries [91].

In contrast to mean arterial pressure, there is a growing body of evidence that pulse pressure could play an important role in alterations of vascular structure. Indeed, Fischer and co-workers [92] correlated the increase in connective tissue content of atherosclerotic vessels with the magnitude of pressure pulsations to which the vessels were exposed. Leung and co-workers [93] demonstrated that cyclic stretching of vascular muscle cells in vitro accelerates their synthesis of collagen and glycosaminoglycans. Sottiurai and co-workers [94] reported that cyclic stretching of smooth muscle in vitro decreases the number of intracellular myofilaments and increases the amount of rough endoplasmic reticulum. Coarctation of the thoracic aorta in monkey [95] and dog [96] reduces pulse pressure, but not necessarily mean arterial pressure, distal to the coarctation. The reduction in pulse pressure is associated with decreased motion of the aortic wall [95] and a reduction in DNA and collagen content [97]. Taken together, these findings suggest that alterations of pulsatile circumferential stress may influence cellular and extracellular components in the vessel wall and affect vascular growth [98]. The role of pulse pressure has been confirmed by the Rotterdam Elderly Study [99] in humans. This study demonstrates that the mean intima-media thickness of the common carotid artery was correlated with the amplitude of pulse pressure, after adjustment for differences in age, sex, body surface area, serum lipids, smoking and fibrinogen.

Another approach was to study the differential effects of antihypertensive treatments on the prevention of vascular hypertrophy, according to their effects on pulse pressure and mean arterial pressure. For example, hydralazine (vasodilator) and cilazapril (angiotensine 1 converting enzyme inhibitor) are equally effective in reducing pulse pressure and preventing hypertrophy in cerebral arterioles of stroke-prone spontaneously hypertensive rats (SHRSP), although hydralazine is less effective in reducing mean arterial pressure [2]. Christensen et al. [3] also considered the possible role of pulse pressure by measuring mean arterial pressure and pulse pressure in awake spontaneously hypertensive rats that had been treated with perindopril or captopril (both angiotensin I converting enzyme inhibitors), isradipine (calcium channel blocker), hydralazine and metoprolol (beta-1 blocker). The correlation between blood pressure and media/lumen ratio of small mesenteric arteries was stronger for pulse pressure than for systolic, mean or diastolic blood pressure. Ligation of the internal carotid artery prevents hypertrophy and normalizes pulse pressure, but not systolic pressure and mean arterial pressure, in pial arterioles of SHRSP [98]. Furthermore, there is not a significant correlation among cross-sectional area of the vessel wall and mean arterial pressure whereas there is a strong correlation between cross-sectional area and pulse pressure [98]. These findings suggest that reduction of pulse pressure during hypertensive treatment may be a factor in prevention of altered

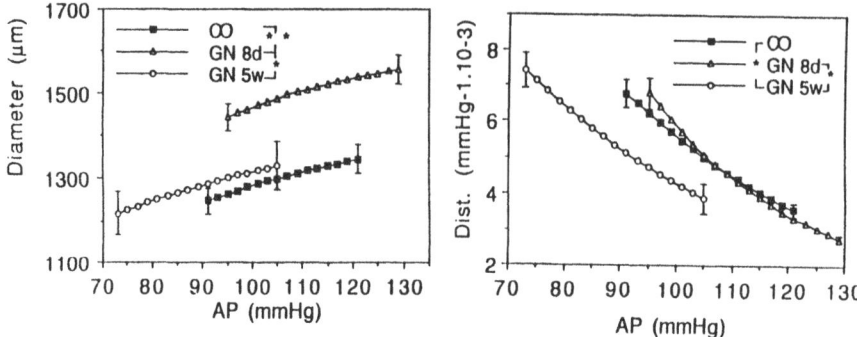

Figure 3. Diameter-pressure and distensibility-pressure relationships of the abdominal aorta in three groups of 3 month old Wistar rats. Rats were treated with guanethidine for 8 days (GN 8d; *n* = 10) or 5 weeks (GN 5w; *n* = 10) in order to increase lability of blood pressure without changing mean arterial pressure and pulse pressure, or with saline (Co; *n* = 20). Distensibility-pressure diameter curve was significantly shifted to the left in rats treated with guanethidine for 5 weeks, and distensibility for 100 mmHg was significantly reduced as compared to control rats. From Lacolley [101].

vascular structure during chronic hypertension. However further work is needed in order to determine the mechanisms whereby pulse pressure can contribute to arterial wall hypertrophy.

An excessive lability of tensile stress may favor the alterations of wall material seen with ageing and hypertension, but, to our knowledge, no evidence that variability per se is a factor of vessel damage has been reported. Absolute long and short-term blood pressure variabilities have been reported to be greater in hypertensives than in normotensives [100] and 24-h variability of blood pressure could be more closely related to the severity of target-organ damage than casual blood pressure, in hypertensives [4]. It remains to be determined whether an excessive lability of blood pressure represents, per se, a factor of arterial wall damage. Lacolley et al. [101] reported preliminary data showing a decrease in aortic distensibility in Wistar rats, in which an increased lability of blood pressure was induced by chronic guanethidine treatment (Figure 3).

Although it is not the scope of this chapter to review wall stress changes due to atherosclerosis, hypertension is a potientating factor for the development of atherosclerosis and the effects of structural atherosclerotic changes on circumferential stress deserve to be taken into account. Hypertension is a potientating factor for the fracture of the surface of an atherosclerotic plaque, a common cause of acute myocardial infarction and unstable angina. A number of studies have described the sequence of events leading from plaque rupture to luminal thrombosis and to myocardial necrosis [102–104]. Different mechanisms have been proposed, for explaining plaque rupture, including shear stress injury [105], transient collapse of the stenosis [106], rupture of the vasa vasorum [107], turbulent plaque injury [108] and mechanical shear stress [109]. Subintimal structure, rather than stenosis severity, may be critical in determining overall plaque stability, explaining why coronary angiography has not been reliable method for predicting future myocardial infarction [110]. Richardson and colleagues [111] have identified stress-concentration regions by finite element modeling, which correlate with locations of plaque rupture in autopsy specimens. Lee and colleagues [110], by modeling the plaque and the artery, have shown that reducing the fibrous cap thickness dramatically increases peak circumferential stress in the plaque, whereas increasing the stenosis severity actually decreases peak stress in the plaque.

Acute arterial changes due to an increase in shear stress

Shear stress acutely modulates arterial diameter through the phenomenon of flow-dependent vasodilation. If increases in shear stress really induce the adaptive vascular dilation, one can assume an autoregulatory mechanism of wall shear as follows. Wall shear stress, when increased during a sustained increase in blood flow, induces the adaptive enlargement of the vessel radius, which acts as negative feedback to reduce the stress itself (Equation 10). If the wall shear stress fully controls the enlargement and reduction of the vessel diameter, the stress will be maintained constant at the control level for any sustained blood flow changes. This autoregulatory mechanism can provide a reasonable basis to explain flow-radius relationships in the vascular system [112].

Chronic arterial changes due to changes in shear stress

Shear stress modulates the growth of vessel caliber. The significant effect of blood flow or shear stress on the growth of vessel caliber was initially pointed out by Thoma (1893), who observed in chicken embryos that the pathways of the fastest blood velocity became the main arteries while those with slower velocity atrophied. This effect, controlling the vessel diameter during angiogenesis, was clearly distinguished from that of the circumferential stress due to the transmural pressure, which induced the changes in the wall thickness. Later studies on arteriovenous fistulas and on the collateral circulation also show that increased blood flow induces blood vessel dilation [113]. Guyton and Hartley [114], who restricted blood flow in carotid artery of the rat pup, observed that this vessel showed both a smaller diameter and less medial tissue mass than the contralateral control artery. In addition, Langille and co-workers [115] showed that reductions in blood flow produced by ipsilateral external carotid artery ligation elicited growth inhibition of arterial wall tissues in immature rabbits and no significant change in vessel mass or wall constituents in adult rabbit. Whether long term adaptation of vessel wall to shear stress is more dependent upon pulsatile velocity than mean velocity remains controversial [114, 115]. Shear stress may play a significant role not only on the physiological adaptation of the vascular wall but also on the pathogenesis of the atherosclerosis. Fry and co-workers [116] demonstrated that increased wall shear stress caused by increased blood flow velocity enhanced protein permeability across the endothelial layer of the arterial wall; moderately elevated stress induced intimal hyperplasia of a physiological nature and moderate increases in the arterial diameter, although excessive stress caused erosion of the endothelium followed by histopathological changes resembling the early lesions of atherosclerosis. Caro et al. [37, 117] suggested that low wall shear, on the contrary, may adversely affect the rate of mass transport of lipids across the arterial wall, consistently with the development of atherosclerotic lesions at the site of low wall shear in bifurcations. These authors postulated control of the transport by the diffusion boundary layer; wall shear rate will enhance flux if diffusion across the boundary layer is the rate-limiting process by a steepening effect on the concentration gradient driving the process [117]. Glagov & Zarins [118] strongly suggested from human artery studies and experimental models, that lowered mean wall shear stress induces such focal thickening to restore wall shear to normal baseline levels of 15–20 dyn/cm^2. In addition, total wall thickness in normal arteries tends to maintain a constant relation to lumen diameter for homologous segments, and intimal thickening appears to participate in this process. Contrarily to what is observed in atherosclerotic lesions, there is no circumscribed lipid accumulation and no necrosis in this intimal thickening, but an organization into fibrocellular layers, lending further support to their role in an adaptive process to altered wall shear and tensile stress [119]. The controversy whether low or high shear stress would affect the development of atherosclerostic lesions may be viewed as the impossibility of measuring exactly the level of shear known to vary largely at the site of complex lesions, in humans.

The consequences of shear stress abnormalities on the structure and function of the arterial wall have mainly been studied In the field of atherogenesis. In these studies, hypertension was most often considered as a potentiating factor. However the abnormalities of shear stress during chronic hypertension deserve to be studied independently of atherogenesis. Several rheological abnormalities have been reported in hypertension, mainly the elevation of whole blood viscosity [120, 121]. The hyperviscosity magnitude observed in hypertensive patients was found to be inversely related to shear rate [122] In addition, increased red blood cell aggregation and disaggregation shear rate and shear stress were observed in hypertensive patients when compared to normotensive subjects [123].

A better knowledge of the relationships between shear stress abnormalities and tensile stress abnormalities should help to understand the structural and functional alterations cf large and small vessels in hypertension.

References

1. Darne B, Girerd X, Safar M, Cambien F, Guize L. Pulsatile versus steady component of

blood pressure: a cross-sectional analysis and a prospective analysis on cardiovascular mortality. Hypertension 1989; 13: 392–400.

2. Hadju MA, Heistad DD, Baumbach GL. effects of antihypertensive treatment on mechanics of cerebral arterioles in rats. Hypertension 1990; 17: 308–16.

3. Christensen KL. Reducing pulse pressure in hypertension may normalize small artery structure. Hypertension 1991; 18: 722–7.

4. Parati G, Pomidossi G, Albini F, Malaspina D, Mancia G. Relationship of 24-hour blood pressure mean and variability to severity of target-organ damage in hypertension. J Hypertens 1987; 5: 93–98.

5. Nichols WW, O'Rourke MF. McDonald's blood flow in arteries. London/Melbourne/Auckland: Edward Arnold, 1990.

6. Milnor WR, Principles of hemodynamics. In: Milnor WR, editor. Cardiovacular physiology. New York: Oxford University Press, 1990: 171–215.

7. Cox RH. Mechanics of canine iliac artery smooth muscle in vitro. Am J Physiol 1976; 230: 462–70.

8. Dobrin PB, Rovick AA. Influence of vascular smooth muscle on contractile mechanics and elasticity of arteries. Am J Physiol 1969; 217: 1644–52.

9. Dobrin PB. Mechanical properties of arteries. Physiol Rev 1978; 58: 97–460.

10. Reneman RS, van Merode T, Hick P, Muytens AMM, Hoeks APG. Age related changes in carotid artery wall properties in men. Ultrasound Med Biol 1986; 12: 465–71.

11. Arcaro G, Laurent S, Jondeau G, Hoeks A, Safar M. Stiffness of the common carotid artery in treated hypertensive patients. J Hypertens 1991; 9: 947–54.

12. Cox RH. Determination of series elasticity in arterial smooth muscle. Am J Physiol 233 (Heart Circ Physiol 2) 1977; H248–H55.

13. Attinger FML. Two-dimensional in vitro studies of femoral arterial walls of the dog. Circ Res 1968; 22: 829–40.

14. Gow BS. Circulatory correlates: vascular impedance, resistance, and capacity. In: Bohr DF, Somlyo AP, Sparks HV, editors. Handbook of physiology. The cardiovascular system. Vascular smooth muscle. Bethesda: Am Physiol Soc, 1980, Sect 2, Vol II, Ch 14: 353–408.

15. Hoeks APG, Brands PJ, Smeets F, Reneman RS. Assessment of the distensibility of superficial arteries. Ultrasound Med Biol 1990; 16: 121–8.

16. Tardy Y, Meister JJ, Perret F, Brunner HR, Arditi M. Non invasive estimate of the mechanical properties of peripheral arteries from ultrasonic and photoplethysmographic measurements. Clin Physiol Meas 1991; 12: 39–54.

17. Kelly RP, Hayward CS, Ganis J, Daley J, Avolio A, O'Rourke M. Non invasive registration of the arterial pressure pulse waveform using high fidelity applanation tonometry. J Vasc Med Biol 1989; 1: 142–9.

18. Saba PS, Roman MJ, Pini R, Spitzer M, Pickering T, Devereux R. The carotid pressure waveform is related to carotid and left ventricular anatomy. Am J Hypertens 1992; 5: 38A.

19. Girerd X, Mourad JJ, Boutouyrie P, Safar M, Laurent S. Incompressibility of the arterial wall: a noninvasive evaluation in man. J. Hypertension 10(suppl 6): S111–S114, 1992.

20. Lawton RW. Some aspects of research in biological elasticity. Introductory remarks. In: Remington JW, editor. Tissue Elasticity. Washington, DC: Am Physiol Soc, 1957: 1–11.

21. Patel DJ, Fry DL. In situ pressure-radius-length measurements in ascending aorta of anaesthetized dogs. J Appl Physiol 1964; 19: 413–6.

22. Patel DJ, Greenfield JC, Fry DL. In vivo pressure-length-radius relationship of certain blood vessels in man and dog. In: Attinger EO, editor. Pulsatile blood flow. Int Symp, Philadelphia, PA: McGraw-Hill, 1963; 293–306.

23. Dobrin PB, Doyle JM. Vascular smooth muscle and the anisotropy of dog carotid artery. Circ Res 1970; 27: 105–19.

24. Dobrin PB. Vascular mechanics. In: American Physiological Society, Handbook of Physiology, Section 2, The cardiovascular system, Vol 3, Baltimore. 1983: 65–102.

25. Stehbens WE. Hemodynamics and the blood vessel wall. Springfield: Charles C. Thomas, 1979.
26. Carton RW, Dainauskas J, Clark JW. Elastic properties of single elastic fibers. J Appl Physiol 1962; 17: 547–51.
27. Remington JW, Hamilton WF, Dow P. Some difficulties involved in the prediction of the stroke volume form the pulse wave velocity. Am J Physiol 1945; 180: 83–95.
28. McDonald DA. Blood flow in arteries. London: Edward Arnold, 1974.
29. Doyle JM, Dobrin PB. Stress gradients in the walls of large arteries. J Biomech 1973; 6: 631–9.
30. Simon BR, Kobayashi AS, Strandness E, Wierderhielm CA. Reevaluation of arterial constitutive relations. Circ Res 1972; 30: 491–500.
31. Wolinsky H, Glagov S. Lamellar unit of aortic medial structure and function in mammals. Circ Res 1967; 20: 99–111.
32. Hedin U, Sjolund M, Hultgardh-Nilsson B, Thyberg J. Changes in expression and organization of smooth muscle specific alpha actin during fibronectin-mediated modulation of arterial smooth muscle cell phenotype. Differentiation 1990; 44: 222–31.
33. Bottger BA, Hedin U, Johansson S, Thyberg J. Integrin-type receptors of rat arterial smooth muscle cells: isolation, partial characterisation and role In cytoskeletal organisation and control of differential properties. Differentiation 1989,41: 158–7.
34. Saouaf R, Takasaki I, Eastman E, Chobanian A, Brecher P. Fibronectin biosynthesis in the rat aorta in vitro. J Clin Invest 1991; 88: 1182–9.
35. Bayliss LE. The rheology of blood. In: American Physiological Society Handbook of Physiology, Section 2, Circulation, Vol 1, Washington, 1962.
36. Fung YC. Biomechanics: Mechanical properties of living tissues. New-York: Springer-Verlag; 1981.
37. Caro CG, Pedley JG, Schroter RC, Seed WA. The mechanics of the circulation. Oxford: Oxford University Press, 1978.
38. Schretzenmayr A. Uber kreislaufregulatarische Vorgange an den grossen Arterian bei der Muskelarbeit. Pfluegers Arch 1933; 232: 743–8.
39. Smiesko V, Kokik J, Dolezel S. Role of endothelium in the control of arterial diameter by blood flow. Blood Vessels 1985; 22: 247–51.
40. Olensen SP, Clapham DE, Davies PF. Hemodynamic shear stress activates a K^+ current in vascular endothelial cells. Nature 1988; 331: 168–70.
41. Pohl U, Holtz J, Busse R, Bassenge E. Crucial role of endothelium in the vasodilator response to increased flow in vivo. Hypertension 1986; 8: 34–44.
42. Rubanyi GM, Romero JC, Vanhoutte PM. Flow-induced release of endothelium-derived relaxing factor. Am J Physiol 1986; 250: H1145–H49.
43. Koller A, Kaley G. Prostaglandins mediates arteriolar dilation to increased blood flow velocity in skeletal muscle microcirculation. Circ Res 1990; 67: 529–34.
44. Bevan JA, Joyce EHN,Wellman GC. Flow dependent dilation in a resistance artery still occurs after endothelium removal. Circ Res 1988; 63: 980–5.
45. Bevan JC, Joyce EH. Flow-induced resistance artery tone balance between constrictor and dilator mechanisms. Am J Physiol 1990; 258: H663–H8.
46. Berne RM, Levy MN. Cardiovascular physiology. St Louis: CV Mosby, 1972: 41–99.
47. Womersley JR. Method for the calculation of velocity, rate of flow and viscous drag in arteries when the pressure gradient is known. J Physiol 1955; 127: 553–63.
48. Hale JF, McDonald DA, Womersley JR. Velocity profiles of oscillating arterial flow, with some calculations of viscous drag and the Reynold number. J Physiol 1955; 128: 629–40.
49. Ku DN, Giddens DP, Zarins CK, Glagov S. Pulsatile flow and atherosclerosis in the human carotid bifurcation: positive correlation between plaque location and low and oscillating shear stress. Arteriosclerosis 1985; 5: 293–302.
50. Klanchar M, Tarbell JM, Wang DM. In vitro study of the influence of radial wall motion on wall shear stress in an elastic tube model of the aorta. Circ Res 1990; 66: 1624 35.

51. Sandor B. Fundamentals cf cyclic stress and strain. Madison: University of Wisconsin, 1972.
52. Prokop EK, Palmer RF, Wheat MW. Hydrodynamic forces in dissecting aneurysms. Circ Res 1970; 27: 121–7.
53. Mayer S. Studien zur Physiologie des Herzens und der Blutgefasse: 5. Abhandlung: uber spontane Blutdruckschwankungen. Sber Akad Wiss Wien 1876; 74: 281–307.
54. Penaz J. Mayer waves: history and methodology. Automedica 1978; 2: 135–141.
55. Malliani A, Pagani M, Lombardi F, Cerutti S. Cardiovascular neural regulation explored in the frequency domain. Circulation 1991; 84: 482–92.
56. Furchgott RF, Zawadzki JV. The obligatory role of endothelial cell in the relaxation of arterial smooth muscle by acetylcholine. Nature 1980; 288: 373–6.
57. Vanhoutte PM. The endothelium-dependent modulation of vascular smooth muscle tone. New Eng J Med 1988; 319: 512–3.
58. Rees DD, Palmer RJ, Schultz R, Hodson HF, Moncada S. Characterization of three inhibitors of endothelial nitris oxide synthase in vitro and in vivo. Br J Pharmacol 1990; 1 0 1: 746–52.
59. Hutcheson IR, Griffith TM. Release of endothelium derived relaxing factor is modulated both by frequency and amplitude of pulsatile flow. Am J Physiol 1991; 261: H257–H62.
60. Rubanyi GM. Endothelium-dependent pressure-induced contraction of isolated canine carotid artery. Am J Physiol 1988; 255: H783–H8.
61. Griffith T, Hutcheson 1, Randall M, Edwards D. Role of flow in endothelium-mediated responses. In: Mulvany MJ, Aalkjer C, Heagerty AM, Nyborg NCB, Strandgaard S, editors, Resistance arteries, structure and function. Amsterdam: Excerta Medica, 1991: 204–7.
62. Bevan JA,, Joyce EH, Wellman GC. Flow dependent dilation in a resistance artery still occurs after endothelium removal. Circ Res 1988; 63: 980–5.
63. Bevan JA, Joyce EH. Flow-induced resistance artery tone: balance between constrictor and dilator mechanisms. Am J Physiol 1990 258: H663–H669.
64. Laurent S, Lacolley P, Brunel P, Laloux B, Pannier B, Safar M. Flow-dependent vasodilation of the brachial artery in essential hypertension. Am J Physiol 1990; 258: H1004–11.
65. Girerd X, Arcaro G, Laurent S, Laloux B, Safar M. Etude de la vasodilatation flux-dépendante au niveau de l'artere fémorale chez l'hypertendu et le normotendu. Arch Mal Coeur 1991; 84: 1075–9.
66. Busse R, Mulsch A, Bassenge E. Shear stress-dependent nitric oxide release controls neuro-and myogenic vasoconstriction. In: Mulvany MJ, Aalkjer C, Heagerty AM, Nyborg NCB, Strandgaard S, editors, Resistance arteries structure and function. Amsterdam: Excerta Medica, 1991: 221–5.
67. Folkow B. Intravascular pressure as a factor regulating the tone of the small blood vessels. Acta Physiol Scand 1949; 86: 211–22.
68. Burrows ME, Johnson PC. The response of cat mesenteric arteries to arterial pressure reduction. Arch Int Pharmacodyn Ther 1978; 236: 290–1.
69. London G, Pannier B, Laurent S, Lacolley P, Safar M. Brachial artery diameter changes associated with cardiopulmonary baroreflex activation in humans. Am J Physiol 1990; 258: H773–H7.
70. Laurent S, Juillerat L, London GM, Nussberger J, Brunner H, Safar M. Increased response of brachial artery diameter to norepinephrine in hypertensive patients. Am J Physiol 1988; 255: H36–H43.
71. Lacolley P, Laurent S, Boutouyrie P, Girerd X, Beck L, Safar M. Sympathetic activation decreases arterial compliance through a direct effect on the arterial wall. 14th Scientific Meeting of the International Society of Hypertension, 1992: S–59.
72. Yamori Y, Mano M, Nara Y, Horie R. Catecholamine-induced polyploidization in vascular smooth muscle cells. Circulation 1987; 75(suppl I): 1–92–5.
73. Geisterfer AAT, Peach MJ, Owens G. Angiotensin II induces hypertrophy, not hyperplasia of cultured rat aortic smooth muscle cells. Circ Res 1988; 62: 749–56.

74. Folkow B. 'Structural factor' in primary and secondary hypertension. Hypertension 1990; 16: 89–101.
75. Schwartz SM, Majesky MW, Dilley RJ. Vascular remodeling in hypertension and athero-sclerosis. In: Hypertension: pathophysiology, diagnosis and management. Laragh JH, Brenner BM, editors. New York: Raven Press, 1990: 521–39.
76. Mulvany MJ, Hansen PK, Aalkjer C. Direct evidence that the greater contractility of resistance vessels in spontaneously hypertensive rat is associated with an increased number of smooth muscle cell layers. Circ Res 1978; 43: 854–64.
77. Folkow B, Hallbaeck,M, Lundgren Y, Weiss L. Background of increased flow resistance and vascular reactivity in spontaneously hypertensive rats. Acta Physiol Scand 1974; 91: 103–15.
78. Wolinski H. effect of hypertension and its reversal on the thoracic aorta of male and female rats. Circ Res 1971; 28: 622–36.
79. Berry CL, Greenwald SE. Effect of hypertension on the static mechanical properties and chemical composition of the rat aorta. Cardiovasc Res 1976; 10: 437–51.
80. Folkow B, Grimby G, Thulesius 0. Adaptive structural changes of the vascular walls in hypertension and their relation to the control of peripheral resistance. Acta Physiol Scand 1958; 44: 255–72.
81. Friberg P, Wahlander H, Nordlander M. Structural and functional adaptations within the myocardium and coronary vessels after antihypertensive therapy in spontaneously hypertensive rats. J Hypertens 1986; 4(suppl 3): S519–S21.
82. Aalkjer C, Heagerty AM, Petersen KK, Swales JD, Mulvany MJ. Evidence for increased media thickness, increased neuronal amine uptake, and depressed excitation-contraction coupling in isolated resistance vessels from essential hypertension. Circ Res 1987; 61: 181–6.
83. Schwartzkopff B, Motz W, Knauer S, Frenzel H, Strauer B. Morphometric investigation of intramyocardial arterioles in right septal endomyocardial biopsy of patients with arterial hypertension and left ventricular hypertrophy. J Cardiovasc Pharmacol 1992; 20(Suppl 1): S12–S7.
84. Horwitz D, Clineschmidt BV, Vanburen G, Omaya AK. Temporal arteries from hypertens-ive and normotensive man. Circ Res 1974; (suppl 1): 1–109–15.
85. Avolio AP, Deng Fa-Quan, Li WQ, et al. Effects of aging on arterial distensibility in populations with high and low prevalence of hypertension: comparison between urban and rural communities in China. Circulation 1985; 71: 202–10.
86. Mulvany MJ. Biophysical aspects of resistance vessels studied in spontaneous and renal hypertensive rats. Acta Physiol Scand 1988; 133(suppl 571): 129–38.
87. Baumbach GL, Dobrin PB, Hart MN, Heistadt DD. Mechanics of cerebral arterioles in hypertensive rats. Circ Res 1988; 62: 56–64.
88. Laurent S, Hayoz D, Trazzi S, et al. Isobaric compliance of the radial artery is increased in patients with essential hypertension. J Hypertens 1993; 11: 89–98.
89. Mulvany MJ. A reduced elastic modulus of vascular wall components in hypertension ? Hypertension 1992; 20: 7–9.
90. Learoyd MB, Taylor MG. Alterations with age in the viscoelastic properties of human arterial wall. Circ Res 1966; 18: 278–92.
91. Boutouyrie P, Laurent S, Benetos A, Girerd X, Hoeks A, Safar M. Opposing effects of aging on distal and proximal large arteries in hypertensives. J Hypertens 1992; 10(suppl 6): S87–S91.
92. Fischer GM, Swain ML, Cherian K. Increased vascular collagen and elastin synthesis in experimental atherosclerosis in the rabbit. Variation in synthesis among multiple vessels. Atherosclerosis 1980; 35: 11–20.
93. Leung DY, Glagov S, Mathews MB. Cyclic stretching stimulates the synthesis of matrix components by arterial smooth muscle cells in vitro. Science 1976; 191: 475–7.
94. Sottiurai VW, Kollros P, Mathews MB, Zarins CK, Glagov S. Morphologic alteration of smooth muscle cells by cycling stretching. J Surg Res 1983; 35: 490–7.

95. Lyon RT, Runyon–Hass A. Davis HR, Glagov S, Zarins CK. Protection from atherosclerosis lesion formation by reduction of artery wall motion. J Vasc Surg 1987; 5: 59–67.

96. Hollander W, Kramsch DM, Farelant M, Madoff IM. Arterial wall metabolism in experimental hypertension of coarctation of the aorta of short duration. J Clin Invest 1968; 47: 1221–9.

97. Bomberger RA. Zarins CK, Taylor KE, Glagov S. Effects of hypotension on atherogenesis and aortic wall composition. J Surg Res 1980; 36: 745–60.

98. Baumbach GL, Siems JE, Heistadt DD. Effects of local reduction in pressure on distensibility and composition of cerebral arterioles. Circ Res 1991; 68: 338–51.

99. Bots M, Hofman A, de Bruyn AM. de Jong PTVM, Grobbe DE. Isolated systolic hypertension and vessel wall thickness of the carotid artery. The Rotterdam Elderly Study.. Arteriosclerosis and Thrombosis 1993; 13: 64–9.

100. Mancia G, Ferrari A, Gregorini L. et al. Blood pressure and heart rate variabilities in normotensive and hypertensive human beings. Circ Res 1983; 53: 96–104.

101. Lacolley P, Glaser E, Challandes P. Brisac A-M, Safar M, Laurent S. Effects of sympathetic denervation on mechanical properties of rat large arteries. Arch Mal Coeur 1991; 84: S13.

102. Fuster V, Badimon L, Cohen M, Ambrose JA, Badimon JJ, Chesebro J. Insights into the pathogenesis of acute ischemic syndromes. Circulation 1988; 77: 1213–20.

103. Davies MJ. A macro and micro view of coronary vascular insult in ischemic heart disease. Circulation 1990; 8Z(suppl II) II-38–II-46.

104. Falk E. Coronary thrombosis: Pathogenesis and clinical manifestations. Am J Cardiol 1991; 68: 28B–35B.

105. Gertz SD, Roberts WC. Hemodynamic shear force in rupture of coronary arteria atherosclerotic plaques. Am J Cardiol 1990; 66: 1368–72.

106. Binns RL, Ku DN. Effect of stenosis on wall motion: a possible mechanism of stroke and transient ischemic attack. Arteriosclerosis 1989; 9: 842–7.

107. Barger AC, Beeuwes R, Lainey LL, Silverman KJ. Hypothesis: vasa vasorum and neovascularization of human coronary arteries: A possible role in the pathophysiology of atherosclerosis.. N Eng J Med 1991; 88: 8154–8.

108. Loree HM, Kamm RD, Atkinson CM, Lee RT. Turbulent pressure fluctuations on surface of model vascular stenoses. Am J Physiol 1991; 261: H644–H50.

109. Vito RP, Whang MC, Giddens DP, Zarins CK, Glagov S. Stress analysis of the diseased arterial cross-section. ASME Adv Bioeng Proc 1990; 19: 273–6.

110. Loree HM, Kamm RD, Stringfellow RG, Lee RT. Effects of fibrous cap thickness on peak circumferential stress in model atherosclerotic vessels. Circ Res 1992; 71: 850–8.

111. Richardson PD, Davies MJ, Born GVR. Influence of plaque configuration and stress distribution on fissuring of coronary atherosclerotic plaques. Lancet 1989; 2: 941–4.

112. Kayima A, Togawa T. Adaptive regulation of wall shear stress to flow change in the canine carotid artery. Am J Physiol 1980; 239: H14–H21.

113. Liebow AA. Situations which lead to changes in vascular patterns. In: Handbook of Physiology. Section 2, The cardiovascular system, Washington DC, 1963, American Physiological Society; pp 1251–76.

114. Guyton JR, Hartley CJ. Flow restriction of one carotid artery in juvenile rats inhibits growth of arterial diameter. Am J Physiol 1985; 248: H540–H46.

115. Langille BL, Bendeck MP, Keeley FW. Adaptations of carotid arteries of young and mature rabbits to reduced carotid blood flow. Am J Physiol 1989; 256: H931–H939.

116. Fry DL. Acute vascular endothelial changes associated with increased blood flow velocity gradients. Circ Res 1968; 22: 165–97.

117. Caro CC, Nerem RM. Transport of 14 C-4-cholesterol between serum and wall in the perfused dog common carotid artery. Circ Res 1973; 32: 187–205.

118. Glagov S, Zarins CK. Is intimal hyperplasia an adaptive response or a pathologic process? Observations on the nature of nonatherosclerotic intimal thickening. J Vasc Surg 1989; 10: 571–3.

119. Margitic SE, Bond MG, Crouse JR, Furberg CD, Probstfield JL. Progression and regression of carotid atherosclerosis in clinical trials. Arteriosclerosis and Thrombosis 1991; 11: 443–51.
120. Dintenfass L, Bauer GE. Dynamic blood coagulation and viscosity and degradation of artificial thrombi in patients with hypertension. Cardiovasc Res 1970; 4: 50–60.
121. Zannad F, Voisin P, Brunotte F, Bruntz JF, Stolz JF, Gilgenkrantz JM. Hemorheological abnormalities in arterial hypertension and their relation to cardiac hypertrophy. J Hypertens 1988; 6: 293–7.
121. Levenson J, Simon AC, Cambien FA, Beretti C. Cigarette smoking and hypertension: factors independently associated with blood hyperviscosity and arterial rigidity. Arteriosclerosis 1987; 7: 572–7.
122. Razavian S, Del Pino M, Simon A, Levenson J. Increase in erythrocyte disaggregation shear stress in hypertension. Hypertension 1992; 20: 247–52.

2. Hypertension and the conduit and cushioning functions of the arterial tree

MICHAEL F. O'ROURKE

Introduction

The diagnosis of hypertension is an unsatisfactory one, since it depends not on a pathological abnormality, but on measurement of a physiological variable, arterial pressure [1, 2]. This varies within each heart beat, throughout the respiratory cycle, and throughout the 24-hour period of each day. The diagnosis is determined clinically by measuring pressure by a cuff sphygmomanometer in the brachial artery, yet it is known that this pressure (at least for the highest or systolic value) is often quite different to that in other arteries – especially in the ascending aorta, and in the left ventricle of the heart [3, 4]. Further, it is known that the relationship between systolic pressure in central and peripheral arteries varies with heart rate, with exercise, and with drug therapy, as well as with aging and disease [5–8].

The diagnosis of hypertension usually implies elevation of both systolic and diastolic pressure, but may be referred to as diastolic hypertension when diastolic pressure only is raised, or isolated systolic hypertension when only systolic pressure is raised [9]. Contrary to earlier reports, it is now accepted that systolic pressure is a better predictor than diastolic pressure, of morbidity and mortality in all forms of hypertension [9–12].

In the light of these difficulties, it is not surprising that a more fundamental approach might be sought to the underlying problem of hypertension, and to the mechanisms whereby ill effects are brought about. This chapter will describe such an approach.

Arterial function

The arterial system can be seen as having two separate components – the conduit arteries, and the resistive arterioles – and to have two distinct functions – to distribute blood to bodily tissues according to need (conduit function) and to cushion the flow pulsations generated by intermittent ventricular ejection (cushioning function) [2]. The low resistance arteries are

M. E. Safar and M. F. O'Rourke (eds.), The arterial system in hypertension. pp. 27–37.
© 1993 Kluwer Academic Publishers. Printed in the Netherlands.

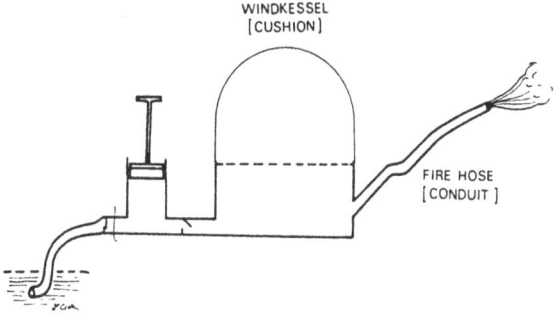

Figure 1. The arterial system was likened by Stephen Hales (1733) to the contemporary fire engine whose air filled dome or 'Windkessel' acted as cushion, and whose fire hose acted as conduit. The Windkessel smoothed out the intermittent spurts from the pump so that water was delivered through the hose in a steady stream. The Windkessel represents arterial distensibility, the fire hose the distributing arteries, and the nozzle the peripheral resistance. From: Ref [2] with permission.

vitally important in both functions, while the arterioles, by sustaining autonomic-nerve mediated vasoconstrictor tone, maintain mean arterial pressure, and permit blood to be distributed to different tissues according to their needs.

In the classic treatise by Stephen Hale on blood pressure, first published in the 1733 [13], the arterial system was likened to the contemporary fire engine device, where cushioning function was served by an inverted air-filled dome or 'Windkessel' and the arterial conduit function was served by the fire hose itself, and with the smallest arteriolar resistance vessels likened to the fire hose nozzle (Figure 1).

The Windkessel provides a good simple model of the arterial system, and describes effectively the principal alterations in peripheral resistance, and in vascular compliance, that are seen in hypertension (Figure 2). When resistance only is increased, the mean arterial pressure is elevated, with the same change in pressure pulsation about this, and so equal increase in both systolic and diastolic pressure. When however increased resistance is associated with decreased compliance (increased stiffness of the arterial system), mean pressure is elevated to the same degree, but pressure oscillation is increased such that systolic pressure is disproportionately increased, while diastolic pressure may be near normal [1, 2].

The Windkessel is a good simple model for describing the elementary disturbance of conduit and cushioning function as seen in hypertension. It is however an oversimplification – because it considers all compliance to be lumped at one spot (the Windkessel itself) and with conductance confined to the non-compliant fire hose. The arterial system actually combines both the cushioning and conduit functions. The arteries cushion flow pulsations as they distribute blood to the periphery – there is no separate Windkessel [2, 3].

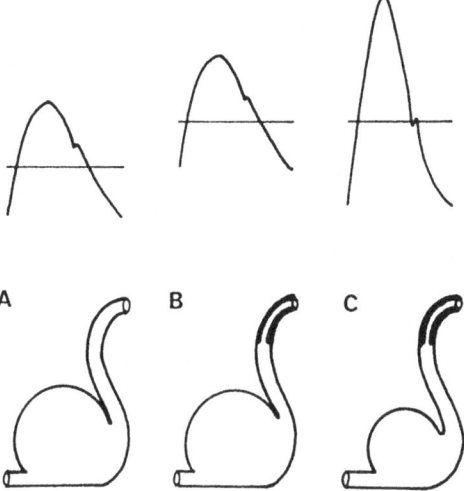

Figure 2. Effects of increased resistance and decreased compliance on arterial pressure waves (top) in three 'Windkessel' models of the arterial system (bottom). (A) Normal compliance, normal resistance. (B) Normal compliance, increased resistance. (C) Reduced compliance, increased resistance. Mean arterial pressure is represented by the solid line From: Ref [2] with permission.

A more realistic model of the arterial tree is a simple tube which terminates at the peripheral resistance, but whose distributed elastic properties permit generation of a pressure wave which travels along the tube. This model too might be regarded as an oversimplification of the arterial tree, but it is a vast improvement on the Windkessel [14]. In the model (Figure 3) as in life, the wave takes a finite time to travel along the tube such that there is delay in the foot of the wave at different sites between the proximal and distal part of the tube. Further, high resistance at the tube's end (which represents the peripheral resistance) creates wave reflection, with generation of a retrograde wave. This is responsible for appearance of secondary fluctuations on the pulse (as seen in life), and difference in amplitude of the pressure wave itself between central and peripheral arteries (also as seen in life) [2, 3].

In such a tubular model (Figure 3) increase in peripheral resistance increases mean pressure just as in the Windkessel, but decrease in compliance can be seen to create two separate effects which correspond to the separate phenomena which are seen in life. These are illustrated in Figure 3 which shows the form of a pressure wave generated at the input of a simple elastic tubular model for the same flow input. In the first case, flow ejection creates a single systolic pressure wave, while wave reflection from the periphery generates a smaller secondary diastolic wave; the pattern is very similar to what one normally sees in the ascending aorta of the young human adult. In

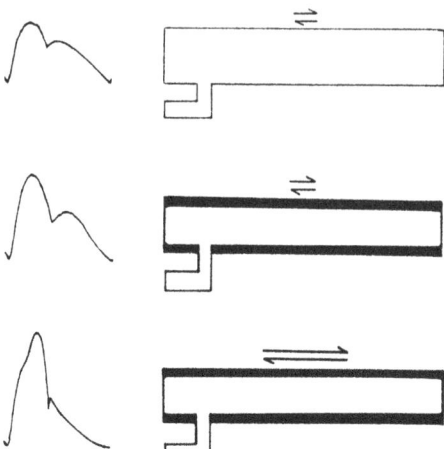

Figure 3. Simple tubular models of the systemic arterial system. *Top* – normal distensibility and normal pulse wave velocity; *Centre* – decreased distensibility but normal pulse wave velocity; *Bottom* – decreased distensibility with increased pulse wave velocity. At left are the amplitude and contour of the pressure waves that would be generated at the origin of these models by the same ventricular ejection. Decreased distensibility per se increases pressure wave amplitude only, but increased wave velocity causes the reflected wave to return during ventricular ejection, rather than during ventricular diastole, causing augmentation to late systolic pressure. From: Ref [14] with permission.

the second case, compliance of the tube is decreased without any change in timing of wave reflection.

This generates a wave of greater amplitude (just as it does in the Windkessel, and shown in Figure 2), but the diastolic wave remains, and is of similar relative amplitude as before. In the third case, decreased compliance (increased stiffness) is combined with increased velocity of the arterial pulse wave. The input systolic pressure wave is increased, just as before, but increased wave velocity results in early appearance of the reflected wave which now boosts the systolic pressure further, while causing pressure to fall steeply without any secondary fluctuation throughout diastole. This is just the type of appearance seen in the ascending aorta of experimental animals when arterial pressure is artificially elevated (Figure 4), and in human subjects with arteriosclerosis or hypertension (Figure 5). Indeed, such an appearance was noted as characteristic of hypertension (in young subjects) by Frederick Mahomed in his sphygmographic studies conducted twenty years before the Riva-Rocci cuff was introduced [15].

These fundamental principles and these simple models help to explain the hemodynamic findings in human hypertension, and assist in understanding ill effects of the process, and the logical approach to therapy [2, 3, 8].

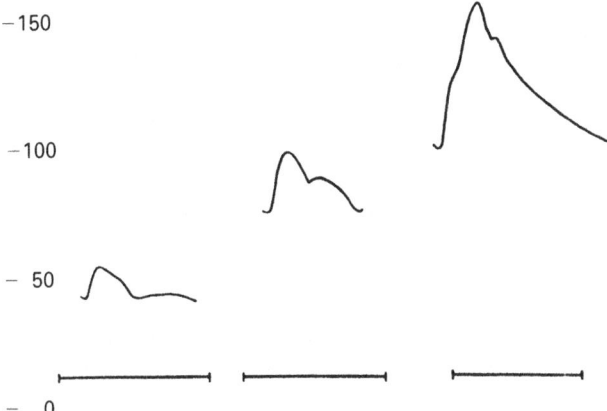

Figure 4. Effect of increasing pressure on contour of pressure waves in the ascending aorta of a rabbit. Diastolic waves are apparent at lower pressures but absent when arterial pressure is abnormally high. With hypertension, the diastolic wave is replaced by a late systolic pressure peak. From: Ref [16] after data rearranged from Wetterer (1954), with permission, American Heart Association Inc.

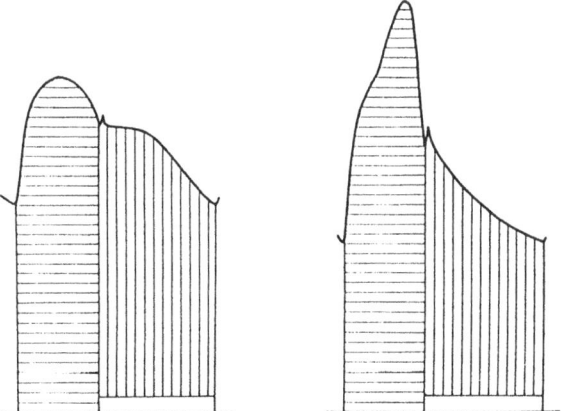

Figure 5. Typical ascending aortic pressure waves in a young human adult (*left*) and in a middle-aged adult (*right*). The horizontally hatched area is the pressure generated during cardiac ejection, while the vertically hatched area is the pressure maintained during cardiac diastole. From: Ref [2] with permission.

Pathophysiological mechanisms in hypertension

The basic problem of essential hypertension is increased peripheral resistance, with consequent elevation in mean arterial pressure. This may be due to increased tone, and decreased calibre of individual resistance vessels, or to vascular rarefaction, and decreased total number of resistance vessels [2, 3, 9]. The former process is dominant in young hypertensive subjects, the latter in the elderly [8]. Increased arterial pressure throws greater tension on elastic load bearing components of the arterial wall. As previously discussed by Laurent on p. 8, these exhibit non linear stress/strain relationships, such that the arteries are less compliant (more stiff) at the higher pressure. Further, wave velocity increases concurrently with stiffness – the two are directly related through the Moens-Korteweg equations [3]. It follows that while with hypertension, the basic problem is created by elevated peripheral resistance and elevated mean pressure, secondary problems follow in consequence of increased arterial stiffness and increased wave velocity – and are manifest as increase in pulse pressure with disproportionate increase in systolic pressure [3, 8].

These principles were formulated by our group in Sydney in the 1960s and were illustrated by change in pressure contour in experimental animals during infusion of sympathomimetic agents and through determination of ascending aortic pressure/flow relationships as ascending aortic impedance [1, 16, 17; Figure 6].

Figure 6 shows these changes in schematic form, and illustrates alterations in the ascending aortic pressure wave and in ascending aortic impedance modulus which is seen in hypertension. The figure displays in the time domain (with the pressure wave) and in the frequency domain (with the impedance plot) how increased peripheral resistance, with consequent increased aortic stiffening and early wave reflection, alter arterial hemodynamics in hypertension.

Figure 6 shows (above) the ascending aortic pressure wave under normal circumstances (at left), and with hypertension (at right) for the same left ventricular ejection wave, illustrated centre. Increased peripheral resistance increases mean arterial pressure. Increased aortic stiffness increases amplitude of the pressure wave at the time of peak flow. Early wave reflection causes a boost to late systolic pressure in consequence of the reflected wave moving from diastole into systole; this is associated of course with disappearance of the diastolic wave. These alterations caused by change in resistance, aortic stiffness, and early wave reflection, are shown in the figure by the arrows at points 1, 2, and 3. As previously noted, these features of the pressure wave in hypertension were first used by Mahomed in 1874 to characterise the condition of high blood pressure in studies with the sphygmograph [15].

Changes in ascending aortic impedance modulus are shown in the lower part of Figure 6. The lower curve illustrates the normal impedance modulus

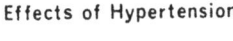

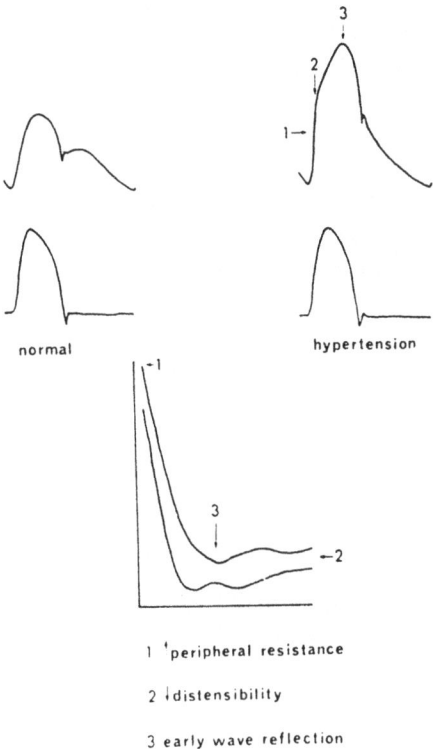

Figure 6. Diagrammatic illustration of hypertensive effects on the ascending aorta pressure wave with the same ascending aortic flow wave (*top panels*) and on modulus of ascending aortic impedance (*bottom*). Increased peripheral resistance explains increased mean pressure (top) and increased impedance modulus at zero frequency (bottom). Increased proximal aortic stiffness explains more rapid rate of rise of pressure to a high anacrotic 'shoulder' (top) and increased characteristic impedance (bottom), while the earlier return of wave reflection explains the late systolic peak of pressure (top) and shift of impedance curves to the right (bottom). From: Ref [1].

pattern while the upper curve shows the effects of hypertension. The same three mechanisms are shown by the arrows at point 1 (increased resistance), 2 (increased aortic stiffness), and 3 (early return of wave reflection). Increased peripheral resistance (1) elevates the level of impedance modulus at zero frequency and so shifts the early part of the curve upwards. Increased aortic stiffness (2) increases characteristic impedance and elevates impedance modulus at higher frequencies. Early wave reflection (3) shifts the whole curve to the right, with the discreet minima and maxima of impedance modulus occurring at higher frequencies than under control conditions.

Changes in the arterial pressure wave with hypertension are characteristic and were first described over one hundred years ago. The changes in impedance modulus were predicted in the 1960s [16, 17] and were subsequently described by Merillon et al in Paris [18, 19], and by Ting, Yin and colleagues in Taipei and Baltimore [20–22]. These studies are further discussed by Latham in the following chapter.

These recent studies [18–22] have confirmed that in human subjects with hypertension, increased peripheral resistance is associated with increased aortic characteristic impedance (expressed in terms of flow velocity) and increased aortic pulse wave velocity, together with evidence of early wave reflection from peripheral sites. Merillon et al. showed that all the changes could be reversed by infusion of a vasodilator agent such as nitroprusside [19] while Ting et al. showed that peripheral resistance and wave reflection are actually increased by beta-blockade [22]. Safar and co-workers in Paris have pointed to the different effects of anti-hypertensive agents on arterial distensibility [23, 24]. These are discussed elsewhere in this book (see Chapters 12–14).

Ill effects of hypertension

In the past, ill effects of hypertension were related to increase in peripheral resistance and to increase in mean arterial pressure. Since diastolic pressure is closer than systolic to mean pressure, diastolic pressure was considered a better guide than systolic to mean pressure and to abnormalities of arteriolar tone. This view appeared to gain authority from seminal works on clinical cardiovascular medicine, such as Mackenzie's text [25], and certainly did apply to the acute hypertensive emergencies that were so common in the past but that are so rare in modern practice [12, 26, 27]. Such emergencies include eclampsia, hypertensive encephalopathy and acute renal failure in malignant hypertension. These emergencies arise from an acute elevation in peripheral resistance which, through elevation of mean pressure, induces damage to the walls of small blood vessels with swelling of the wall and encroachment on the lumen. This further increases peripheral resistance, thus inducing a vicious circle [28]. Arterial compliance is of little relevance to this situation. Smirk & Alstad [29] were the first to show how this type of problem is reversed by use of ganglion blocking drugs which reduce peripheral resistance and drop mean and diastolic pressure. Byrom [28] attributed benefit to reduction of the tearing stress in the walls of small blood vessels. This problem can be viewed as one of disturbed conduit function of the arterial tree, with the main problem in the arterioles and small arteries.

In modern times, this type of problem however is not the usual cause of morbidity and mortality for persons whose blood pressure is high. Recent studies have confirmed the greater relevance of chronically elevated systolic pressure for the common complications of heart failure, myocardial infarction and stroke – and these usually occur in older patients whose systolic blood pressure is known to have been elevated for many years [11, 12]. Such knowledge directs attention to factors which determine systolic pressure and which affect the cushioning function of the arterial system. Attention has of course been focused on this subject with the success of the SHEP Study [30] in the USA, and the STOP Hypertension Study [31] in Europe. Both targeted systolic hypertension in elderly patients and both showed substantial reduction in morbidity and morbidity from cardiovascular events and from all causes.

These recent therapeutic trials draw attention to factors which alter the cushioning function of arteries, which elevate systolic arterial pressure, and which might be expected to reduce systolic pressure most effectively. Ironically, it appears that the drugs which were selected for use in the SHEP and STOP hypertension trials – diuretics and beta- blocking agents – may be the least effective for this condition. Diuretics have little or no effect on arterial compliance and no effect on wave reflection, whereas beta-blockers may decrease compliance and actually increase wave reflection [8, 20]. Calcium antagonists and ACE inhibitors (and nitrates) have more favourable effects on compliance and reduce wave reflection [8, 26]. These agents are more logical for use in the elderly where increase in systolic pressure is largely due to impaired arterial compliance and to early return of wave reflection from peripheral sites. Definitive long term studies have yet to be performed with such agents.

A vicious circle has thus been identified in malignant hypertension, whereby increased peripheral resistance increases mean arterial pressure, and this through damage to the walls of small arteries and arterioles causes oedema and inflammation with further increase in resistance and further increase in mean arterial pressure [28, 32].

Another vicious cycle affects the larger arteries and disturbs cushioning function, thus causing progressive increase in systolic blood pressure, in creased wall stress and damage to the arterial walls [2]. This process is a more chronic one and relates to the fatiguing effects of cyclic stress over years of arterial pulsation [1–3, 33] (Figure 7). Fatigue and fracture of the non living, inert elastin fibres of the arterial wall causes the wall to dilate, for more stress to be applied to the remaining elastin fibres, and for stress to be transferred to less extensible collagenous fibres in the wall. The La Place effect contributes as well. Higher systolic pressure causes faster fatigue and fracture. This causes further stiffening of the wall and higher systolic pressure [2, 3, 8]. Fundamental principles suggest that this process cannot be prevented, but it can be slowed by reducing peak systolic stress on central arteries (as by calcium antagonists, ACE inhibitors and nitrates) and by reducing the number of fatiguing cycles (as through use of beta-blocking agents).

Conclusion

It has been customary to focus attention in arterial hypertension on peripheral resistance, on factors which increase this, and on drugs which reduce

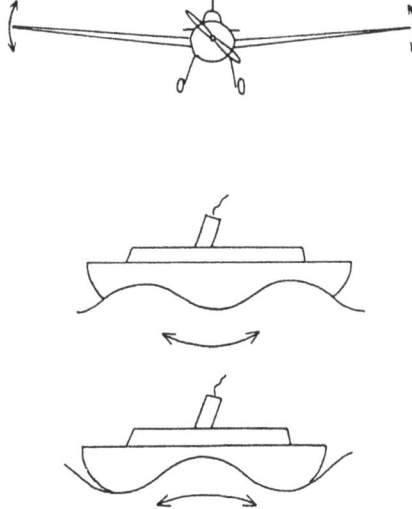

Figure 7. Cyclic stress causing fatigue and ultimately fracture in physical materials. From: Ref [2] after Sandor [33].

resistance. Recognition of increased systolic pressure as the most important challenge in hypertension today, draws attention to the cushioning function of arteries, and to the principal factors – arterial compliance and wave reflection which determine this. Optimal therapeutic interventions depend on understanding underlying mechanisms which determine mean pressure, and which determine pulsatile pressure, and a knowledge of how best to manipulate these.

References

1. O'Rourke MF. Pulsatile arterial haemodynamics in hypertension. Aust NZ J Med 1976; 6(Suppl 2): 40–8.
2. O'Rourke MF. Arterial function in health and disease. Edinburgh: Churchill Livingstone, 1982.
3. Nichols WW, O'Rourke MF. McDonald's blood flow in arteries. 3rd ed. London: Arnold, 1990.
4. O'Rourke MF, Avolio AP, Kelly RP. The arterial pulse. Baltimore: Lea & Febiger, 1991.
5. Gallagher D, Karamanoglu M, Herok G, Avolio A, Baird D, O'Rourke M. Peripheral pressure measurements may be unreliable for calculation of cardiac properties with change in heart rate. Aust NZ J Med 1993; 23: 112.
6. Rowell LB, Brengelmann GL, Blackmon JR et al. Disparities between aortic and peripheral pulse pressures induced by upright exercise and vasomotor changes in man. Circulation 1968; 37: 954–64.
7. Kelly RP, Gibbs H, O'Rourke MF, et al. Nitroglycerin has more favorable effects on the left ventricular afterload than apparent from measurement of pressure in a peripheral artery. Eur Heart J 1990; 11: 138–44.

8. O'Rourke MF. Arterial stiffness, systolic blood pressure, and logical treatment of arterial hypertension. Hypertension 1990; 15: 339–47.

9. Kaplan N. Clinical hypertension. Baltimore: Williams & Wilkins, 1990.

10. Garland C, Barrett-Conner E, Suarez L, Criqui MH. Isolated systolic hypertension and mortality after age 60 years. A prospective population-based study. Am J Epidemiol 1983; 365–76.

11. Rutan GH, Kuller LH, Neaton JD, Wentworth DN, McDonald RH, McFate-Smith W. Mortality associated with diastolic hypertension and isolated systolic hypertension among men screen for multiple risk factor intervention trial. Circulation 1988; 77: 504–14.

12. Birkenhager WH, de Leeuw PW. Impact of systolic blood pressure on cardiovascular prognosis. J Hypertension 1988; 6: (Suppl 1) S21–S24.

13. Hales S. 1733. Statical essays containing haemastaticks. History of Medicine Series. Library of New York Academy of Medicine 1964; No. 22. New York: Harper Publishing.

14. O'Rourke MF, Avolio AP, Nichols WW. Left ventricular-systemic arterial coupling in humans and strategies to improve coupling in disease states. In: Yin FCP. Ventricular vascular coupling. New York: Springer, 1987, 1–19.

15. Mahomed F. The aetiology of Bright's disease and the prealbumenuric stage. Med Chir Trans 1874; 57: 197–228.

16. O'Rourke MF. Arterial haemodynamics in hypertension.Cir Res 1970; 26 & 27: II,123–33.

17. O'Rourke MF. Taylor MG. Input impedance of the systemic circulation. Cir Res 1967; 20: 365–80.

18. Merillon JP, Motte G, Masquet C, Azancot I, Guiomard A, Gourgon R. Relationship between physical properties of the arterial system and left ventricular performance in the course of aging and arterial hypertension. Eur Heart J 1982; 3(Suppl A): 95–102.

19. Merillon JP, Fonterier GH, Lerallut JF, et al. Aortic input impedance in normal man and arterial hypertension: its modification during changes in aortic pressure. Cardiovasc Res 1982; 16: 646–56.

20. Ting CT, Brin KP, Lin Sj, et al. Arterial hemodynamics in human hypertension.J.Clin Invest 1986; 78: 1462–71.

21. Ting CT, Chang MS, Wang SP, Chiang BN, Yin FCP. Regional pulse wave velocities in hypertensive and normotensive humans.Cardiovasc Res 1990; 24: 865–72.

22. Ting CT, Chou CY, Chang MS, Wang SP, Chiang BN, Yin FCP. Arterial hemodynamics in human hypertension effects of adrenergic blockade. Circulation 1991; 84: 1049–57.

23. Safar ME. Management of hypertension in the elderly. New Engl J Med 1980; 303: 1234.

24. Safar ME, Bouthier JA, Levinson JA, Simon AC. Peripheral large arteries and the response to antihypertensive treatment. Hypertension 1983; 5(Suppl III): 63–8.

25. Mackenzie J. Principles of diagnosis and treatment of heart affections. 3rd ed. London: Oxford 1926.

26. O'Rourke MF, Safar ME, Dzau V, et al. Arterial vasodilation: mechanics and therapy. London: Edward Arnold/Philadelphia: Lea & Febiger, 1992.

27. Dunstan H. Isolated systolic hypertension: a long-neglected cause of cardiovascular complications. Am J Med 1989; 86: 368–9.

28. Byrom F. The hypertensive vascular crisis – an experimental study. London: Heineman, 1969.

29. Smirk FH, Alstad KS. Treatment of arterial hypertension by peta- and hexamethonium salts. Br Med J 1951; 1: 1217–28.

30. S.H.E.P. Cooperative Research Group. Prevention of stroke by antihypertensive drug treatment in older persons with isolated systolic hypertension: final results of the Systolic Hypertension in the Elderly Program. J Am Med Assoc 1991; 265: 3255–64.

31. Dahlof B, Lindholm LH, Hansson L, Schersten B, Ekbom T, Wester PO. Morbidity and mortality in the Swedish Trial in Old Patients with Hypertension / (STOP Hypertension). Lancet 1991; 338: 1281.

32. Pickering G. High blood pressure. London: Churchill, 1968.

33. Sandor Fundamentals of cyclic stress and strain. Madison: University of Wisconsin 1972.

3. Wave reflections and the pathophysiology of hypertension

RICKY D. LATHAM and DAVID M. SLIFE

Introduction

Cardiovascular research pioneers recognized the changes that occur in the arterial pulse wave as it travels from the heart to the periphery. In 1928 Dr. Carl Wiggers wrote:

> In its passage to the periphery, this fundamental wave is altered in contour in several ways, viz: (a) by the depression of waves through friction and damping, (b) by the introduction of natural or free vibrations in different regions of the arterial system, (c) by the amplification or annihilation of centrifugal by reflected waves having the same or opposite phases respectively, and (d) by the transmission of vibrations and waves through the arterial system at differing velocities [1].

The initial evaluation of the arterial pulse was by characterizing it by palpation and it was noted that the palpable quality of an arterial pulse would change with certain disease states [2, 3]. Stokes described the change in the peripheral pulse of a patient with an aneurysm as a double impulse. Sir William Osler described the peripheral pulse in patients with arteriosclerotic disease as hard and resistant, and plainly perceptible to the finger in the intervals of the beats.

The advent of sphygmomanometry in the early part of this century had the effect of turning clinical attention away from pulse contour and character toward simply the numerical quantity of systolic and diastolic blood pressure [4]. The later development of invasive catheterization techniques and solid-state high-fidelity micromanometers led to a renaissance of investigative interest in the character of arterial waveforms in health and disease [5, 6]. The changes in pulse wave velocity and wave reflections that occur with increasing age or hypertension have significant effects on the arterial waveform [2, 7]. This chapter will focus on wave reflections and their influence on the arterial pulse in normal and hypertensive conditions.

M. E. Safar and M. F. O'Rourke (eds.), The arterial system in hypertension. pp. 39–53.
© 1993 *Kluwer Academic Publishers. Printed in the Netherlands.*

Definitions and mathematics

The existence of wave reflections in the arterial system is suggested by (1) the amplification of the pressure pulse as it travels distally and (2) the disparity in flow and pressure waveforms [8]. Waves in a closed system will reflect at sites of geometric or viscoelastic discontinuity. Thus, in a uniform, nonbranching tube with unchanging diameter or elasticity there would be no wave reflection. This is not the case for the typical mammalian arterial system, however, which has multiple branch points and changes in elasticity from proximal to distal segments. At every point in the circulation where there is a "mismatch" in local pulsatile resistances, from parent to daughter vessels, there will be a reflection of the incident wave [8, 9].

Therefore, at any point in the circulation, the measured pressure (P_m) or flow (Q_m) waveform is the sum of forward (P_f, Q_f) and backward (P_b, Q_b) waves [10]:

$$P_m = P_f + P_b \tag{1}$$

$$Q_m = Q_f + Q_b \tag{2}$$

The resistive pulsatile load may be expressed in terms of *impedance*. A full treatment of arterial impedance is beyond the scope of this text. Briefly, the mathematical technique of Fourier analysis is used to express pressure and flow waves as a series of sinusoidal waves of increasing frequency determined by the fundamental harmonic (or heart rate). Corresponding harmonic amplitudes of pressure are divided by flow to derive a modulus of impedance, and the corresponding phase angles are subtracted to determine the *phase* of impedance Ψ. The average of the higher harmonic values of the modulus gives the *characteristic impedance, Z_c*.

The reflection coefficient, Γ, of a tube with characteristic impedance, Z_c, into two tubes with a combined impedance of Z_D, is given by:

$$\Gamma = \frac{1 - (Z_c/Z_D)}{1 - (Z_c/Z_D)} = \frac{Z_D - Z_c}{Z_D - Z_c} \tag{3}$$

Additionally, the reflection coefficient may be expressed as the ratio of backward to forward waves:

$$\Gamma = \frac{P_b}{P_f} = \frac{-Q_b}{Q_f} \tag{4}$$

Note that pressure waves reflect positively and flow waves reflect negatively.

The forward and reflected waves are in a constant state of interaction. The wave envelopes have regions of peak and minimum amplification determined by the phase relationship between forward and reflected waves [9]. This phase relationship is determined by a multitude of factors, including a propagation coefficient, distance to site of reflection and the reflection coefficient at the terminus.

$$\Gamma = a + jb \tag{5}$$

This complex coefficient λ, is determined by a component, a, related to changes in amplitude and one b, relating to the speed of wave travel.

'*Effective length*' is the *apparent* length of the system that is determined from the quarter-wavelength formula and the input impedance spectrum [8, 11, 12]. Reflections occur at multiple sites along the systemic tree and from peripheral vascular beds all at varying distances from the input (aortic valve). The oscillations of incident and reflected waves result in an interaction that is either a summation or cancellation depending on the phase shift that occurs at the reflection site. The points of minimum peak amplitudes in the resultant wave are referred to as nodes and occur at even integral multiples one quarter wavelength from the terminus of a tube. The net sum behaves mathematically as a discrete reflection form some site at a distance, L_{eff} from the input. Thus, the length, L, to a reflecting site and a node is:

$$L = n\frac{\lambda}{4} \tag{6}$$

where n = any odd integer and λ is wavelength ($\lambda = 2\pi/b$). This formula may be rewritten in terms of wave velocity, c, and frequency, f_{min}:

$$L_{eff} = \frac{c}{4f_{min}} \tag{7}$$

The usual method of determining the effective length is to use the frequency of the first minimum of the modulus of impedance for f_{min}. Many limitations to the use of this formula have been reviewed elsewhere, but it is important to note that L_{eff} varies with the frequency-dependency of Γ.

Another mathematical method for estimating the distance, L, to a dominant reflection site uses the waveform contour itself. The summation effect of reflected waves alters the mid-to-late systolic arterial pulse contour in middle-aged man [13, 14]. The distance time from the foot of the incident wave to the inflection point in mid-systole represents the time, Δtp, for the wave to travel to and return in summation from an apparent reflection point (Figure 1).

With knowledge of the speed of wave travel, c, the distance to the reflects site can be determined:

$$L = \frac{c\Delta tp}{2} \tag{8}$$

L determined in this fashion generally correlates acceptably with that calculated from the quarter-wavelength formula (see above).

Wave velocity may also be evaluated as a function of the traveling velocities

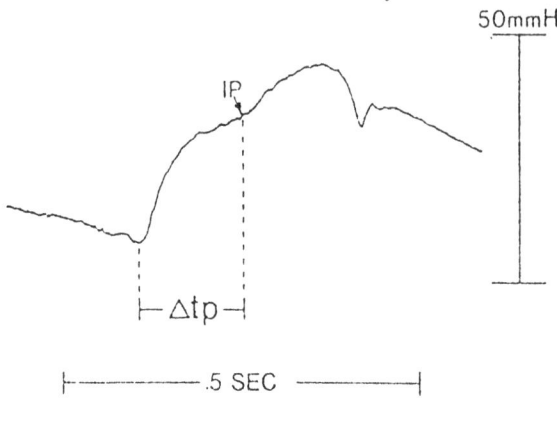

Figure 1. Typical arterial pulse contour in middle-aged man. IP indicates the systolic inflection point, Δ*tp* is the transmission time of the reflected wave. From Latham et al. [14] with permission.

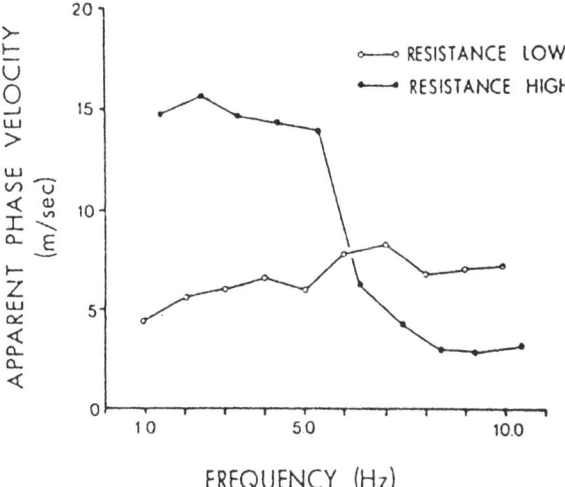

Figure 2. Effect of reflections on C_{app} in distal portion of latex tube model. Open circles refer to low terminal resistance, closed circles represent high resistance. From Latham et al. [14] with permission.

of individual frequency components. This velocity is dependent upon phase-shift along the distance travelled. This velocity; called the apparent phase velocity, C_{app} may be calculated as [15]:

$$C_{app} = \frac{2\pi f \Delta Z}{\Delta\phi} \tag{9}$$

where ΔZ is the distance between two points of interest and $\Delta\phi$ is the difference in phase between corresponding harmonics at those two points of interest. C_{app} is plotted as a function of frequency and the mean of higher harmonic values should correspond to the foot-to-foot velocity. Reflections will affect this plot and care must be taken in the interpretation of mean C_{app} [14, 15] (Figure 2).

Pressure and flow waves can be described in their forward and backward components with the use of the characteristic impedance, Z_c [10]. Backward (reflected) pressure and flow (P_b, Q_b) are given by:

$$P_b = \frac{P_m - Z_c^* Q_m)}{2} \tag{10}$$

$$Q_b = \frac{(Q_m - P_m/Z_c)}{2} \tag{11}$$

The principal sites of wave reflection have been studied extensively [14, 16, 17, 18]. It is now generally agreed, that reflections occur from the arteriolar bed in the periphery [2, 4, 8] as well as from major branch points in large arteries [6, 14]. Vasodilating agents certainly affect the former and may also alter the impedance mismatching at major branch points. The net result is a decrease in wave reflections.

Evaluation of reflections

Measurement of the pulse contour may be performed by either invasive [19, 20] or noninvasive techniques [21, 22, 23]. Early invasive modalities generally used fluid-filled catheter systems. Extensive interrogations of the vascular system in man lay the foundation for understanding the influence of wave reflections on the pulse contour [24, 25]. Fluid-filled systems, however, presented a number of limitations that have been reviewed elsewhere [5, 9]. Basically, fluid catheters are prone to some artifact due to air bubbles in the line, catheter whip, etc. They also have an intrinsic time delay to account for pulse transmission time to the external transducer. Thus, these systems are less than ideal for frequency-dependent analyses.

In the early mid 1970s, high-fidelity micromanometric catheterization made its debut [5]. The new technology also allowed placement of multiple micromanometers on a single catheter [14, 17, 19]. Later, catheter-mounted electromagnetic flow transducer permitted simultaneous recording of pressure and flow waveforms. Thus, frequency-dependent analyses of the vascular pressure-flow relationship could be better defined [20]. Numerous studies investigating the aortic input impedance have since been performed [6, 20, 26, 27].

It was appreciated by early investigators that arterial reflected waves markedly altered the waveform. The wave contour may be changed by enhancing reflections peripheral resistance pharmacologically or with bilateral femoral compression [20]. In animal studies the effect of intra-aortic occlusion on reflections may be seen more clearly [16]. In this case, the amplitude of change and timing are dependent upon distance from the site of measurement (in proximal aorta) (see Figure 3).

Additionally, the location at which the pulse contour is measured is also important. Figure 4 reveals aortic pressures recorded in a young patient with cardiomyopathy and low mean blood pressure. The high-fidelity recording from the aortic root does not show a prominent mid-to-late systolic peak of

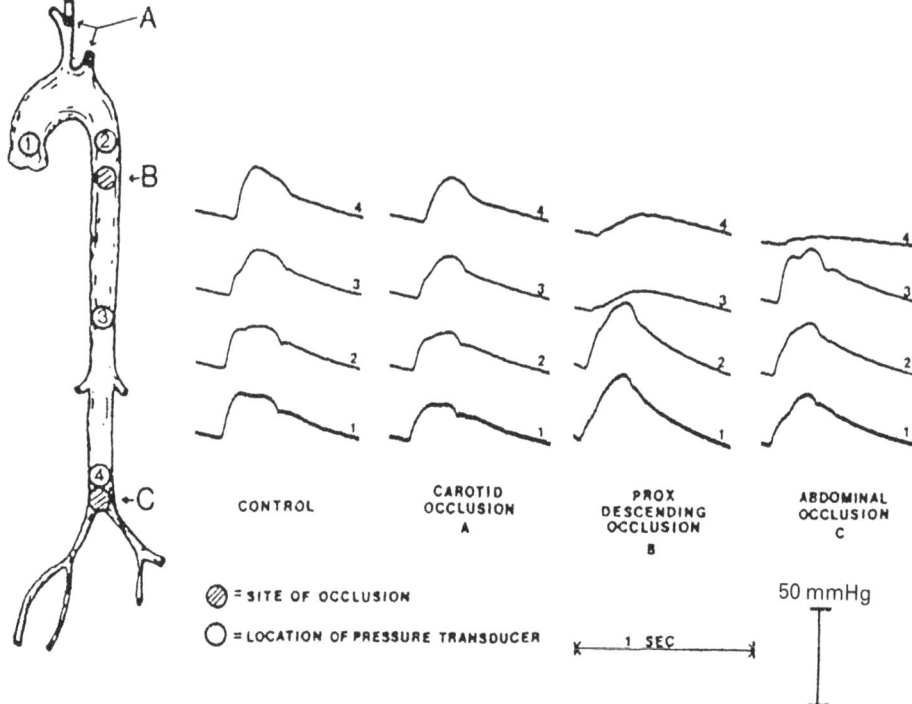

Figure 3. Simultaneous pressures along the baboon aorta with occlusion at various locations. From Latham et al. [15] with permission.

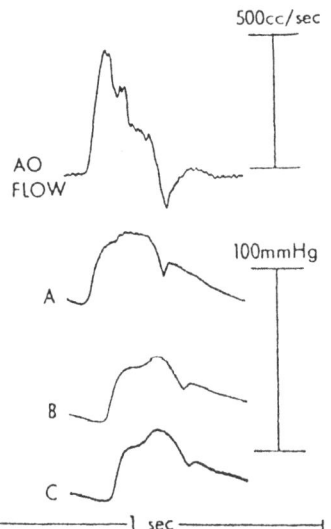

Figure 4. Pressure and flow in a young patient with cardiomyopathy. AO flow and pressure 'A' were simultaneously recorded in the aortic root. Pressures 'B' and 'C' were recorded simultaneously in the proximal descending aorta.
From Latham et al. [15] with permission.

NORMOTENSIVE   HYPERTENSIVE

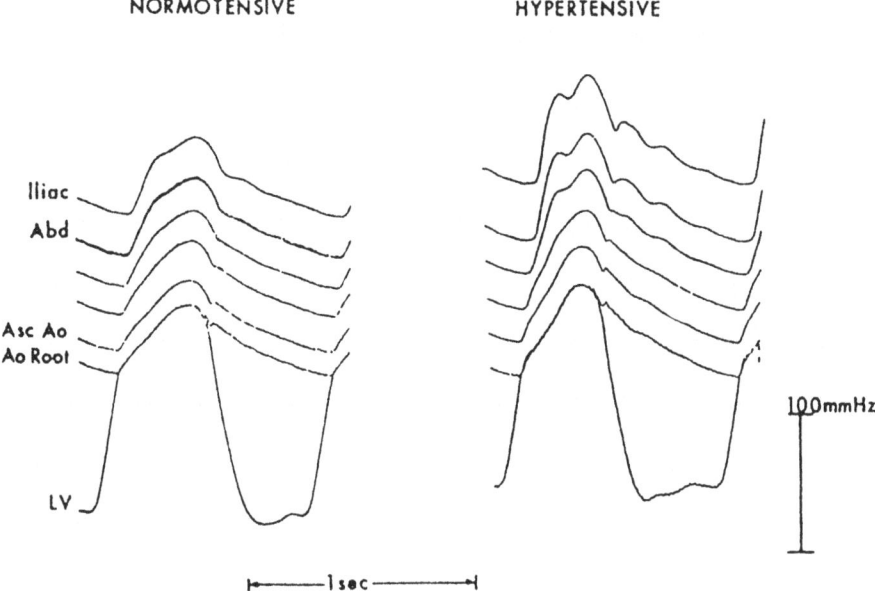

Iliac
Abd

Asc Ao
Ao Root

LV

100mmHz

|———1 sec———|

Figure 5. Simultaneous pressures along the baboon aorta at 5-cm intervals. From [15] with permission.

a reflected wave, perhaps leading one to conclude reflections are diminished in this disorder. However, when the catheter is advanced to the proximal descending aorta a definite reflected wave can be seen to alter the systolic contour. This implies strong attenuation of the returning wave prior to reaching the aortic root, but still visible when evaluated with more distal sensors.

The regional variance in amplitude of reflections may be seen in Figure 5. In this study, a multisensor catheter recorded simultaneous pressures from the femoral artery to the aortic root in normotensive and hypertensive baboons [27]. The reflection and re-reflected waves create an undulating perturbation to the waveform contour most prominent distally, with some attenuation to proximal segments.

Murgo et al. have described three types of waveforms recorded in the proximal aorta [20] (Figure 6). A type A beat is one generally found in middle-aged man and is characterized by a mild-to-late secondary systolic peak. In contrast, the type C beat is characterized by an early systolic peak and is usually found in younger patients. Type B beats represent an intermediate stage. Hypertensive subjects generally have an exacerbated mid-to-late secondary peak and the inflection point occurs earlier in systole (shorter Δtp). These changes are the result of many factors, including an increased peripheral resistance, a stiffening of the large arteries (thus less attenuation of reflected waves), and higher pulse transmission times.

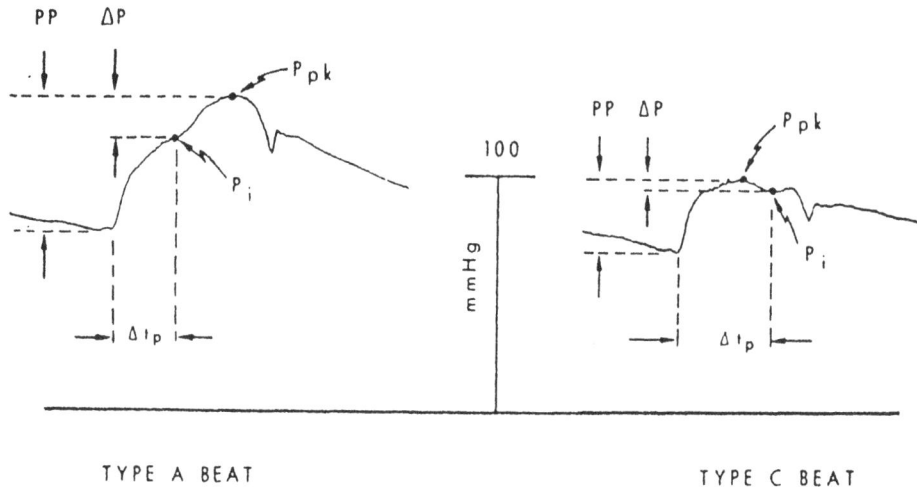

TYPE A BEAT   TYPE C BEAT

Figure 6. Three types of waveforms in man. From [20] with permission.

Noninvasive methods of recording the arterial pulse had their beginning with shygmographs developed by EJ Marey in the 19th century [3]. He made use of both air-filled and mechanical systems. In the later half of the 20th century engineering technology advances have provided micromanometers for applanation tonometry [21, 22] and Doppler ultrasound techniques [23]. Additionally, sophisticated vascular echo systems provide high resolution imaging of arterial diameters [28]. A more extensive discussion of these techniques may be found further in this chapter.

Flow wave contours are generally triangular-shaped in the ascending aorta with zero flow in diastole. The flow waveform in more peripheral arteries reveal diastolic fluctuations due to reflections from the peripheral vascular beds. It should be noted, however, that the overall amplitude of the flow waveform decreases toward the periphery due to the Windkessel behavior of the arterial tree and increasing total vascular cross-sectional area of distal beds [9].

The noninvasive methods do lend themselves to an evaluation of pulse contour changes significantly influenced by wave reflections. The high-fidelity capability of a micromanometer, specially mounted for applanation tonometry, permits recording high frequency information comparable to invasive recordings. In fact, in a study reported by Kelly (1989) tonometric and intra-arterial pressure recordings submitted to Fourier analysis revealed excellent correlations in moduli amplitudes, phase and percentage power of each harmonic [21] (Figure 7).

Early noninvasive pulse recordings with sphygmographs progressed to trials using air or fluid-filled capsules placed over the pulse. A diaphragm in the external volume capsule deflects with displacement of air or fluid with

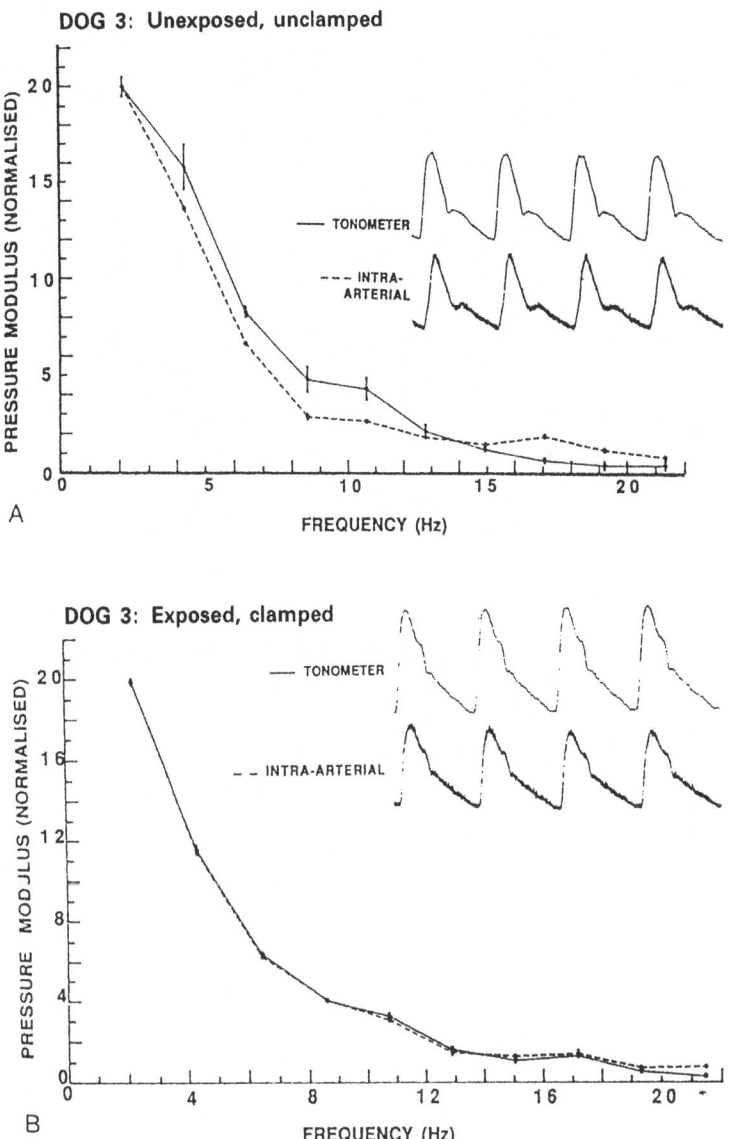

Figure 7. Simultaneous recordings of pressure by tonometry and an indwelling catheter expressed as modulus amplitudes from Fourier analysis. From [3] with permission.

each pulse [29, 30, 31]. The principle difficulty with this technique is that the volume signal recorded is different in wave shape from the intra-arterial pulse. It has been noted that radial volume displacement is not directly proportional to intra-arterial pulse [3]. There are also technical problems with this method including the size of the devices that cover a broad area of

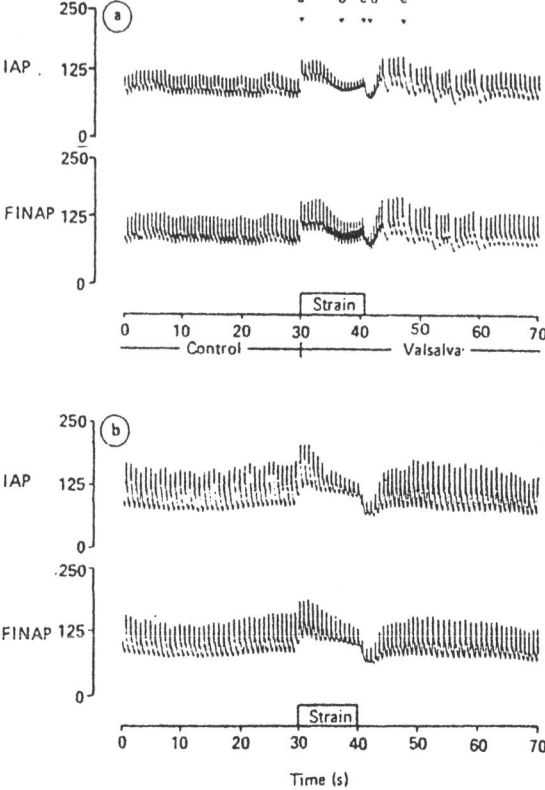

Figure 8. Two recordings of the Valsalva maneuver, showing a classical (*upper panel*) and a typical (*lower panel*) response. Note correlation between noninvasive finger pressure, FINAP, and intra-arterial recordings, IAP. From [36] with permission.

skin and force required to secure them in place often result in movement artifact [30].

Other techniques exist to noninvasively record the pressure pulse. Plethysmography, for example, frequently involves a technique utilizing a light source (on finger or ear lobe) and a photodetector. The methodology shares similar limitations related to assumptions made on the relationship between pressure and volume as stated above [32].

Another innovation uses the Penaz method to continuously record digital blood pressure [33]. The technique gives an accurate, calibrated, continuous digital pressure that faithfully records transients [34, 35, 36]. We have used this technique for recording continuous pressure in unusual environments such as during parabolic flight [36]. The pulse contour, however, may not faithfully represent those of more proximal intra-arterial recordings and has not been useful for evaluation of central wave reflections (Figure 8).

Reflections and pathophysiology

A discussion of wave reflections and the pathophysiology of hypertension should be prefaced with the acknowledgement that reflected waves in the systemic circulation are not the etiology of hypertension. Rather, the alterations in the arterial pulse contour due to augmentation by reflected waves are secondary effects to the changes in peripheral resistance and vascular elasticity resulting in an increased global reflection coefficient. It is true that the increased dP/dt and pulse amplitude may have adverse influence on cardiac function and vascular wall integrity but these end-organ responses are multifactorial, related to steady as well as pulsatile loading effects.

In discussing the pulse contour it is important to define the different components of the pressure waveform. The pressure wave is generated by the pulsatility of cardiac ejection into the arterial tree. It is classically described as consisting of two components: (1) mean arterial pressure defined as the product between cardiac output and peripheral resistance, (2) the pulsatile component corresponding to the values of the systolic and diastolic pressure levels. The mean pressure is affected by the cardiac output and the vascular resistance or the change in the caliber of the cross-sectional area of the small arteries. The pulsatile component or the pulse pressure is altered by the ventricular ejection, arterial distensibility, and the timing of reflected waves.

The systolic pressure waveform is the summation of an incident wave and a reflected wave coming from the peripheral level. The timing of the reflected waves is determined by the arterial distensibility and the reflection site distance from the aortic root. The wave can be broken down into two component pulse waves, reflected forward and backward from the periphery.

These reflected waves can be manipulated by physiologic maneuvers by changing the timing and amplitude of the reflections. This was demonstrated by use of the Valsalva and Mueller maneuvers [6, 12] (Figure 9). The amount of returning reflection at the level of the aortic root was increased due to an increase in amplitude of the mid-to-late systolic peak. The negative pleural pressure causes an increase in the transmural gradient across the intrathoracic aortic wall, which stiffens the proximal aorta resulting in less attenuation of the returning reflections and a decrease in the arterial distensibility.

A study in normal man showed that a change in the timing and amplitude of the reflected wave may also be seen with increasing age. Murgo (1980) showed that in a older age group the reflected waves were seen in late systole and contributed to an increase in the pulse pressure [20].

Other changes occurring to the pressure waveform with aging include an increase in systolic pressure to a greater extent than the rise in diastolic pressure giving a larger pulse pressure. The pulse pressure may be seen to increase with age with a steeper slope than that of the mean pressure. The increase in pressure seen with the elderly is due to the elevation in the mean pressure by an increase in the peripheral resistance and the pulse pressure is dependent on the arterial stiffness and possibly wave reflection changes.

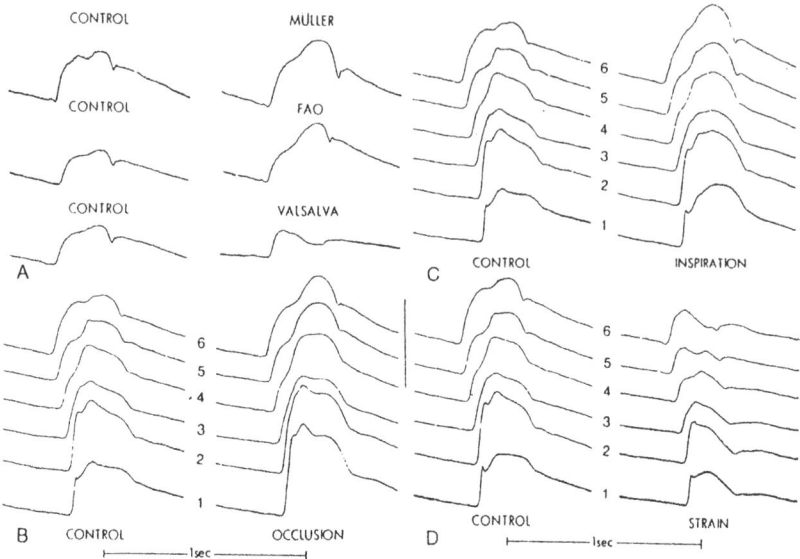

Figure 9. Simultaneous pressures recorded along the aorta in man during control, Valsalva and the Mueller maneuver. From [14] with permission.

It may be an exaggeration of this phenomenon that may account for the large number of patients with systolic hypertension only or systolic/diastolic hypertension with the diastolic component being the lesser of the two.

The mechanisms proposed for the explanation of the systolic and the systodiastolic hypertension seen in the elderly is a decrease in the arterial distensibility (compliance of the arteries) and a change in the reflected wave. In studies evaluating the systemic arterial compliance and its relationship to systemic hypertension, it was found that the same mean pressure in men with systolic hypertension and in controls of the same age that the arterial compliance was reduced in the patients with systemic hypertension [38]. The level of systolic hypertension inversely correlates with the systemic arterial compliance [37].

Arterial wave reflection may also contribute to or cause systolic hypertension. If an increase in stiffness of the arterial wall increases the pulse wave velocity enough It will to earlier return in systolic of the reflected pressure waves. With the addition of the forward and backward waves this alone may increase the systolic pressure enough to cause hypertension. This is an example of reflected waves returning earlier as seen in the Mueller maneuver described above with an increase in arterial stiffness. Examples of the reflected wave returning early and causing hypertension are disease states such as coarctation, traumatic amputation of lower extremities) and atherosclerosis obliterans of the lower extremities [38].

It has been shown that peripheral resistance is normal in the earliest stages of the natural history of hypertension and elevated in later stages [38]. A characterization of the arterial dynamic effects in hypertension only in terms of peripheral resistance neglects the pulsatile loading properties of the systemic tree. Studies have shown that pulsatile load, formulated in terms of aortic input impedance, is elevated in hypertension [39]. Additionally the frequency of the first minimum of the modulus of impedance, f_0, tends to be shifted to the right [39].

Not all investigations agree with these findings, however, and some have not found significant elevations in the characteristic impedance compared to normals [26, 40]. Nevertheless, the increase in characteristic impedance suggests an increase in the local stiffness of the ascending and thoracic aorta and the rightward shift in f_0 suggests an overall increase in the stiffness of the entire systemic arterial tree [41].

Changes observed in pulsatile load with hypertension imply a significant increase in arterial wave reflections [26, 39]. It has been shown that the ratio of backward to forward components of the incident pressure wave is increased in subjects with hypertension [39]. If pulse wave velocity is increased most of these enhanced reflections will occur during systole. The increase in reflections during systole may have a detrimental effect on cardiac function [42].

Reflections may also have long-term deleterious effects on cardiac or vascular structural morphology [8]. We do know there is a significant functional cost with an increase in reflected wave amplitudes. It has been shown that in hypertensive states an increase in pulsatile power is *not* necessarily associated with an increase in actual available power for transmission to peripheral vascular beds [43]. Vasodilators, by reducing peripheral resistance and arterial reflections, have the effect of improving pulsatile power transmission.

It should be emphasized that it is because arteries stiffen with increasing age and/or hypertension that wave reflections are enhanced in these conditions. With the increase in pulse wave velocity in these conditions pulse contour augmentation occurs more centrally [41]. Thus, there is less amplification in the pressure pulse from central to peripheral sites. These differences are important since pharmacological agents have different vasoactive effects on central versus peripheral arteries and assessment of efficacy is usually isolated to noninvasive means of more peripheral vessels.

In conclusion, as arteries stiffen with hypertension arterial pulse wave contours are altered by enhanced wave reflections. The augmented pressure waves may have deleterious effects on vascular or cardiac morphology. Investigations of pulse contours may tell us a great deal about the underlying changes in vascular morphology and vasomotor tone. The future promises improved noninvasive technologies to interrogate the arterial pulse which may reinforce capability for following efficacy of pharmacological therapy.

References

1. Wiggers CJ. The pressure pulses in the cardiovascular system. New York: Longmans, Green and Co., 1928: 73.

2. O'Rourke MF. Arterial function in health and disease. Edinburgh: Churchill Livingstone, 1982.
3. O'Rourke MF, Kelly RP, Aviolo AP. The arterial pulse. Philadelphia: Lea & Febiger, 1992.
4. O'Rourke MF. The arterial pulse in health and disease. Am Heart J 1971; 82: 867.
5. Brown BR, Anderson BT, Queen JG, Murgo JP. New techniques in cardiac catheterization: the advantages of multisensor catheters. Analyzer 1975; 5: 13–8.
6. Murgo JP, Westerhof N, Giolma JP, Altobelli SA. Manipulation of ascending aortic pressure and flow wave reflections with the Valsalva maneuver-relationship to input impedance. Circ 1981; 63: 122–32.
7. Van den Bos GC, Westerhof N, Randall OS. Pulse wave reflection: can it explain the differences between systemic and pulmonary pressure and flow waves? Circ Res 1982; 51: 479–85.
8. Milnor, W. Hemodynamics. 2nd ed. Baltimore: Williams and Wilkins, 1990: 204–20.
9. Nichols WW, O'Rourke MF. McDonald's blood flow in arteries. London: Edward Arnold, 1990.
10. Westerhof N, Sipkema P, Van denBos GC, Elizinga G. Forward and backward waves in the arterial system. Cardiov Res 1972; 6: 648–56.
11. Sipkema P, Westerhof N. Effective length of the arterial system. Ann Biomed Eng 1975; 3: 296.
12. Latham RD, Sipkema R, Westerhof N, Rubal BJ. Aortic input impedance during Mueller maneuver: an evaluation of 'effective length' J Appl Physiol 1988; 65(4): 1604–10.
13. O'Rourke MF, Yaginuma T. Wave reflections and the arterial pulse. Arch Intera Med 1984; 144: 366–71.
14. Latham RD, Westerhof N, Sipkema P, Rubal BJ, Reuderink P, Murgo JP. Regional wave travel and reflections along the human aorta. Circ 1985; 72: 1257–69.
15. Latham RD. Pulse propagation in the systemic arterial tree. In: Westerhof N, Gross D, editors. Vascular dynamics. Plenum Publishing Corp, 1989; 49–67.
16. Latham RD. Arterial dynamics: a comment on arterial wave reflection. In: HEDJ Ter Keurs. Tyberg JV. editors. Mechanics of Circulation. Boston: Martinus Nijhoff, 1987: 261–4.
17. Latham RD, Rubal BJ, Westerhof N, Sipkema P, Walsh RA. Nonhuman primate model for regional wave travel and reflections along aortas. Am J Physiol 1987; 253: H299–H306.
18. O'Rourke MF. Pressure and flow waves in systemic arteries and the anatomical design of the arterial system. J Appl Physiol 1967; 23: 139.
19. Latham RD. Technique of micromanometric catheterization of the descending aorta in man: a method to study regional arterial dynamics. Heart Vessels 1987; 3: 166–9.
20. Murgo JP, Westerhof N, Giolma JP, Altobell SA. Aortic input impedance in normal man: relationship to pressure waveforms. Circ 1980; 62: 105–16.
21. Kelly RP, Haywood C, Ganis J, Daley J, Aviola A, O'Rourke M. Non-invasive registration of the arterial pressure waveform using high fidelity applanation tonometry. J Vasc Med Biol 1989; 1(3): 142–9.
22. Drzewiecki GM, Melbin J, Noordergraaf A. Arterial tonometry: review and analysis. J Biomech 1983; 16(2): 141–53.
23. Levenson JA, Peronneau PP, Simon AC. Pulsed Doppler: determination of diameter, blood flow velocity and volume flow of brachial artery in man. Cardiov Res 1981; 15: 164.
24. Luchsinger PC, Snell RE, Patel DJ, Fry DL. Instantaneous pressure distribution along the human aorta. Cir Res 1964; 15: 510.
25. Mills CJ, Gabe IT, Gault JH, et al. Pressure-flow relationships and vascular impedance in man. Cardiov Res 1970; 4: 405.
26. Merillow JP, Fontenier GJ, Lenallut JF, et al. Aortic input impedance in normal man and arterial hypertension: its modification during changes in aortic pressure. Cardiov Res 1982; 16: 646–56.
27. Latham RD, Rubal BJ, Sipkema P, et al. Ventricular/vascular coupling and regional arterial

dynamics in the chronically hypertensive baboon: correlation with cardiovascular structural adaptation Circ Res 1988; 63: 798–811.

28. Mooser V, Etienne JD, Farine PA, et al. Non-invasive measurement of internal diameter of peripheral arteries during the cardiac cycle. J Hypertension 1988; 6(Suppl 4): S179–S81.

29. Robinson B. The carotid pulse. II: Relation of external recordings to carotid, aortic and brachial pulses. Br Heart J 1963; 25: 61–8.

30. Freis ED, Heath WC, Luchsinger PC, Snell RE. Changes in the carotid pulse which occur with age and hypertension. Am Heart J 1966; 71 (6): 757–65.

31. Lieberman JS. Instrumental methods in the study of vascular disease. Am Heart J 1980; 99: 517–27.

32. Drzewiecki GM, Melbin J, Noodergraaf A. Analytical comparison of transcutaneous pulse recordings. In Hansen EW, editor, 10th Annual Northeast Bioengineering Conference. New Hampshire: Hartmouth, 1982: 121–6.

33. Wesseling KH, Settels JJ, Van der Hoeven MA, Nigboer JA, Butijn MWT, Dorlas JC. Effects of peripheral vasoconstriction on the measurement of the blood pressure in the finger. Cardio 1985; 19: 139–45.

34. Egmond J van, Hasenbos M, Crul JF. Invasive versus noninvasive measurement of arterial pressure. Br J Anesth 1985; 57: 434–44.

35. Imholz BPM, van Montfrans GA, Settels JJ, van der Hoeven GM, Karemaker JM, Wieling W. Continuous noninvasive blood pressure monitoring; reliability of Finapres™ device during the Valsalva maneuver. Cardiov Res 1988; 22: 390–7.

36. Karemaker JM, Latham RD. Parabolic flight profile determines the effects of microgravity on the cardiovascular system. The Physiologist 1991; 34(4): 237.

37. Simon ACh, Levenson JA, Safar ME. Hemodynamic Mechanisms of and therapeutic approach to systolic hypertension. J Cardiov Ph 1985; 7: S22–S27.

38. Freis, ED. Hemodynamics of hypertension. Physiol Rev 1960; 40: 27–54.

39. Ting CT, Brin KP, Lin SJ, et al. Arterial hemodynamics in human hypertension, J Clin Invest 1986; 78: 1462–71.

40. Nichols WW, Conti CR, Walker WE, Milnor WR. Input impedance of the systemic circulation in man. Circ Res 1977; 40: 451–8.

41. O'Rourke MF. Arterial stiffness, systolic blood pressure, and logical treatment of arterial hypertension. Hypertension 1990; 15: 339–47.

42. Latson TW, Yin FCP, Hunter WC. The effects of finite wave velocity and discrete reflections on ventricular loading. In: Yin F, editor. Ventricular/vascular coupling: clinical, physiological and engineering aspects. New York: Springer-Verlag Inc., 1986; 334–83.

43. Li JK Jr. Increased arterial pulse wave reflections and pulsatile energy loss in acute hypertension. Angilogy 1989; 40: 730–5.

4. Structure and function of the arterial system in hypertension

COLIN L. BERRY and JORGE A.SOSA-MELGAREJO

Introduction

Arteries act as conduits for blood, but this is not their only function; much of their specialized structure is dependent on the essential physiological role they have to play in the circulation. They develop under two sets of influences: genetic factors mainly control the morphological pattern of the circulation, and haemodynamic factors control the form of the vessel wall. The haemodynamic factors, permit wall modifications that preserve certain mechanical properties [1–5]. The necessity to preserve these properties, an essential part of the wall function, determines much of the vascular response to hypertension and probably the interindividual variation in vessel wall thickness, in direct relationship to individual blood pressure, as mentioned in Chapter 1.

Architecture and ultrastructure of the normal arterial wall

The basic morphological plan of large arteries is presumably a biologically sound one; it is highly conserved from lower vertebrates and has persisted for more than 350 million years. How does the structure of the wall relate to its function? The walls of arteries are well organized connective tissue structures composed of cell and matrix arranged in the three transmural zones or tunicae, the intima, media and adventitia.

Tunica intima

The intima consists of a narrow region bounded on the luminal side by a single continuous layer of endothelial cells and peripherally by a fenestrated sheet of elastic fibres, the internal elastic lamina. In the subendothelium, smooth muscle cells and various components of the extracellular connective

M. E. Safar and M. F. O'Rourke (eds.), The arterial system in hypertension. pp. 55–72.
© 1993 *Kluwer Academic Publishers. Printed in the Netherlands.*

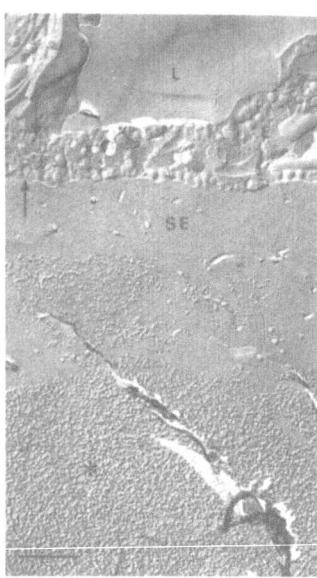

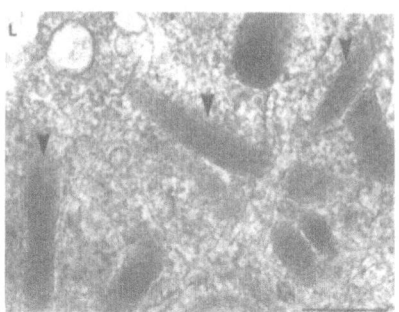

Figure 2. The cytoplasm of an endothelial cell with Weibel-Palade bodies (arrow heads). L = Lumen. Bar = 0.3 μm.

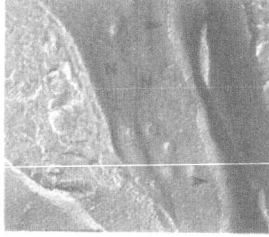

Figure 1. Freeze-fracture replica of the endothelium (E), subendothelium (SE) and elastic lamellae (*). Note that some pinocytic vesicles (arrows) are open to the lumen (L) and others to the subendothelium. Bar = 0.5 μm.

Figure 3. Freeze-fracture picture of endothelial cells with nexus junctions (N) and tight junctions (arrowheads), which can be seen running vertically and also around the the nexus junction. Bar = 0.3 μm.

tissue matrix are present (Figure 1). Although the intima contributes little to the mechanical properties of arteries, there are aspects of its morphology that are relevant to the response to increasing blood pressure.

Endothelial cells clearly interact with each other and the media. They are flat, elongated in the direction of blood flow and with a nucleus causing a focal luminal protrusion. Numerous pinocytic vesicles are seen close to the plasma membrane and present a flask-shaped invagination of the luminal and abluminal cell membrane. The cytoplasm of endothelial cells contains Weibel-Palade bodies (Figure 2) in addition to usual intracellular organelles [6]. Intermediate filaments of vimentin type are present in the endothelial cells, sometimes abundant and present as fascicles, or as whorls filling the cell cytoplasm. Excess of this type of filaments has been regarded as a regressive change associated with aging and disease [7]. By careful inspection, actin filaments are also identified in endothelial cells. Most of them can be observed close to the cell membrane and few in the cytoplasm.

Adjacent endothelial cells are interconnected by tight junctions and nexus junctions (Figure 3) [8, 9]. Nexus junctions are membrane specializations that provide a cell-to-cell low resistance conduction pathway for coordination of tissue function. They are composed of nonselective channels which allow passage of ions, nucleotides and other small molecules with molecular masses up to 1200 Da [10]. The presence of nexus junctions between arterial endothelial cells may be related to metabolic co-operation in this cell layer. It is also possible, that nexus junctions have a role in transmitting some signals to the underlying smooth muscle cells. Coupled endothelial cells in arteries may act as a unit and this interaction, along with that of myoendothelial contacts [11], may help explain the ability of an intravascular hormone to affect vascular tone without gaining direct access to all cells of the vascular wall.

Tight junctions serve to prevent the free passage of molecules across an endothelium. In the region of a tight junction, the plasma membrane of two adjacent endothelial cells are fused. For complete sealing, the junction has to extend as a continuous band or belt around the entire circumference of a cell. How effectively a tight junction acts as a seal depends on the number of strands in the junction. The greater their number, the less permeable the junction and on this basis, they may be categorized from very leaky to very tight. In some arteries, endothelial cells have up to 5 continuous strands. However, in most capillaries (except capillaries of the blood brain barrier) the strands are staggered and often discontinuous. Tight junctions are relatively labile structures which may widen under the influences of haemodynamic factors such as high blood pressure [12, 13] and possibly of vasoactive agents [14].

Tunica media

The tunica media is the main load bearing component of the arterial wall. In 1893 Thoma stated that 'the growth in thickness of a vessel wall is proportional to the tension in the wall, which itself is determined by the diameter of the vessel lumen and by the blood pressure'. As already indicated this statement forms the basis of our understanding of the relationships between structure and mechanical function in arteries.

The mechanical properties of elastic arteries depend largely on this coat which is composed of numerous layers of strong concentrically arranged, elastic lamellae which alternate with interlamellar zones (Figure 4). The zones are formed by sheets of smooth muscle cells containing fine elastic fibers and ground substance rich in mucopolysaccharides. One lamella and an adjacent interlamellar zone form a lamellar unit [15]. In man, there are about 40 lamellar units at birth [16] and up to 52 in young adults [17]. The increase in number is accompanied by an increase in thickness of the lamellar units from 8.2 μm at four years of age to 10.6 μm in young adults. Wolinsky and Glagov [15] showed that the number of lamellar units in the media of the adult mammalian aorta is almost proportional to the radius regardless of

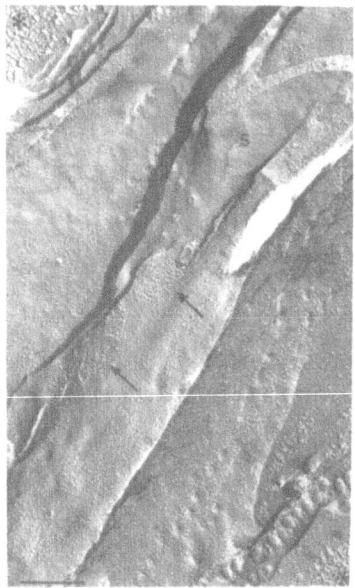

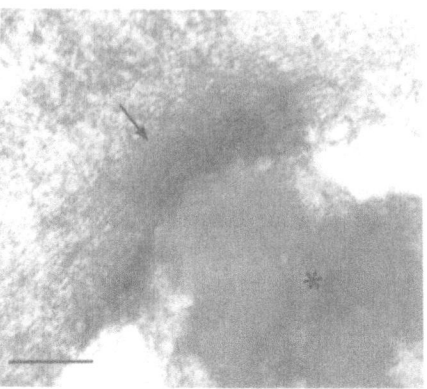

Figure 5. Higher magnification of a peripheral dense body (arrow) revels increased electron density close to the elastic fibre (*). Bar = 0.2 μm.

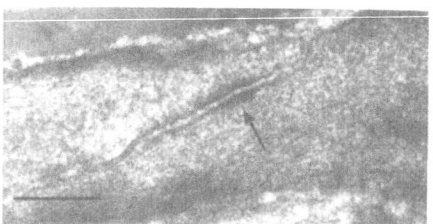

Figure 4. Freeze-fracture preparation of the aortic media showing a smooth muscle cell (S) with nexus junctions (arrows). C = Collagen; (*) = Elastic tissue. Bar = 0.3 μm.

Figure 6. Intermediatejunction (arrow) between two smooth muscle cells. Note the electron dense material under the plasma membranes. Bar = 0.3 μm.

the species or variations in the wall thickness. Hence, the average tension per lamellar unit of the media is remarkably constant regardless of the radius or the species (2000 ± 400 dyn/cm).

Smooth muscle cells in the arterial wall form a multifunctional component. They produce active contraction and are able to synthesize collagen fibers, elastic fibers and other components of the extracellular matrix. Vascular smooth muscle cells are capable of considerable proliferative activity after injury and in certain pathological states. Vascular muscle cells contain: thick (myosin), thin (actin) and intermediate (10 nm) filaments. The filamentous organization of actin and myosin are compatible with a sliding filament mechanism of contraction as in skeletal and cardiac muscle [18]. The major intermediate filament proteins present in vascular smooth muscle cells is vimentin [19]. Smooth muscle cells of the arterial wall are also heterogeneous as far as their contents of vimentin and desmin are concerned [20, 21]. More desmin positive cells are present in the aorta towards the iliac arteries than at the arch [22, 23]. These filaments are associated with the typical structures of the vascular smooth muscle cells, dense bodies and dense bands.

Dense bodies are electron dense structures scattered in the sarcoplasm of smooth muscle cells. They are elongated and lie parallel to the myofilaments. The material of the dense bodies appears similar to the material forming the dense bands which are attached to the cell membrane [24]. The distribution of myofilaments and the occurrence of dense bands are probably an essential part of the mechanism which allows for the remarkable amount of shortening a smooth muscle cell can undergo; they may also account for the wide range of changes in the shape of the cell profile [25]. The cytoplasmic side of the muscle cell membrane is heavily encrusted with electron dense material forming the so-called peripheral dense bodies or dense bands (Figure 5) [26]. Force transmission from contractile apparatus to the cell membrane in smooth muscle cells occurs mainly via the insertion of bundles of actin filaments into the dense bands [26].

Intercellular contacts in vascular smooth muscle are basically of two types [27]. Firstly, intercellular junctions where the muscle cells show cell membrane or cytoplasmic modifications at the area of cell contact, these include nexus junctions and intermediate junctions. Secondly, cell contacts where there is no membrane or cytoplasmic modification such as simple appositions and interdigitations.

Nexus junctions between smooth muscle cells show the same general features described for the endothelial cells. These intercellular junctions are usually rounded or elongated and have their major axis parallel to the length of the cell (Figure 4). It has been demonstrated that nexus junctions between vascular smooth muscle cells are not only instrumental in conducting impulses, but they also provide mechanical coupling between these cells [28]. Obviously such electrical and mechanical coupling is essential if the contraction of these cells is to be co-ordinated. In addition to force transmission between smooth muscle cells and the surrounding stroma, sites of direct adherence between smooth muscle cells allow transmission of stress directly from one cell to another [26, 29]. In response to this load, smooth muscle cells produce scleroproteins which are arranged in a way which distributes the load in the wall. The sites of direct adherence, called intermediate junctions, are symmetrical structures formed by two electron dense areas that match each other in adjacent smooth muscle cells (Figure 6).

Simple appositions are the most common type of contacts observed between vascular smooth muscle cells (Figure 7) [30]. Little is known about the possible function of simple appositions, but their frequency and the fact that the intercellular space is often less than 10 nm are reasons for considering them as true cell contacts [31]. It is also likely that cell adhesion molecules are present at this type of contact.

Interdigitations are elaborate contacts between smooth muscle cells with

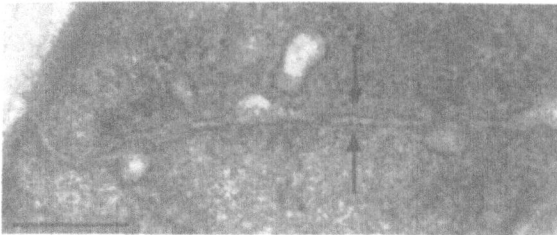

Figure 7. Simple apposition (arrows) between two smooth muscle cells. The presence of the closely related vesicles suggests that material exocytosed from one cell was perhaps being endocytosed by the other across the contact. Bar = 0.3 μm.

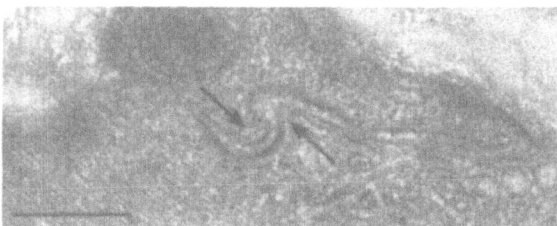

Figure 8. Interdigitations (arrows) between two smooth muscle cells. Bar = 0.3 μm.

cell processes from one cell that penetrate into invaginations of another (Figure 8). It has been suggested that these anchoring apparatuses may be important in the transmission of force between cells [25].

Adventitia

The tunica adventitia merges gradually with the surrounding tissue and consists mainly of bundles of collagen (Figure 9) and fibroblasts. Blood vessels, nerves and occasional elastic fibres are also present.

Myoendothelial contacts

Following the discovery in 1980 of endothelium dependent vasodilatation by Furchgott & Zawadzki [32] vascular endothelium has been recognized as an important functional unit in the regulation of vascular smooth muscle tone. It does so primarily by the release of vasodilator and vasoconstrictor substances, termed endothelium-derived relaxing factor and endothelium - derived contracting factor [33–36]. Other examples of interaction between cells of the intima and media of the vessel wall are the regulation of smooth muscle proliferation by endothelium-derived growth factors [37] and growth inhibitors [38] and the regulation of smooth muscle lipoprotein metabolism by endothelial cells [39].

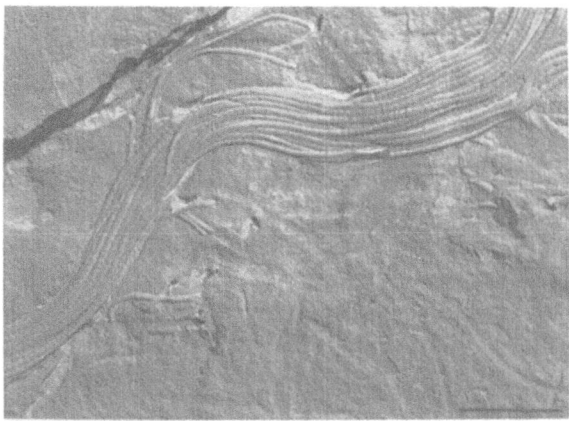

Figure 9. Freeze-fracture replica of collagen bundles of the adventitia. Bar = 1 μm.

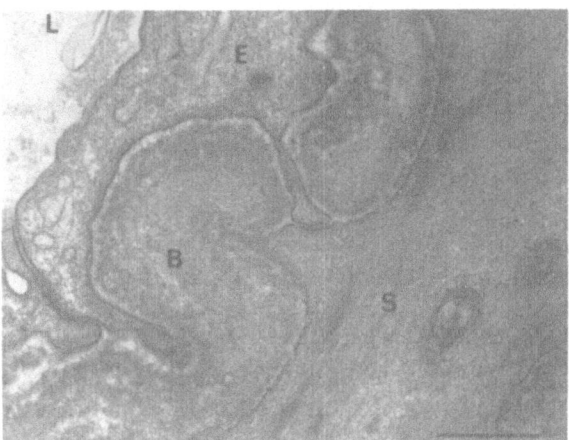

Figure 10. An arteriole from human kidney in which a process from an endothelial cell (E) extends through the basal lamina (B) to make a contact with a smooth muscle cell (S) [42]. Bar = 0.5 μm.

Structurally, it has been particularly well documented for the microcirculation [40–43] and to a lesser extent for larger vessels [11, 44], that endothelium and smooth muscle cells frequently extend processes to form heterocellular zones of contacts, the myoendothelial contacts.

Myoendothelial contacts have been thought to be the mediators of blood-borne humoral signals involved in the control of cerebral [45] or peripheral [40] vascular tone. They are also considered to be involved in the myogenic response of vascular smooth muscle [46]. The presence of abundant nexus junctions between endothelial cells suggests that they may have a role in

transmitting some signal to underlying smooth muscle cells. Coupled endothelial cells in arteries may act as a unit and this interaction, along with that
of myoendothelial contacts, may help to explain the ability of an intravascular
hormone to affect vascular tone without gaining direct access to all cells of
the vascular wall. The myoendothelial contacts have an appropriate morphology to facilitate the operation of the intima and media as a unit (Figure 10).

In a thick walled vessel such as the thoracic aorta, tension is highest in
the endothelium and decreases considerably toward the outer part of the
tunica media. The myoendothelial contacts are thus localized at sites of
maximal stress and may be the morphological basis for the postulated tension
sensor in the vessel wall [42].

Modifications for the arterial system in hypertension

For the arterial wall, high blood pressure represents an increase in stress
(force per unit area), which strains the elements within the wall. Whatever
the mechanism initiating the increased stress, hypertension is associated with
an increase in thickness of arterial and arteriolar walls which leads to a
decrease in arterial compliance and to an increase in peripheral resistance.
The relevant changes for each tunicae will be considered in turn.

Tunica intima

The increase in thickness of the intima is predominantly due to the effect of
hyperplasia of subendothelial cells, predominantly smooth muscle cells. This
hyperplasia is associated with an increase in intimal content of extracellular
matrix proteins, particularly collagens. Although the number of endothelial
cells does not change, there is an increase in their rates of production
and degradation. This, suggests an increase in regeneration turnover of
endothelium in hypertension, which is associated with a functional increase
in permeability.

Cell-to-cell contacts between endothelial cells change in hypertension. The
ratios of the area of tight junctions and nexus junctions to lateral endothelial
membrane surface has been studied using thin-sectioning and freeze-fracture
electron microscopy [47]. In all experimental models studied, there has been
a significant increase in tight junction/lateral membrane surface area ratios.
This is due, in part, to the presence of many small linear branching aggregates
of intramembrane particles seen in freeze fracture. Similar structures have
been reported to occur during cell junction development in embryonic tissue
and in vitro cell systems and have been considered to represent early steps
of tight junction assembly. Their presence in aortic endothelium during
hypertension may implicate neoformation of cell junctions. It is also possible,
however, that they represent steps in tight junction disassembly rather than
assembly. In either case, it is likely that these structures contribute to the

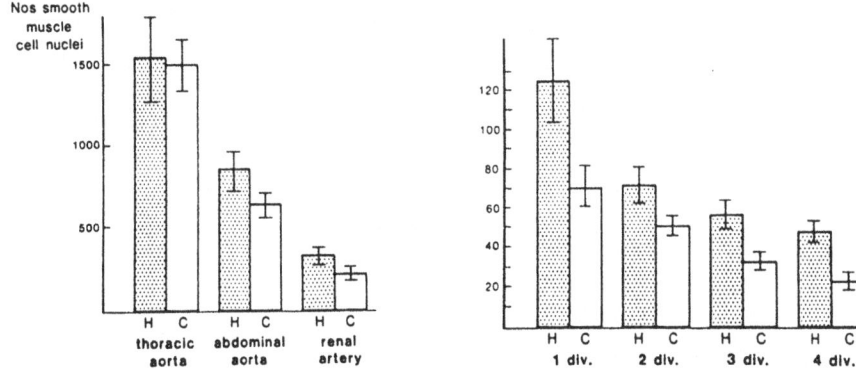

Figure 11. Counts of medial smooth muscle cell nuclei in an arterial cross-section. The higher counts of medial smooth muscle cells in the abdominal aorta and the renal artery in hypertensive rats (H) are significant ($p < 0.01$). C: normotensive control rats [51].

Figure 12. Cross-sectional areas of the media in intrarenal 6 l arteries according to their number of division from the renal artery. In all intrarenal arteries there are significant ($p < 0.005$) increases of medial mass in hypertensive rats (H), when compared with normotensive (C) [51].

increased tight junction/lateral membrane surface area ratios in hypertension. An increase in tight junction density in aortic endothelium may represent an adaptive change to hypertension; however, it is conceivable that when these junctions are mostly discontinuous (due to assembly and/or disassembly) they do not result in an efficient barrier [47]. This may contribute to the increase permeability of endothelium in hypertension.

Morphometry of nexus junctions between endothelial cells has revealed consistent structural changes in nexus junction configuration. These changes are in the form of bizarrely shaped nexus junctions common in all models of hypertension. These studies have also demonstrated a non significant change in the nexus junction/lateral membrane surface area ratios in any of the experimental groups.

Tunica media

The increase in arterial wall thickness seen in hypertension is due predominantly to the change in medial thickness. This increase in medial thickness is related to an increase in both smooth muscle mass and extracellular collagen content. Elastin content probably increases slightly in absolute value [48] but its relative value does not change [49, 50]. The mechanism of increase in smooth muscle mass probably depends on the type of arterial wall studied. Although it has been discussed that in the wall of large elastic arteries such as the aorta, the increase is due predominantly to hypertrophy of smooth muscle cells, we [51] have observed, in the DOCA-salt model (Figure 11), hyperplasia of smooth muscle cells.

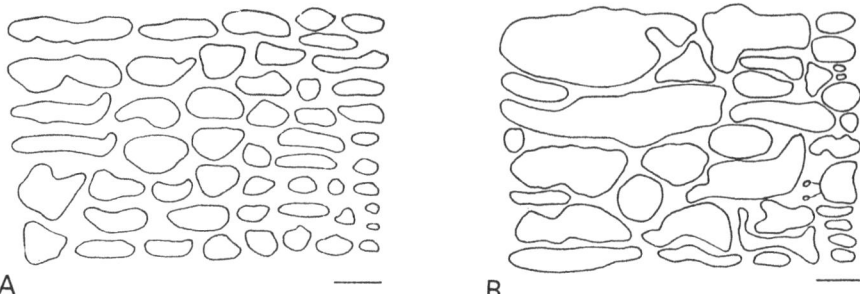

Figure 13. Drawing of the profiles of nexus junctions from the control (*A*) and hypertensive (*B*) thoracic aorta. The nexus junctions are arranged so that the longitudinal axis of the cells ' run horizontally. Two satellite nexuses are connected by a line f to the main nexus junction [53]. Bar = 0.3 μm.

The increase in relative and absolute content of extracellular matrix proteins in the arterial wall in hypertension depends partly on the model and the assay used. In the experimental renovascular model of hypertension in rats, the relative and absolute values of collagen content increased consistently without a marked change in the relative amount of elastin in the aortic wall. A similar observation has been made in spontaneously hypertensive rats of the Okamoto strain. In contrast, in the DOCA-salt model, we have reported a significant increase in the elastic content within the aortic wall [48]. In the same experimental model, Ooshima demonstrated an increase in the biosynthesis of collagens by smooth muscle cells in the aortic wall [52]. Apparently, the synthesis of scleroproteins can be modified during the hypertensive states by factors more complex than the direct increase in stress-strain relationship at cellular level.

In small calibre arteries and arterioles, hypertension is predominantly associated with a hyperplasia of smooth muscle cells (Figure 12). This hyperplasia is also associated with an increase in collagen biosynthesis and in arterioles, can lead to the successive stratification of cells, producing the classical 'onion skin' characteristic of the hypertensive microangiopathy. Cell-to-cell contacts between smooth muscle cells also change in hypertension. The tunica media bears most of the stress in the vessel wall, therefore links between cells and between cells and the stroma are expected to be affected by increase of wall tension.

Our studies have demonstrated nexus junctions which, in hypertensive states, are larger and more numerous than in normotensive vascular smooth muscle. Proliferation of small and irregularly shaped nexus junctions (Figure 13) are seen in contrast with the more regularly organized nexus junctions encounter in the normotensive media [53]. Thus, the observation that both the number of nexus junctions and the surface area of plasma membrane occupied by them is greater in hypertensive smooth muscle cells than in normal vascular muscle, suggests an 'increased' intercellular communication. This may contribute to the increased response of hypertensive vascular smooth muscle to agonists.

We have observed that a high blood pressure decreases the density of intermediate junctions, involved in cell adhesion [54]. This may be compensated by the augment in nexus junctions, which also provide some form of mechanical attachment.

The number of cell-to-stroma contacts (defined as the association of dense bands with the elastic fibers) fell significantly in hypertension [55]. This suggests that cell-to-stroma contacts may respond in the same way as the intermediate junctions to a chronic increase in tangential tension within the vessel wall. Why this reduction in the number of contacts which allow the transmission of forces from cell to stroma occurs is unclear.

All these findings suggests that hypertension produces a tunica media where the muscle cells have increased intercellular communication and decreased intercellular adhesion. This may affect its mechanical integrity.

Vasa vasorum

The aortic media is nourished by diffusion from the endothelial surface and by vasa vasora from the adventitial side. Ingress from the aortic lumen is apparently sufficient to nourish the inner 0.5 mm of the media. This zone encompasses about 30 medial lamellae [56]. Aortic medias composed of more than 30 layers contain vasa vasora between the thirtieth layer and the adventitia. Distention of large arteries during each cardiac cycle increases vessel diameter 8–10% and increases vessel length about 1%; these changes are associated with narrowing of the wall thickness. Furthermore, the pressure exerted directly against the vessel wall produces a compressive stress in the radial direction. This radial stress and the narrowing of the wall that accompanies circumferential deformation all compress the structures contained within the wall including the vasa vasora. Elevated blood pressure increases this compression but also raises perfusion pressure in the vasa. Nevertheless, experimental evidence indicates that hypertension decreases flow through the vasa vasora [57]. Which may impair arterial wall nutrition [58].

Myoendothelial contacts in hypertension

Tozzi et al. [59] have demonstrated that a functionally complete endothelium is necessary for the production of scleroproteins by the muscle cells in vascular remodeling. We have observed, in normotensive vessels, myoendothelial contacts with simple appositions, but in hypertensive states the myoendothelial contacts have electron dense material in the form of a loosely woven submembranous mat on the cytoplasmic side of the muscle cell involved

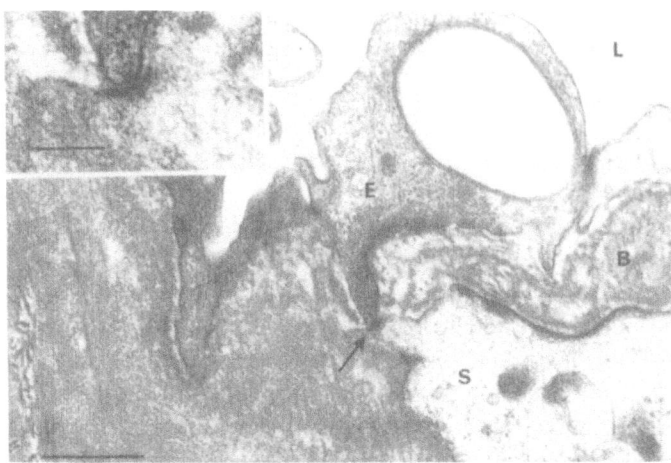

Figure 14. Myoendothelial contact in a human kidney arteriole (arrow). Note the increased electron density. L = Lumen; E = Endothelium; S = Smooth muscle; B = Basal lamina [42]. Bar = 0.5 μm. Insert, Bar = 0.1 μm. Reproduced from Sosa-Melgarejo et al. [42] by courtesy of *Virchows Archiv A.*

(Figure 14) [42]. This type of contact, with increased cytoplasmic electron density, has some resemblance to intermediate junctions [60] and may provide strong intercellular cohesion.

Myoendothelial contacts are potential sites for electrical and metabolic communication between elements of the intima and media, ensuring that the vessel wall works as a unit. The demonstrated necessity of intact endothelium for smooth muscle cell response to load [59] may depend on this type of contact.

Functional implications of arterial adaptation to hypertension

Arterial wall thickening in hypertension is an adaptive process which attempts to normalize the stress at the level of each contractile unit within the wall. Adult arteries adapt to chronic pressure increases in a manner similar to that seen in the wall thickening that accompanies developmental increases in blood pressure during growth. However, growing elastic arteries thicken by adding lamellar units to the vessel wall, whereas a fixed number of lamellar units will thicken following the onset of hypertension.

It has been demonstrated that hypertrophy and hyperplasia of smooth muscle cells amplifies the functional contractile response to vasoactive agents [61]. We think this response is related to the increase in intercellular communication via increase in nexus junction density and nexus junction area

[53, 54]. For a similar nervous or hormonal signal leading to vasoconstriction in a normotensive model, more effectors respond in hypertension, where muscle generates more force. In vivo, an increase response to catecholamines has been demonstrated in hypertensive patients when compared with normotensive controls.

Folkow [62] proposed that wall thickening encroaches on the lumen of resistance vessels and provides a mechanical advantage for constriction when smooth muscle is stimulated. Part of this mechanical advantage is due to stimulation of a greater mass of muscle. In addition, however, thickened arteries or arterioles narrow their lumen more for a given level of constriction than do normal vessels. For example, if a normal and hypertrophied artery with the same outer diameter constrict, both vessels will thicken as diameter decreases. This thickening occurs simply because the mass of tissue is unchanged as circumference decreases. However, the relative change in internal diameter of the thickened artery exceeds that of the normal vessel. If both vessels constrict to reduce their external radius by one-half, the hypertrophied vessel achieves a final diameter that is more than 30 percent less than that of the normal artery. It is also important to remember that resistance varies inversely to the fourth power of internal radius. This means a resistance difference of only about 10 percent becomes a fourfold resistance difference after constriction.

In general, most of the differences induced in the properties of arteries by increased blood pressure are not due to changes in chemical composition, but rather to differences in wall thickness [63]. Our data show that at a given degree of distention of the vessel, the increase in collagen present in pathologically altered vessels is associated with a decrease in the proportion bearing stress. In normal vessels, a given degree of distention is probably associated with a fixed absolute amount of collagen bearing stress. The pathological changes in vessels only 'dilute' the stress bearing component; they do not contribute to it [64]. In other words, 'new' collagen in a vessel is analogous to a scar in the skin, it does not help the tissue to function properly.

Similarity between hypertension, the aging process and arteriosclerosis

The ill effects of hypertension on the arterial system are similar to those of aging and arteriosclerosis, and are explicable on the same basis of increase impedance

Aging

The more evident effect of advancing senescence on the cardiovascular system appears to be alterations in the anatomy and dynamic properties of the aorta and systemic vasculature. It has long been known that aging is associated with increased wall thickness and reduced elasticity of the aorta. This is accompanied by an increase in diameter and volume of the aorta, which also becomes elongated and tortuous. In the aortic root, the degree of dilatation may be such that the aortic valve cusps are inadequate for occlusion of the orifice, resulting in some degree of valvular incompetence. The aortic rigidity and peripheral vasculature resistance are increased, the impedance to left ventricular ejection is greater.

The aging process leads to structural changes of the arterial wall which are similar to those observed in hypertension, in fact Pickering [65] has described hypertensive chronic vascular disease as an accelerated form of aging. Medial thickness increases with age, as does intimal thickness. In the aortic tunica media, the aging process is more of a hypertrophic than a hyperplastic phenomenon. The collagen content of the media increases with age as in hypertension, whereas the elastic tissue is degraded. Schlattman and Becker [66] also found an age-related increase in elastic fragmentation and fibrosis. The incidence of cystic mucoid degeneration in the aortic media has been found to rise with age [66, 67]. This rise is greater in hypertensive patients.

Arteriosclerosis

Arteriosclerosis denotes thickening and loss of elasticity of arterial walls. The pathogenesis is likely to be multifactorial and lesions are likely to evolve in stages.

In large arteries, structural changes of the walls play an important role in the relationship between hypertension and the development of atheroma. Although the biological events which relate atheroma to hypertension are not completely defined, two mechanical factors seem to be important in this relationships. Firstly, the increased permeability of the endothelium to macromolecules; secondly, the decreased filtration of the macromolecules through the thicker and collagenous intimal and medial layers of the arterial wall. These phenomena are related and lead to an increase accumulation of lipids in the intimal layer and to the formation of plaques. Other phenomena may also play a role in atherogenesis associated with hypertension. Damaged endothelium, could activate platelet aggregation and release of growth factors. Activation of the endothelial layer could be related to increase in blood velocity associated with sympathetic nervous system activation accompanying some hypertension.

Conclusions

The modification of arterial wall structure in response to hypertension is determined by the need to preserve mechanical properties essential for arterial function. This adaptive response has complex and deleterious consequences. Artery wall thickening will contribute to the progression and entrenchment of hypertension by increasing vascular flow resistance. It is also certain that wall thickening will affect atherogenesis and that loss of two-phase activity will promote aneurysm formation; furthermore, a rigid arterial tree (decreased strain) will evidently increase cardiac work.

Acknowledgement

Supported in part by the Medical Research Council of Great Britain and Consejo Nacional de Ciencia y Tecnologia of Mexico.

References

1. Berry CL. Organogenesis of the arterial wall. In: Camilleri JP, Berry CL, Fiessinger JN, Bariety J, editors. Diseases of the arterial wall. London: Springer-Verlag, 1989: 55–70.
2. Berry CL, Sosa-Melgarejo JA, Greenwald SE. The relationship between wall tension, lamellar thickness and intercellular junctions in the fetal and adult aorta its relevance to the pathology of dissecting aneurysm. J Pathol 1993; 169: 15–20.
3. Glagov S, Zarins CK, Giddens, Ku N. Mechanical Factors in the pathogenesis, localization and evolution of atherosclerosis. In: Camilleri JP, Berry CL, Fiessinger JN, Bariety J, editors. Diseases of the arterial wall. London: Springer Verlag, 1989: 217–34.
4. Doyle JM, Dobrin PB. Stress gradients in the walls of large arteries. J Biomech 1973; 16: 631–9.
5. Apter JT, Rabinowitz M, Cumming MT. Correlation of visco-elastic properties of large arteries with microscopic structure. Circ Res 1966; 19: 104–21.
6. Wagner DD, Olmstead JB, Marder VJ. Immunolocalization of von Willebrand protein in Weibel-Palade bodies of human endothelial cells. J Cell Biol 1982; 95: 355 60.
7. Ghadially FN. Ultrastructural Pathology of the cell and matrix. 3rd ed. London: Butterworths, 1988.
8. Huttner I, Gabbiani G. Vascular endothelium: recent advances and unanswered questions. Lab Invest 1982; 47: 409–11.
9. Cowin P, Kapprell H-P, Franke WW. The complement of desmosomal plaque proteins in different cell types. J Cell Biol 1985; 101: 1442–54.
10. Davies PF. Biology of disease: vascular cell interactions with special reference to the pathogenesis of atherosclerosis. Lab Invest 1986; 55: 5–24.
11. Sosa-Melgarejo JA, Berry CL. Myoendothelial contacts in the thoracic aorta of rat fetuses. J Pathol 1992; 166: 311–6.
12. Huttner I, Boutet M, Rona G, More RH. Studies on protein passage through arterial endothelium: III. Effect of blood pressure levels on the passage of fine structural protein tracers through rat arterial endothelium. Lab Invest 1973; 29: 536–46.
13. Nagy Z, Mathieson G, Huttner I. Opening of tight junctions in cerebral endothelium: II. Effect of pressure pulse induced acute arterial hypertension. J Comp Neurol 1979; 185: 579–86.
14. Thorgeirsson G. Robertson AL. The vascular endothelium – pathobiologic significance. A review. Am J Pathol 1978; 93: 803–48.
15. Wolinsky H, Glagov S. A lamellar unit of aortic medial structure and function in mammals. Circ Res 1967; 20: 99–111.
16. Grunstein M. Uber den Bau der grosseren menschlichen Arterien in verschidenen Alter-sstufen. Arch Mikr Anat 1896; 47: 583–654.

17. Knieriem HJ, Hueber A. Quantitative morphological studies of the human aorta. Beitr Path Anat 1970; 140: 280–97.
18. Somlyo AP. Ultrastructure of vascular smooth muscle. In: Bohr DF, Somlyo AP, Sparks HV, editors. Handbook of physiology, section 2: the cardiovascular system, Vol II: vascular smooth muscle. Bethesda: American Physiological Society, 1980: 33–67.
19. Gabbiani G, Schmid E, Winter S, et al. Vascular smooth muscle cells differ from other smooth muscle cells: predominance of vimentin filaments and a specific alpha-type actin. Proc Natl Acad Sci USA 1981; 78: 298–302.
20. Kocher O, Skalli O, Bloom WS, Gabbiani G. Cytoskeleton of rat aortic smooth muscle cells. Normal conditions and experimental intimal thickening. Lab Invest 1984; 50: 645–62.
21. Kocher O, Skalli O, Cerutti D, Gabbiani F, Gabbiani G. Cytoskeletal features of rat aortic cells during development. An electron microscopic, immunohistochemical, and biochemical study. Circ Res 1985; 56: 829–38.
22. Osborn M, Caselitz J, Weber K. Heterogeneity of intermediate filament expression in vascular smooth muscle: a gradient in desmin positive cells from the rat aortic arch to the level of the arterial iliac communis. Differentiation 1981; 20: 196–202.
23. Schmid E, Osborn M, Rungger-Brandle E, Gabbiani G, Weber K, Franke WW. Distribution of vimentin and desmin filaments in smooth muscle tissue of mammalian and avian aorta. Exp Cell Res 1982; 137: 329–40.
24. Geiger B, Volk T, Volverg T. Molecular heterogeneity of adherens junctions. J Cell Biol 1985; 101: 1523–31.
25. Gabella G. Structure of smooth muscle. In: Bulbring E, Brading AF, Jones AW, Tomita T, editors. Smooth muscle. An assessment of current knowledge. London: Edward Arnold, 1981: 24–31.
26. Gabella G. Structural apparatus for force transmission in smooth muscle cells. Physiol Rev 1984; 64: 455–77.
27. Sosa-Melgarejo JA, Berry CL. Intercellular contacts in the media of the thoracic aorta of rat fetuses treated with B-aminopropionitrile. J Pathol 1991; 164: 159–65.
28. Henderson RM, Duchon G, Daniel EE. Cell contacts in duodenal smooth muscle layers. Am J Physiol 1971; 221: 564–74.
29. Staehelin LA, Hull BE. Junctions between living cells. Scient Am 1978; 2 38: 140–52.
30. Sosa-Melgarejo JA, Berry CL. Contact relationships between vascular smooth muscle cells. An in-vivo and in-vitro study. J Pathol 1989; 157: 213–7.
31. Daniel EE, Daniel VP, Duchon G, et al. Is the nexus necessary for cell to cell coupling of smooth muscle? J Membr Biol 1976; 28: 207–39.
32. Furchgott RF, Zawadzki JV. The obligatory role of endothelial cells in the relaxation of arterial smooth muscle by acetilcholine. Nature 1980; 288: 373–6.
33. Palmer RMJ, Ferrige AG, Moncada S. Nitric oxide release accounts for the biological activity of endothelium-derived relaxing factor. Nature 1987; 327: 524–6.
34. Snydner SH, Bredt DS. Biological roles of nitric oxide. Sci Am 1992; 266: 28–35.
35. Yanagisawa M, Kurihara H, Kimura S, et al. A novel potent vasoconstrictor peptide produced by vascular endothelial cells. Nature 1988; 332: 411–5.
36. Simonson MS, Dunn MJ. Endothelins: a family of regulatory peptides. Hypertension 1991; 17: 856–63.
37. Di Corletto PE, Bowen Pope DF. Cultured endothelial cells produce a platelet-derived growth factor-like protein. Proc Natl Acad Sci USA 1983; 80: 1919–23.
38. Castellot JJ, Vhoay J, Lormeau J-C, Petitou M, Sache E, Karnovsky MJ. Structural determinants of the capacity of heparin to inhibit the proliferation of vascular smooth muscle cells. II. Evidence for a pentasaccharide sequence that contains a 3- O-sulfate group. J Cell Biol 1986; 102: 1979–84.
39. Davies PF, Truskey GA, Warren HB, O'Connor SE, Eisenhaure BH. Metabolic co-operation between vascular endothelial cells and smooth muscle cells in co-culture: changes in low density lipoprotein metabolism. J Cell Biol 1985; 101: 871–9.

40. Rhodin JAG. The ultrastructure of mammalian arterioles and precapillary sphincters. J Ultrastruct Res 1967; 18: 181–223.

41. Rhodin JAG. Ultrastructure of mammalian venous capillaries, venules and small collecting veins. J Ultrastruct Res 1968; 25: 452–500.

42. Sosa-Melgarejo JA, Berry CL, Dodd S. Myoendothelial contacts in the small arterioles of human kidney. Virchows Archiv A 1988; 413: 183–7.

43. Sosa-Melgarejo JA, Berry CL. Myoendothelial contacts in arteriolosclerosis. J Pathol 1992; 166: 311–16.

44. Spagnoli LG, Villaschi S, Neri L, Palmieri G. Gap junction in myo-endothelial bridges of rabbit carotid arteries. Experientia 1982; 38: 124–5.

45. Dahl E. The innervation of the cerebral arteries. J Anat 1973; 115: 53–63.

46. Johnson PC. The myogenic response. In: Bohr DF, Somlyo AP, Sparks HV Jr. editors. Handbook of Physiology; section II. The cardiovascular system; vol 2: Vascular smooth muscle. Bethesda: American Physiological Society, 1980: 409–42.

47. Huttner I, Costabella PM, Chastonay CD, Gabbiani G. Volume, surface, and junctions of rat aortic endothelium during experimental hypertension. Lab Invest 1982; 46: 489–504.

48. Berry CL, Greenwald SE. Effects of hypertension on the static mechanical properties and chemical composition of the rat aorta. Cardiovasc Res 1976; 10: 437–51.

49. Wiener J, Loud AD, Giacomelli F, Anversa P. Morphometric analysis of hypertension induced hypertrophy of rat thoracic aorta. Am J Pathol 1977; 88: 619–34.

50. Levy BI, Michel JB, Salzman JL et al. Effect of chronic inhibition of converting enzyme on mechanical and structural properties of arteries in rat renovascular hypertension. Circ Res 1988; 63: 227–39.

51. Berry CL, Henrichs KJ. Morphometric investigation of hypertrophy in the arteries of DOCA-hypertensive rats. J Pathol 1982; 136: 85–94.

52. Ooshima A, Fuller GC, Cardinale G, Spector S, Udenfriend S. Collagen biosynthesis in blood vessels of brain and other tissues of the hypertensive rat. Science 1975; 190: 898–900.

53. Berry CL, Sosa-Melgarejo JA. Nexus junctions between vascular smooth muscle cells in the media of the thoracic aorta in normal and hypertensive rats. A freeze-fracture study. J Hypert 1989; 7: 507–13.

54. Sosa-Melgarejo JA, Berry CL, Robinson NA. Effects of hypertension on the intercellular contacts between smooth muscle cells in rat thoracic aorta. J Hypert 1991; 9: 475–80.

55. Sosa-Melgarejo JA, Robinson N, Berry CL. Changes in number and type of cell to cell and cell to stroma contacts in vascular smooth muscle cells in hypertension. Path Res Pract 1989; 185–1: 152A.

56. Wolinsky H, Glagov S. Nature of species differences in the medial distribution of aortic vasa vasorum in mammals. Circ Res 1967; 20: 409–21.

57. Heistad DD, Marcus ML, Law EG, Armstrong ML, Ehrhardt JC, Abbound FM. Regulation of blood flow to the aortic media in dogs. J Clin Invest 1978; 62: 133–40.

58. Martin JF, Booth RF, Moncada S. Arterial wall hypoxia following hyperfusion through the vasa vasorum is an initial lesion in atherosclerosis. Eur J Clin Invest 1990; 20: 588–92.

59. Tozzi CA, Poiani GJ, Harangozo AM, Boyd CD, Riley DJ. Pressure-induced connective tissue synthesis in pulmonary artery segments is dependent on intact endothelium. J Clin Invest 1989; 84: 1005–12.

60. Geiger B, Avnur Z, Volverg T, Volk T. Molecular domains of adherens junctions. In: Edelman GM, Thiery JP, editors. The cell in contact, Adhesions and junctions as morphogenetic determinants. New York: Wiley, 1985: 461–89.

61. Mulvany MJ. Do resistance vessel abnormalities contribute to the elevated blood pressure of spontaneously hypertensive rats? Blood vessels 1983; 20: 1–22.

62. Folkow B. Physiological aspects of primary hypertension. Physiol Rev 1982; 62: 347–504.

63. Berry CL, Greenwald SE, Rivett J. Static mechanical properties of the developing and mature rat aorta. Cardiovasc Res 1982; 9: 669–78.

64. Greenwald SE, Berry CL. The effect of alterations in scleroprotein content on thestatic elastic properties of the
arterial wall. Adv Physiol Sci 1980; 8: 203–12.
65. Pickering GW. Hypertension. London: Churchill, 1968.
66. Schlatmann TJ, Becker AE. Histological changes in the normal ageing aorta: implications for dissecting aortic aneurysm. Am J Cardiol 1977; 39: 13–20.
67. Carlson RG, Lillehei CW, Edwards JE. Cystic medial necrosis of the ascending aorta in relation to age and hypertension. Am J Cardiol 1970; 25: 411–5.

5. Cyclic guanosine monophosphate, smooth muscle tone and mechanical properties of large arteries

MARIE CHRISTINE MOURLON-LE GRAND and
BERNARD I.LÉVY

Introduction

Cyclic nucleotides have been investigated since the late 1950s as potential regulators of cellular functions [1]. The biological role of cyclic nucleotides in the regulation of vascular smooth muscle activity is not still clearly defined. Information on the regulatory role of cyclic AMP (cAMP) is far more prevalent than that of cyclic GMP (cGMP), probably because studies began about fifteen years prior to those on cGMP, and many more investigators are presently studying cAMP than cGMP. However, metabolism of cGMP is important to study due to (i) its physiological role mainly related to the vasoactive functions of endothelium and (ii) its involvement in vasodilation induced by nitrates. In this chapter, we are focusing on the role of cGMP in smooth muscle cells relaxation especially in large arteries and its implication in the mechanical properties of the arterial wall.

BIOCHEMISTRY of cGMP

Discovery and role of cyclic GMP

Following the initial discovery of cGMP in 1963 [2], several years passed before investigators began to extensively study the formation, metabolism, and action(s) of cGMP in cells. At this time of its 'career', cGMP was considered as a cAMP antagonist, or at least an intracellular second messenger whose function was to oppose the actions of cAMP [3] since cAMP was already known to be an important mediator of . . . smooth muscle relaxation, cGMP was believed to be a mediator of contraction [4]. This new concept allowed to think that, by their opposite actions, these two cyclic nucleotides could regulate the smooth muscle function. However, further studies showed later that vasodilator drugs caused a marked accumulation of cGMP, but not cAMP, in vascular tissue. This leads to the following question: 'Could cGMP possibly be involved in smooth muscle relaxation?'

M. E. Safar and M. F. O'Rourke (eds.), The arterial system in hypertension. pp. 73–87.
© 1993 *Kluwer Academic Publishers. Printed in the Netherlands.*

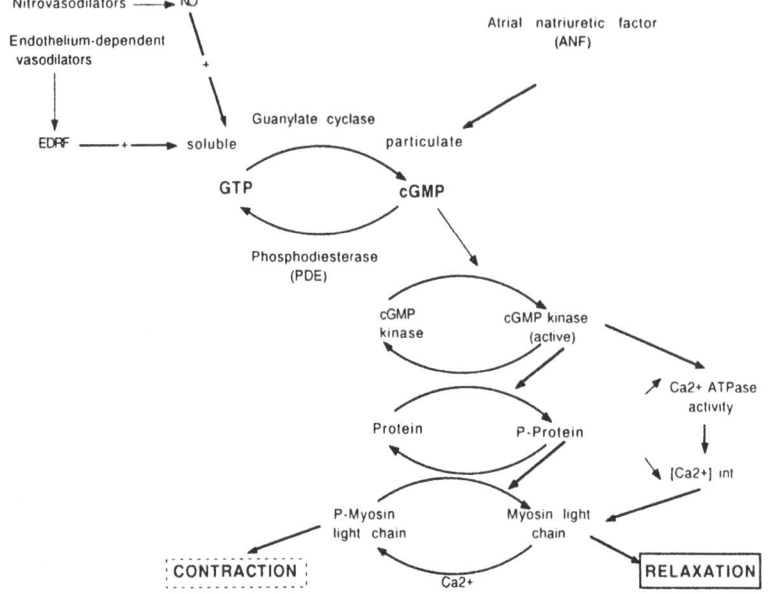

Figure 1. Schematic illustration of the mechanism of action of different classes of vasodilators on cyclic GMP synthesis and vascular smooth muscle relaxation. EDRF. endothelium derived relaxing factor; NO·, nitric oxide.

This question was elucidated in 1977 by several studies [5, 6] showing that vasodilator compounds, especially those containing nitrogen-oxide constituents (nitrovasodilators), stimulated cGMP formation. In most cases, cGMP was associated in both a time- and concentration-dependent fashion with relaxation [7, 8]. Furthermore, Furchgott et al. [9, 10] showed that acetylcholine induced an endothelium-dependent vascular smooth muscle relaxation via the release of a diffusible endothelial factor (EDRF: endothelium-derived relaxing factor) acting on smooth muscle. Besides, several studies [11–13] confirmed that EDRF relaxes vascular smooth muscle through increase in cGMP.

The chemical nature of EDRF has been a subject of intense investigation. It was identified in 1987 as an unstable free radical that is very likely the nitric oxide (NO·) [14–17]. Several studies confirmed that cGMP, but not cAMP, is the mediator of vascular smooth muscle relaxation.

The tissue cGMP accumulation by nitrovasodilators (or similar substances) is the result of the soluble guanylate cyclase activation by these substances, probably mediated by the release of NO· (Figure 1) [18, 19].

Synthesis of cyclic GMP

It is known that the conversion of guanosine triphosphate (GTP) to cyclic GMP is catalyzed by guanylate cyclase. This enzyme is localized in different tissues, in particular in smooth muscle, and appears under at least two isoenzyme forms: one is soluble and cytosolic, the other one, particular, is membrane-associated. The kinetic, physicochemical, and antigenic properties of the cytosolic and membrane-associated isoenzymes are quite different [20]. The soluble guanylate cyclase is a heme-containing enzyme [21, 22] whose interaction with nitric oxide results in an increase of its activity. Thus it was proposed, in 1985, that soluble guanylate cyclase is the 'NO· receptor' [23]. The particular guanylate cyclase, localized in the plasma membrane of cells, binds to and is specifically activated by atrial natriuretic factor (ANF).

Degradation of cyclic GMP

The intracellular metabolism of cGMP is controlled by several enzymes: the phosphodiesterases which transform cGMP in inactive 5′GMP. Among these different phosphodiesterases, some hydrolyzes specifically cAMP while others hydrolyze specifically cGMP. In the present chapter, we will focus on cGMP-dependent phosphodiesterases.

These enzymes present two binding sites for cGMP: the first one functions as a catalytic site hydrolyzing cGMP in inactive 5′GMP; the second one, without hydrolytic activity, represents a specific binding site for cGMP [24]. Five types of phosphodiesterases (PDEs I to V) have been identified in mammals tissues but their nomenclature is not still unanimous; we will use the classification proposed by Beavo & Reifsnyder [25]. Phospho diesterases are preferentially localized in endothelial or smooth muscle cells (Figure 2). Different PDEs either hydrolyze cGMP (Type I and V PDEs), or have an activity positively (Type II PDE) or negatively (Type III PDE) regulated by cGMP. In the vascular smooth muscle, the major types of phospho diesterases are of Type I and Type IV [26] although the Types III and V are also present [27] As shown in Figure 2, cGMP is hydrolyzed by two types of PDEs in vascular smooth muscle cells:
– Type I PDE, Ca^{2+}-Calmodulin dependent, which also hydrolyzes cAMP. Each mole of native holoenzyme binds one mole of calmodulin. The binding of calmodulin is Ca^{2+}-dependent and reversible.
– Type V PDE, specific for cGMP.
Only two types of PDEs have been identified in endothelial cells [28]
– Type II PDE, which hydrolyzes both cGMP and cAMP and is selectively activated by low concentrations of cGMP.
– Type IV
The role of these two endothelial phosphodiesterases has not been yet identified; different selective inhibitors are actually used for a better knowledge of the respective role of these enzymes in smooth muscle (Figure 2).

Cyclic GMP receptors in smooth muscle

To induce a relaxation, cGMP must bind to a receptor. The purification and characterization of one of the major receptor proteins for cGMP, called the

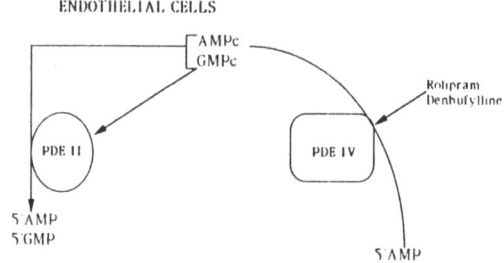

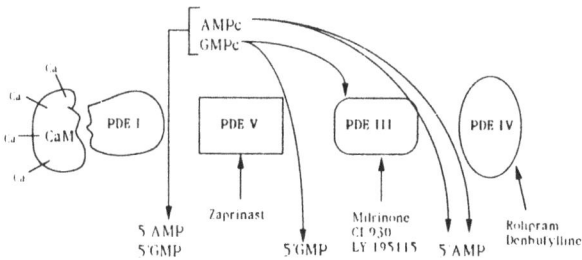

Figure 2. Distribution of different phosphodiesterases and their regulation by specific inhibitors in vascular smooth muscle and endothelial cells.

cGMP-dependent protein kinase (PK_G), have been determined before the first report on the effects of cGMP on smooth muscle relaxation. Nevertheless, the cellular function of PK_G has been less studied than that of cAMP-dependent protein kinase (PK_A) or protein kinase C [29, 30].

The PK_G can be either in a soluble and cytosolic form [31, 32] or in a particular form (platelets [33], smooth muscle [34]). This enzyme contains catalytic, regulator and inhibitor domains. It is localized in different tissues and in high concentrations in vascular smooth muscle suggesting that this enzyme has an important physiological role in this tissue [35]. Nevertheless, its specific activity or amount is less important than that of PK_A (by over 5 to 20-fold) excepted in the aorta where amounts of cAMP- and cGMP-dependent proteins are approximately equal.

De Jonge and Rosen showed that PK_G phosphorylates itself in the presence of adenosine triphosphate (ATP), Mg^{2+} and arginine residues [36, 37]. The mechanism by which cyclic nucleotides stimulate the auto- phosphorylation reaction remains still unknown. Nevertheless, it is interesting to note that cyclic nucleotides which have a low affinity for PK_G (cAMP, cIMP) stimulate the reaction whereas those with a high affinity (cGMP, 8-Br-cGMP) do not stimulate the auto-phosphorylation.

Cyclic GMP binds to PK_G with a high affinity ($K_D = 10^{-9}$ M) and a high specificity to two distinct sites [38]. This binding is necessary for a complete activation of the enzyme although a partial activation could be obtained with

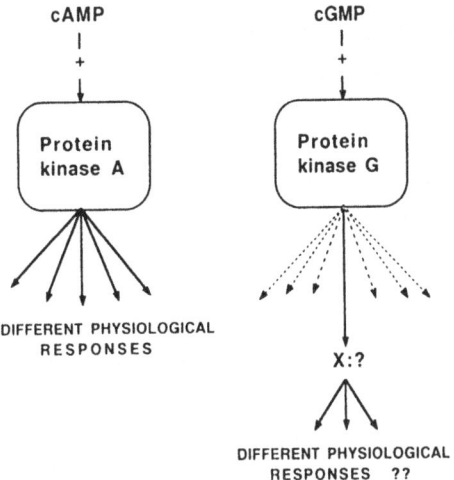

Figure 3. Schematic model describing the mechanism of action of cyclic nucleotides on protein kinases.

saturating levels of cGMP. However, it is unlikely that auto-phosphorylation could not have a major physiological role with a so slow rate of auto-phosphorylation.

The stimulation of PK_G by cGMP induces the phosphorylation of target-proteins [39, 40]. However, their natural substrates into the cells are not well known (Figure 3). Nevertheless, the final effect of the activation of the PK_G is an important decrease of intracellular free calcium which could be actively re-uptaked by sarcoplasmic reticulum and calciosomes and actively released from the cell to the extracellular liquid. The PK_G could phosphorylate the proteins responsible for the uptake of calcium, but it could also have other substrates. The phospholamban-like proteins could be one of these targets [41], it seems established that a protein identified as the 'myosin light chain' is dephosphorylated in response to cGMP [42]. This led to the proposal that the mechanism of relaxation by cGMP involves the dephosphorylation of myosin light chain.

The determination of a specific role for cGMP in a physiological process could be an important step in the understanding of the role of the PK_G and of its potential substrate.

Effect of cyclic GMP on calcium

The works of Schultz et al. [4] and Goldberg et al. [3] showed a connection between two intracellular messengers: cyclic GMP and Ca^{2+}, however it was not clear whether Ca^{2+} affected cGMP levels or whether cGMP affected Ca^{2+} levels, or both. In 1978, Lincoln and Corbin [43] speculated that one major role of cGMP-dependent protein kinase might be the regulation of Ca^{2+} levels.

Studies suggested that the mechanism of action of nitrovasodilators involved enhanced binding or sequestration of Ca^{2+} inside the cell [44]. Lincoln's group suggested that cGMP and Ca^{2+} might in some way 'antagonize' each other in smooth muscle [45]. Studies in several laboratories have now demonstrated that elevations in smooth muscle cell Ca^{2+} concentrations in response to K^+ and to agonists such as angiotensin II were reduced by 8-Br-cGMP [46], atrial natriuretic factor (ANF) [47, 48], and nitrovasodilators [49].

Mechanism of action of cyclic GMP

It is now well established that cGMP induces a relaxation in vascular smooth muscle by lowering free intracellular Ca^{2+}. This results in a dephosphorylation of myosin light chain. Few arguments exist for a direct control of contractile protein function by cGMP, it is more likely that cGMP regulates this function indirectly through Ca^{2+} regulation with different levels of interaction between cGMP and Ca^{2+}.

Possible role of cyclic GMP on sarcoplasmic reticulum

An attractive hypothesis would be that cGMP-dependent protein kinase phosphorylates proteins in the sarcoplasmic reticulum involved in IP_3 action. The inhibition of IP_3-induced Ca^{2+} release may be one possible mechanism by which cGMP could contribute to the inhibition of contraction due to agonists in the aorta.

Cyclic GMP could also have a possible role on phosphatidylinositol turnover but results are still conflicting [50, 51] and the mechanism by which cGMP inhibits the phosphatidylinositol accumulation has not yet been clearly determined.

Possible role of cyclic GMP on calcium influx

Another possible effect of cGMP is on the uptake of Ca^{2+} into the cell. Recently, several workers showed that cGMP-dependent relaxation is associated with decreases in Ca^{2+} uptake in aorta [52, 53]. Therefore, it is likely that at least a part of the mechanism of cGMP-induced relaxation in agonist-contracted aortic smooth muscle could involve both inhibition of Ca^{2+} uptake and of Ca^{2+} release from intracellular stores.

Possible role of cyclic GMP on calcium efflux

The small number of cGMP-dependent protein kinase substrates identified and characterized is an argument to suspect a more generalized mode of action of cGMP in the smooth muscle. cGMP could directly stimulate the Ca^{2+} emux from the vascular smooth muscle cells. The regulation of Ca^{2+}

transport across the plasma membrane may be therefore a potentially important site of action of cGMP.

There are at least four transport systems or 'pumps' in smooth muscle cells able to remove cytosolic Ca^{2+} out of the cells:

– the sarcoplasmic reticulum Ca^{2+}-ATPase, less developed in smooth muscle than in cardiac muscle;
– the plasmic membrane Ca^{2+}-ATPase with a high affinity for Ca^{2+} which is activated by calmodulin;
– the Na^{+}-Ca^{2+} exchange which contributes significantly to the rapid decline in cytosolic Ca^{2+} levels [54];
– the mitochondrial Ca^{2+}-ATPase with a low affinity for Ca^{2+}.

All these transport systems contribute to the maintenance of low levels of free cytosolic Ca^{2+} [55, 56].

Of the protein kinases tested (PK_G, PK_A, PK_C), PK_G was found to be the best activator of Ca^{2+}-ATPase [47]. Thus, it was suggested that Ca^{2+}-calmodulin activated Ca^{2+}-ATPase was a physiological substrate for PK_G in smooth muscle. Nevertheless, Lincoln et al. could not demonstrate that smooth muscle Ca^{2+}-ATPase is phosphorylated by the PK_G; they suggested that the activation of the Ca^{2+}-ATPase by PK_G does not involve the direct phosphorylation of the pump, but rather the phosphorylation of some other component which exerts a regulatory influence. One may speculate that PK_G phosphorylates phospholamban-like proteins which could activate Ca^{2+}-ATPase in an indirect manner. Thus the high affinity Ca^{2+}-ATPase appears to be a probable target for cGMP activation.

A recapitulative scheme of interactions between the different J second messengers in smooth muscle is presented in Figure 4.

cGMP and mechanical properties of the carotid artery in spontaneously hypertensive rats

As reviewed in this chapter, the endothelial factors have an important role in the formation of cyclic GMP in the vascular smooth muscle. Nevertheless, the role of cGMP in experimental and clinical hypertension is not well known. Lüscher and Vanhoutte showed that the endothelium have a predominant role in SHR by the simultaneous release of relaxing (EDRFs) and contracting (EDCFs) factors [57–59]. However, the relation between vasomotor tone, mechanisms of regulation of soluble guanylate cyclase, cGMP metabolism and mechanical properties of arterial wall in SHR are still not clear. Furthermore, there is evidence that the endothelium not only releases relaxant factors but also various vasoconstrictor agents (EDCFs, endothelin(s)) [58–62] that act on the local vasomotor tone.

We recently studied the relationship between the mechanical properties and the vascular tissue cGMP content in anesthetized normotensive Wistar-Kyoto (WKY) rats and in spontaneously hypertensive rats (SHRs) under

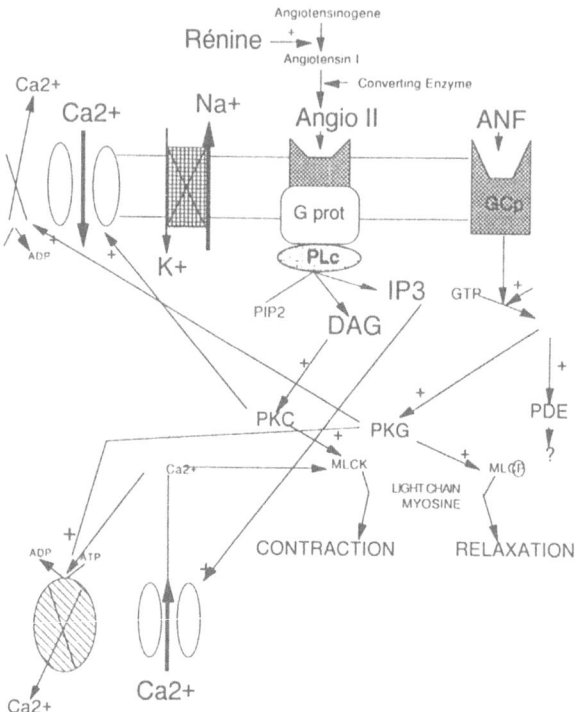

Sarcoplasmic Reticulum

Figure 4. Recapitulative scheme of mechanisms of interaction 'Ca^{2+}/cGMP' in smooth muscle cell. Angio I, II, angiotensin I, II; CE, converting enzyme; CEI, converting enzyme inhibitors; EDRF, endothelium derived relaxing factor; NO, nitric oxide; ANF, atrial natriuretic factor; pGC, particulate guanylate cyclase; sGC, soluble guanylate cyclase; IP$_3$, inositol triphosphate; DAG, diacylglycerol; PLc, phospholipase C; PIP$_2$, phosphatidylinositol bisphosphate; PK$_C$, protein kinase C; PK$_G$, protein kinase G; PDE, phosphodiesterase; MLCK, myosin light chain kinase; MLCP, myosin light chain phosphatase.

basal conditions (with intact endothelium), after the inhibition of the soluble guanylate cyclase by methylene blue, and after the mechanical removal of endothelium (E$^-$). Animals were operated according to the method routinely used in our laboratory and previously described in details [63]. Briefly, the carotid artery is studied 'in situ' and 'in vivo': a removable clamp is first placed at the root of the carotid artery, just down-stream of the aortic arch, then a catheter is introduced into the upper part of the carotid artery. The 'in situ' isolated segment of carotid artery is then connected to a simple system allowing to precisely measure the volume isolated arterial segment for imposed levels of steady controlled transmural pressure. The pressure-volume relationship obtained depends on the static mechanical properties of

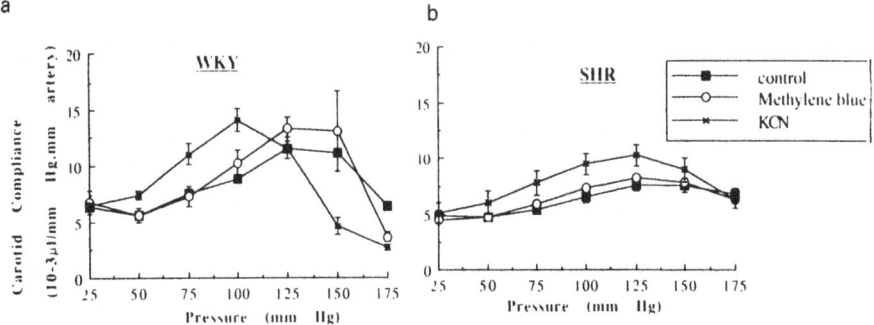

Figure 5. Effect of a local incubation in carotid artery with methylene blue (10^{-5} M for 20 minutes) (open circles) on carotid compliance in normotensive Wistar-Kyoto rats (WKY) (*a*) and spontaneously hypertensive rats (SHR) (*b*) Solid squares, control conditions with endothelium; *x* symbols, after smooth muscle poisoning by potassium cyanide for 30 min. Values are mean ± SEM.

the carotid artery. The carotid compliance (μl/mmHg) is defined, at a given level of transmural pressure, as the slope of the pressure-volume curve.

Local incubation with methylene blue [10^{-5} M for 20 minutes) did not significantly modify carotid compliance compared with control values in WKY rats (Figure 5a) and in SHRs (Figure 5b).

Mechanical removal of the endothelium induced a similar increase in carotid compliance in both strains relative to carotid compliance with intact endothelium ($p < 0.01$) (Figure 6a–b).

Under control conditions with intact endothelium, cyclic GMP level was significantly higher in the carotid arterial wall in SHRs than in WKY rats ($p < 0.02$] (Figure 7).

Local incubation with methylene blue (10^{-5} M for 20 minutes) induced similar reductions of tissue cGMP in normotensive and in hypertensive rats by 88% ($p < 0.001$) and 94% ($p < 0.001$), respectively, as compared to control values.

Endothelium removal induced a significant decrease in cGMP content by 28% in WKY rats ($p < 0.02$] and by 90% in SHRs ($p < 0.001$]. This decrease was significantly larger in SHRs than in normotensive rats ($p < 0.001$).

Furthermore, the after removal of endothelium or after local incubation with methylene blue the arterial tissue cGMP levels were significantly different in WKY rats ($p < 0.001$) but were similar in SHRs.

Under basal conditions, the decrease in carotid compliance and the increase in vasomotor tone in SHRs were paradoxically associated to a high tissue cGMP level. The higher tissue cGMP content in the SHR might reflect a compensatory mechanism as a protection against genetic hyper-reactivity and the increase in tone of the vascular smooth muscle. This result is in agreement with that of Amer et al. [64] who suggested, in 1974, that high

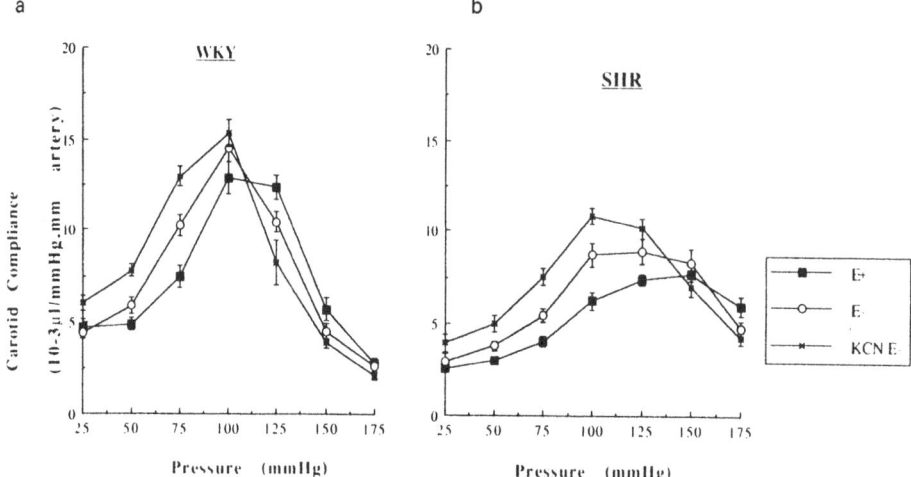

Figure 6. Effect of de-endothelialization of carotid artery on carotid compliance (open circles) in normotensive Wistar-Kyoto rats (WKY) (*a*) and spontaneously hypertensive rats (SHR) (*b*) Solid squares, control conditions with endothelium; *x* symbols, after smooth muscle poisoning by potassium cyanide for 30 min. Values are mean ± SEM.

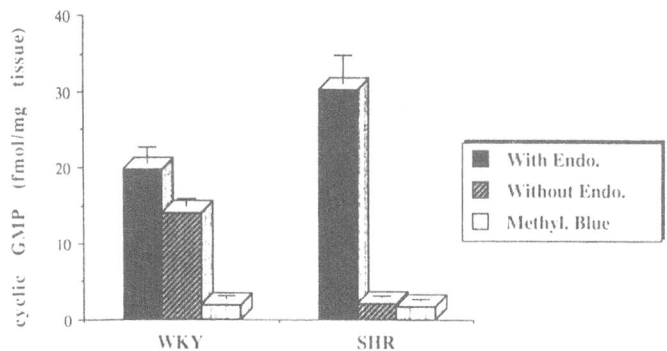

Figure 7. cGMP content in carotid artery in Wistar-Kyoto rats (WKY) (left columns) and spontaneously hypertensive rats (SHR) (right columns) under several conditions: with intact endothelium, without endothelium and after local incubation with methylene blue (10^{-5} M for 20 minutes). Values are mean ± SEM.

levels of arterial cGMP could be responsible for the high smooth muscle tone and increased peripheral resistances in SHRs. In contrast, Otsuka et al. [65] found lower aortic cGMP level in deoxycorticosterone acetate salt rats, aortic stenosis, and renovascular hypertension than in their normotensive controls. These discrepancies could be due to differences in cGMP pathway in genetic and secondary hypertension experimental models and/or to the different vessels studied.

The accumulation of tissue cGMP in the SHR could be explained by:

– an activation of cGMP synthesis pathway via the stimulation of guanylate cyclases [66];

– a decrease of cGMP degradation in inactive 5'GMP via the decrease of the cGMP-dependent phosphodiesterases activity [67,68].

In order to evaluate the relative contribution of both guanylate cyclases (soluble and particulate forms), we incubated methylene blue in the carotid artery.

Inhibition of soluble guanylate cyclase by methylene blue did not induce variation in mechanical properties of the carotid artery but dramatically decreased the tissue cGMP content in both strains. This result suggests that the local production of cGMP is essentially related to the soluble guanylate cyclase activity in normotensive and hypertensive rats.

Mechanical removal of the endothelium from the carotid artery induced a larger decrease in cGMP content in SHRs than in WKY rats. This result suggests that

– the tissue cGMP content is more endothelium-dependent in SHRs than in WKY rats;

– other non endothelial mechanisms could control the cGMP synthesis in the WKY rat.

Therefore, despite a higher vasomotor tone, the 'cGMP pathway' is probably more activated in the arterial wall from spontaneously hypertensive rats than from Wistar-Kyoto rats. Furthermore, the regulation of the cGMP synthesis in the hypertensive rat seems endothelium-dependent. However, in this strain of genetic hypertension, the local hyperproduction of cGMP does not counter balance the vasoconstriction induced by neuro humoral factors and is not able to normalize the vasomotor tone.

To conclude this short review, it may be admitted that multiple sites of action of cGMP are present in various smooth muscle preparations, and that different tissues have different mechanisms whereby cGMP reduces intracellular Ca^{2+}.

A general mechanism can be resumed as follows: 'signals' such as endogenous nitric oxide (EDRF), free radicals or ANF activate the various forms of guanylate cyclase (the 'transducer'). Elevations in cGMP (the 'messenger') affect Ca^{2+} metabolism in the cell, inducing reductions in smooth muscle tone and vasodilation.

In arteries from spontaneously hypertensive rats, the production of cyclic GMP is markedly enhanced, due to the endothelium release of nitric oxyde, and could limit the increase in the tone of smooth muscle cells.

References

1. Robinson GA, Burcher RW, Sutherland EW. In: Cyclic AMP. New York, Academic Press, 1971.
2. Ashman Df, Lipton R, Melicow MM. Price TD. Isolation of adenosine 3'5'-monophosphate

and guanoslne 3'5'-monophosphate from rat urine. Biochem Biophys Res Commun 1963; 11: 330–4.

3. Goldberg ND, Haddox MK, Harple DK, Haden JW. The biological role of cyclic 3'5' guanosine monophosphate. Proc, Futh, Int Congr Pharmac 1973; 5: 146–69.

4. Schultz G, Hardman JG, Schultz K, Baird CE, Sutherland EW. The importance of calcium ions for the regulation of guanosine 3'5'-cyclic monophosphate levels. Proc Nat Acad Sci 1975; 70: 3889–93.

5. Schultz KD, Schultz K, Schultz G. Sodium nitroprusside and other smooth muscle relaxants increase cyclic GMP levels in ductus deferens. Nature 1977; 265: 750–1.

6. Katsuki S, Murad F. Regulation of adenosine cyclic 3'5'-monophosphate and guanoslne cyclic 3'5'-monophosphate levels and contractility in bovine tracheal smooth muscle. Mol Pharmacol 1977; 13: 330–41.

.7 Axelsson KL, Wikberg JGS, Andersson RGG. Relationship between nitroglycerine cyclic GMP, and relaxation of vascular smooth muscle. Life Sci 1979; 24: 1779–86.

8. Gruetter CA, Gruetter DY, Lyon JE. Kadowitz PJ, Ignarro LJ. Relationship between cyclic GMP formation and relaxation of coronary arterial smooth muscle by glyceryl trinitrate, nitroprusside, nitrite and nitric oxide: Effects of methylene blue and methemoglobin. J Pharmacol Exp Ther 1981;219: 181–6.

9. Furchgott RF, Zawadzki JV. The obligatory role of endothelial cells in the relaxation of arterial smooth muscle by acetylcholine. Nature 1980; 288: 373–6.

10. Furchgott RF. Role of endothelium in responses of vascular smooth muscle. Circ Res 1983; 53: 557–73.

11. Holzmann S. Endothelium-induced relaxation by acetylcholine associated with large rises in cyclic GMP in coronary arterial strips. J Cyclic Nucl Res 1982; 8: 409–19.

12. Rapoport Rm, Murad F. Agonist-induced endothelium-dependent relaxation in rat thoracic aorta may be mediated through cGMP. Circ Res 1983; 52: 352–7.

13. Ignarro LT, Burke TM, Wood KS, Wolin MS, Kadowitz PJ. Association between cyclic GMP accumulation and acetylcholine-elicited relaxation of bovine intrapulmonary artery. J Pharmac Exp Ther 1984; 228: 682–90.

14. Palmer RMJ, Ferrrige AG. Moncada S. Nitric oxide release accounts for the biological activity of endothelium-derived relaxing factor. Nature 1987; 327: 524–6.

15. Ignarro LJ, Buga GM, Wood KS, Byrns RE, Chaudhuri G. Endothelium-derived relaxing factor produced and released from artery and vein is nitric oxide. Proc Natl Acad Sci USA 1987; 84: 9265–9.

16. Ignarro LJ, Byrns RE, Buga GM, Wood KS, Chaudhuri G. Pharmacological evidence that endothelium-derived relaxing factor is nitric oxide: use of pyrogallol and superoxide dismutase to study endothelium-dependent and nitric oxide-elicited vascular smooth muscle relaxation. J Pharmac Exp Ther 1988; 244: 181–9.

17. Furchgott RF. Evidence that the endothelium-derived relaxing factor of rabbit is nitric oxide. In: Beven JA, Majewski H, Maxwell RA, Story DF, editors. Vascular neuroeffector mechanisms. Paris: ICSU Press, 1988; 6: 77–84.

18. Arnold WP, Mittal CK, Katsuki S. Murad F. Nitric oxide activates guanylate cyclase and increases guanosine 3'5'-cyclic monophosphate levels in various tissue preparations. Proc Natl Acad Sci USA 1977; 74: 3203–7.

19. Gruetter CA, Barry BK, McNamara DB, Grutter DY, Kadowitz PJ, Ignarro LJ. Relaxation of bovine coronary artery and activation of coronary arterial guanylate cyclase by nitric oxide nitroprusside and a carcinogenic nitrosamine. J Cyclic Nucl Res 1979; 5: 211–24.

20. Mittal CK, Murad F. In: Nathanson JA, Kebabian JW, editors. Handbook of Experimental Pharmacology. Berlin: Springer-Verlag 1982; 58: 225–60.

21. Gerzer R. Bohme F. Hofmann F, Schultz G. Soluble guanylate cyclase purified from bovine lung contains heme and copper. Febs Lett 1981; 132: 71–7.

22. Ohlstein EH, Wood KS, Ignarro LJ. Purification and properties of heme-deficient hepatic soluble guanylate cyclase: effects of heme and other factors on enzyme activation by NO, NO-heme, and protoporphyrin IX. Arch Biochem Biophys 1982; 218: 187–98.

23. Ignarro LJ, Kadowitz PJ. The pharmacological and physiological role of cyclic GMP in vascular smooth muscle relaxation. Ann Rev Pharmacol Toxicol 1985; 25: 171–91.
24. Francis SH, Thomas MK, Corbin JD. Cyclic GMP-binding cyclic GMP-specific phosphodiesterase from lung. In: Beavo J, Houslay MD, editors. Cyclic nucleotide phosphodiesterases: Structure, regulation and drug action 2. 1990: 117–40.
25. Beavo JA, Reifsnyder DH. Primary sequence of cyclic nucleotide phosphodiesterase isozymes and the design of selective inhibitors. Trends Pharm Sci 1990; 11: 150–5.
26. Keravis TM, Wells JN, Hardman JG. Cyclic nucleotide phosphodiesterase activity from pig coron arteries lack of interconvertibility of major forms. Biochem Biophys Acta 1980; 613: 116–29.
27. Coquil JF, Brunelle G, Guedon J. Occurrence of the methylisobutylxanthine-stimulated cyclic GMP binding protein in various rat tissues. Biochem Biophys Res Commun 1985; 127: 226–31.
28. Lugnier C, Schini VB. Characterization of cyclic nucleotide phosphodiesterases from cultured bovine aortic endothelial cells. Biochem Pharmacol 1990; 39: 75–84.
29. Kuo JF, Greengard P. Cyclic nucleotide-dependent protein-kinases VI. Isolation and partial purification of a protein kinase activated by guanosine 3'5'-monophosphate. J Biol Chem 1970; 245: 2493–8.
30. Lincoln TM, Corbin JD. Characterization and biological role of the cGMP-dependent protein kinase. Adv Cyclic Nucl Res 1983; 15: 139–92.
31. Lohmann SM, Walter U, Miller PE, Greengard P, de Camilli P. Immunohistochemical localization of cyclic GMP-dependent protein kinase in mammalian brain. Proc Natl Acad Sci USA 1981; 78: 653–7.
32. Walter U. Distribution of cyclic GMP-dependent protein kinase in various rat tissues and cell lines determined by a sensitive and specific radioimmunoassay. Eur J Biochem 1981; 118: 339–46.
33. Waldmann R, Bauer S, Gobel C, Hofmann F, Jakobs KH, Walter U. Demonstration of cGMP-dependent protein kinase and cGMP-dependent phosphorylation in cell-free extracts of platelets. Eur J Biochem 1986; 158: 203–10.
34. Ives HE, Casnellie JE, Greengard P, Jamieson JD. Subcellular localization of cyclic-GMP-dependent protein kinase and its substrates in vascular smooth muscle. J Biol Chem 1980; 255: 3777–85.
35. Casnellie JE, Schlichter DJ, Walter U, Greengard P. Photoaffinity labeling of a guanosine 3'5'-monophosphate-dependent protein kinase from vascular smooth muscle. J Biol Chem 1978; 253: 4771–6.
36. De Jonge HR, Rosen OM. Self-phosphorylation of cyclic guanosine 3'5'-monophosphate dependent protein kinase from bovine lung. J Biol Chem 1977; 252: 2780–3.
37. Lincoln TM, Flockhart DA, Corbin JD. Studies on the structure and mechanism of activation of the guanosine 3'5'-monophosphate-dependent protein kinase. J Biol Chem 1978; 253: 6002–9.
38. Corbin JD, Ogreid D, Miller JP, Suva RH, Jastorff B, Doskeland SO. Studies of cGMP analog specificity and function of the two intrasubunit binding sites of cGMP-dependent protein kinase. J Biol Chem 1986; 261: 1208–14.
39. Yashida Y, Sun HT, Cai JQ, Imai S. Cyclic GMP dependent protein kinase stimulates the plasma membrane Ca^{++} pump ATPase of vascular smooth muscle via phosphorylation of a 240 KDa protein. J Biol Chem 1991; 266: 19819–25.
40. Furukawa KI, Ohshima N, Tawada-Iwata Y, Shigekawa M. Cyclic GMP stimulates Na^{+}/Ca^{++} exchange in vascular smooth muscle cells in primary culture. J Biol Chem 1991; 266: 12337–41.
41. Raeymaekers L, Hofmann F, Casteels R. Cyclic GMP-dependent protein kinase phosphoryfates phospholamban in isolated sarcoplasmic reticulum from cardiac and smooth muscle. Biochem J 1988; 252: 269–73.
42. Draznin MB, Rapoport RM, Murad F. Myosin light chain phosphorylation in contraction and relaxation of intact rat thoracic aorta. Int J Biochem 1986; 18: 917–28.

43. Lincoln TM, Corbin JD. Hypothesis on the role of the cAMP- and cGMP-dependent protein kinases in cell function. J Cyclic Nucl Res 1978; 4: 3–14.
44. Hester RK., Weiss GB, Fry WJ. Differing actions of nitroprusside and D-600 on tension and ^{45}Ca fluxes in canine renal arteries. J Pharmacol Exp Ther 1979; 208: 155–60.
45. Lincoln TM. Effect of nitroprusside and 8-bromo-cyclic GMP on the contractile activity of the rat aorta. J Pharmacol Exp Ther 1983; 224: 100–7.
46. Rashatwar SS, Cornell TL, Lincoln TM. Effects of 8-bromo-cGMP on Ca^{2+} levels in vascular smooth muscle cells: possible regulation of Ca^{2+}-ATPase by cGMP-dependent protein kinase. Proc Natl Acad Sci USA 1987; 84: 5685–9.
47. Hassid A. Atriopeptin II decreases cytosolic free Ca in cultured vascular smooth muscle cells. Am J Physiol 1986; 251: C681–C6.
48. Cornwell TL Lincoln TM. Regulation of phosphorylase a formation and calcium content in aortic smooth muscle and smooth muscle cells: effects of atrial natriuretic peptide II. J Pharmacol Exp Ther 1988; 247: 524–30.
49. Morgan JP. Morgan KG. Alteration of cytoplasmic ionized calcium levels in smooth muscle by vasodilators in the ferret. J Physiol Lond 1984; 357: 539–51.
50. Takai Y., Kikkawa K. Nishizuka Y. Membrane phospholipid metabolism and signal transduction for protein phosphorylation. Adv Cyclic Nucl Res 1984; 18: 119–158.
51. Resink TJ, Scott-Burden T, Jones CR, Baur U. & Bühler FR. Atrial natriuretic peptide: binding and cyclic GMP response in cultured vascular smooth muscle cells from spontaneously hypertensive rats. Am J Hypertens 1989; 2: 32–9.
52. Collins P, Griffith TM, Henderson AH, Lewis MJ. Endothelium-derived relaxing factor alters calcium fluxes in rabbit aorta: a cyclic guanosine-monophosphate-mediated effect. J Physiol Lond 1986; 381: 427–37.
53. Taylor CJ, Meisheri KD. Inhibitory effects of a synthetic atrial peptide on contractions and ^{45}Ca fluxes in vascular smooth muscle. J Pharmacol Exp Ther 1986; 237: 803–8.
54. Smith JB. Smith L. Extracellular Na^{+} dependence of changes in free Ca^{2+}, $^{45}Ca^{2+}$ efflux, and total cell Ca^{2+} produced by angiotensin II in cultured arterial muscle cells. J Biol Chem 1987; 262: 17455–60.
55. Carafoli E. Plasma membrane Ca^{2+} transport, and Ca^{2+} handling by intracellular stores: an integrated picture with emphasis on regulation. In: Mechanisms of Intestinal Electrolyte transport and Regulation by Calcium. New York: LISS AR. Inc, 1984: 121–34.
56. Carafoli E. The calcium pumping ATPase of the plasma membrane. Ann Rev Physiol 1991; 53: 531–47.
57. Luscher TF. Vanhoutte PM. Hypertension and endothelium-dependent responses. In: Vasodilation. New York: Raven Press, 523–9.
58. Luscher TF, Boulanger CM, Dohi Y. Yang ZH. Endothelium-derived contracting factors. Hypertension 1992; 19: 131–7.
59. Luscher TF, Vanhoutte PM. Dysfunction of the release of endothelium-derived relaxing factor. In: Endothelial Cell Dysfunctions. 1992A: 65–102.
60. Harder DR. Pressure induced myogenic activation of cat cerebral arteries is dependent on intact endothelium. Circ Res 1987; 60: 102–7.
61. Katusic ZS. Shepherd JT, Vanhoutte PM. Endothelium-dependent contraction to stretch in canine basilar arteries. Am J Physiol 1987; 252: H671–H3.
62. Furchgott RF, Vanhoutte PM. Endothelium-derived relaxing and contracting factors. Faseb J 1989; 3: 2007–18.
63. Mourlon-Le Grand MC, Benessiano J, Levy BI. cGMP pathway and mechanical properties of carotid artery wall in WKY rats and SHR: role of endothelium. Am J Physiol 1992; 63: H61–H7.
64. Amer SM, Gomoll AW, Perhach JL, Hugh JR, Ferguson C, McKinney GR. Aberrations of cyclic nucleotide metabolism in the heart and vessels of hypertensive rats. Proc Nat Acad Sci 1974; 71: 4930–4.
65. Otsuka Y, DiPiero A, Hirt E, Brennaman B, Lockette W. Vascular relaxation and cGMP in hypertension. Am J Physiol 1988; 254: H163–H9.

66. Goldberg D, Haddox MK. Cyclic GMP metabolism and involvement in biological regulation. Ann Rev Biochem 1977; 46: 823–96.
67. Harris AL, Lemp BM, Bentley RG, Perrone MH, Hamel LT, Silver PJ. Phosphodiesterase isozyme inhibition and the potentiation by zaprinast of endothelium-derived relaxing factor and guanylate cyclase stimulating agents in vascular smooth muscle. J Pharmacol Exp Ther 1989; 249: 394–400.
68. Weishaar RE. Multiple molecular forms of phosphodiesterase: a review. J Cyclic Nucl Prot Phosph Res 1987; 11: 463–72.

6. Signals regulating arterial contractile function and growth in hypertension
Role of angiotensin II and nitric oxide

JEAN-BAPTISTE MICHEL and JEAN-FRANÇOIS ARNAL

Introduction

Arterial hypertension is accompanied mainly by trophic alterations in the structure of the arterial wall, such as changes in media thickness, increased collagen, loss of elastin and intimal proliferation. These changes are the result of phenotypic alterations in the smooth muscle cells. They are regulated by hemodynamic signals, blood and interstitial-borne signals, and signals from the endothelial cells. They produce alterations in the intracellular second messenger systems, and these transmit the information required to modify gene expression and thus the cell phenotype.

Structural background

The arterial wall is made up of three layers, the innermost intima, the media and the outer adventitia. The adventitia is composed of a loose network of connective tissue. This external layer is involved in the regulation of contractility and growth (vasotrophicity), as it contains nerve terminals releasing a variety of neurotransmitters that act upon the medial smooth muscle cells. It may also be a major factor in the destruction of the arterial wall by such processes as inflammation or immune disease.

The inner layer, the intima, is normally composed of a single layer of endothelial cells and an extracellular basement membrane. The endothelial cells are directly involved in regulating both normal and pathological contractility and trophic changes. Under normal conditions the intima is simply the endothelium. It is of prime importance as the interface between the circulating blood and the arterial wall. It receives signals from the mobile liquid phase and transmits them to the solid, viscoelastic phase of the media. The intima may become considerably thickened in pathological situations such as arteriosclerosis or atherosclerosis. The processes of cell proliferation, sclerosis and lipid deposition lead to a reduction in the diameter of the arterial lumen. Endothelial cell phenotype can varied between the arterial

M. E. Safar and M. F. O'Rourke (eds.), The arterial system in hypertension. pp. 89–105.

system and the capillaries. Capillary endothelium express several antigens that there are not expressed on the cell membrane of arterial endothelium. Capillary endothelium is richer in enzymatic activities such as converting enzyme than arterial endothelium.

The central layer of the arterial wall, the media, is the thickest. Normal media contains a single cell type, smooth muscle cells, lying in a fibrous extracellular matrix composed of glycoaminoglycans, collagen and elastin. The arterial system is generally divided into two sections, compliance arteries and resistance arteries, depending on the structural and mechanical properties of the arterial wall. Compliance, or elastic arteries are the major arteries in which the elastic component of the extracellular matrix is particularly important. The resistance, or smooth muscle arteries are the medium and small diameter arteries in which the media is less well organized, the elastic network is reduced to internal and external elastic layers. As their name suggests, the walls of these arteries contain mostly smooth muscle cells. The smooth muscle cells is the cellular element responsible for contractility and trophic changes in both the capacitance and resistance arteries. In large arteries, compliance function is mainly chronically dependant on the extra-cellular component of the arterial wall and therefore on the secretory function of the smooth muscle cells. But contractile function also participate from the rigidification of the arterial wall in large arteries. Resistance function is mainly dependant on the contractile state of smooth muscle cells in small arteries, but can be also chronically influenced by smooth muscle cells growth. Therefore it is always difficult in an arterial chronic hemodynamic change to clearly analyse the respective role of contractile function and structure.

Smooth muscle cells

The smooth muscle cell is the active component responsible for arterial contraction or relaxation [1]. It is also the key to arterial trophic changes, because of its capacity for hypertrophy and proliferation and its ability to secrete the proteins forming the extra-cellular matrix.

The three properties, contractility, hypertrophy and secretion, are independent of each other. Thus the arterial smooth muscle phenotype can vary in the expression of these three functions, both in physiological situations and during pathological processes such as arterial hypertension, atherosclerosis, or chronically reduced blood flow. There are many examples of these phenotypic changes. During the development of atheroma there is a migration and proliferation of medial smooth muscle cells into the intima. This migration and proliferation is accompanied by phenotypic regression to myofibroblasts, ie, a loss of contractile potential and increased collagen secreting capacity. Similar changes occur when arterial smooth muscle cells are placed in culture; the contractile functions are lost, while the collagen-secreting capacity decreases during the cell proliferation phase and reappears and becomes predominant once the cells reach confluence. These specific regulatory systems and phenotypic changes are far from completely understood.

The contractile proteins within the smooth muscle cells are independent of each other when the cell is completely relaxed, while the formation of cross-links between the actin and myosin molecules leads to contraction. The release of calcium from its intracellular storage sites within the smooth muscle cell into the cytoplasm is the first step in the contractile response, and the subsequent entry of calcium from the extracellular medium via the cell membrane calcium channels keeps the intracellular concentration of free calcium high, thus maintaining the actin- myosin interaction, and hence contraction. This phenomenon is clearly seen in cultures of smooth muscle cells. The cells can be loaded with a fluorescent marker for intracellular free calcium. When they are stimulated by placing angiotensin II and calcium in the culture medium there is a rapid increase in the free intracellular calcium concentration until it reaches a plateau. If the cells are stimulated by angiotensin II alone, without calcium in the medium, there is the same initial increase in intracellular calcium, but the peak is transient and there is no plateau. There are, therefore, two phases in the change in intracellular free calcium concentration. The initial rapid increase corresponds to the release of intracellularly stored calcium, while the plateau is produced by the entry of free calcium from the extracellular medium.

Sites of angiotensin production

The components of the renin-angiotensin system are each produced at specific sites; renin is produced in the kidney, angiotensinogen in the liver, and converting enzyme in the endothelium, while accessory tissues may produce prorenin (ovary and chorion) or angiotensinogen (arterial adventitia). This information, together with the fact that the circulating angiotensin concentration is not simply a function of the plasma renin-substrate reaction, has given rise to the hypothesis [2] that there may be tissue renin-angiotensin systems that are independent of the plasma and renal systems!

Experiments in which isolated limbs were perfused with renin substrate showed the production of angiotensin II and vasoconstriction. But the substrate used in these preliminary experiments was a synthetic tetradecapeptide containing the 14 amino-terminal aminoacid residues of angiotensinogen. This peptide is cleaved by renin into angiotensin I and a tetrapeptide; it is also cleaved directly by converting enzyme. It is therefore absolutely not specific for the renin- substrate reaction in vivo. Other experiments, in which angiotensinogen was used as the substrate for renin under the same experimental conditions of isolated limb or heart perfusion, were negative [3]. In contrast, perfusion of the isolated kidney with angiotensinogen led to angiotensin production [4], vasoconstriction and inhibition of renin secretion. These two models, perfusion of isolated limbs and perfusion of isolated kidney, produced diametrically opposite responses to the perfusion of angiotensinogen. Perfusion of the isolated limb with the natural substrate of renin had no effect, while perfusion of the isolated kidney led to angiotensin production and its physiological effects. The results of these two experiments clearly demonstrate the overwhelming importance of the kidney in the secretion of renin and in the production of tissue angiotensins.

However, the tissue distribution of specific mRNAs indicates that there is extrarenal synthesis of renin by blood vessel walls, and extrahepatic synthesis of angiotensinogen. This has led some workers to suggest that there are renin-substrate reactions that are independent of the production of active renin by the kidney. However, there is no substantiated evidence for the extrarenal conversion of prorenin to active renin. At all the sites that have been shown to have – sometimes large – concentrations of prorenin, the secreted prorenin has been shown to be inactive. Furthermore, the increase in the endogenous level of prorenin that occurs, for example during ovulation, or the perfusion of recombinant prorenin in primates, does not lead to a change in the circulating level of active renin, and to angiotensin production, or to any modification of biological effectors [5]. Lastly, the circulating concentrations of renin activity and angiotensin [6] drop to undetectable levels after bilateral nephrectomy, while the concentration of prorenin drops by only about 50%.

Nevertheless, while it is quite probable that almost all the circulating renin activity comes from the kidney, it is clear that the plasma renin-substrate reaction is not the exclusive source of angiotensin I [7]. A recent series of fascinating experiments by the Rotterdam group [8–13], in which vascular beds were perfused in situ with a stable concentration of ^{125}I-labelled angiotensin I, allowed measurement of the production and metabolism of endogenous angiotensins. The results indicate that the half-life in vivo in man of angiotensin I is extremely short, about 0.6 min in the presence of converting enzyme inhibitor. The distribution volume of exogenous perfused angiotensin I is 12.5 l, about the same as the plasma volume. The total production of angiotensin I by the human body under basal conditions is about 412 pmol/min, while the plasma production under the same conditions is only 76 pmol/min. The plasma produces only about 20% of the total angiotensins; the remaining 80% come from interstitial sites.

The endogenous concentrations of angiotensin I in samples taken at different arterial and venous sites were the same, despite the massive differences in the rate of angiotensin extraction.The kidney removed 85% of the angiotensin I passing through it, while the upper limbs removed 45%, and the lower limbs 70%. Interstitial production and the movement from the interstitial compartment to the blood fluid constantly balanced this removal by the tissues, and thus made a major contribution to the circulating concentration of angiotensin. There is clearly, therefore, an interstitial, extraplasma renin-substrate reaction, which is responsible for 80% of angiotensin production [10]. However, this extra-plasma production is correlated with the plasma renin activity (correlation factor r = 0.85], showing that plasma renin and interstitial renin are not independent [10], but are both completely dependent on the secretion of active renin by the kidney. Thus there is a concomitant loss of both following sodium repletion or bilateral nephrectomy.

The main sites of angiotensin production and active renin secretion are also indicated by immunisation against angiotensin I and against renin [14–16]. Immunisation of animals against renin [16] very effectively blocked the renin-angiotensin system, produced a significant drop in arterial pressure and made the circulating level of angiotensins undetectable. Immunisation against renin resulted in the deposition of immunoglobulins at the site of renin production: the glomerular afferent arterioles. In contrast, immunisation against angiotensin I or II [14, 15] had no major effect on arterial pressure, although even intravenous injection of renin or angiotensin did not increase arterial pressure and the circulating antibody concentration was extremely high. The difference in the efficacity of the two immunological approaches could well be due to the interstitial site of angiotensin production and the dependence of the system on the renal secretion of renin. During immunisation against renin, the immunoglobulins deposited at the site of renin production block renin activity as it is secreted. This leads to a complete blockade of the plasma and interstitial system because they both depend on renal renin. However, immunisation against angiotensin blocks only the plasma production of angiotensin, while interstitial production is not blocked. As a result, this approach has very little effect on blood pressure. Comparison of the two approaches also shows that angiotensins are largely produced in the interstitium, while the system as a whole depends on the renal secretion of active renin.

There is still considerable controversy over the exact nature of angiotensinogen. The main conflict is between the results of physiological experiments on isolated perfused organs, and those of molecular biology studies. Angiotensinogen is synthesized outside the liver, the choroid plexus, kidney, heart, adrenals and artery wall may all produce it. The exact vascular site of its synthesis is still in doubt, the two main possibilities are the peri-aorta brown fat cells and the medial smooth muscle cells.

Unlike renin, angiotensinogen undergoes no specific maturation before becoming the substrate of active renin. This local production can also be regulated. It increases in the liver and heart in response to corticosteroids, and its renal concentration is increased by androgens [17]. Nevertheless, the greatest concentrations of angiotensinogen mRNA detected in these tissues are 10 times lower than the angiotensinogen mRNA concentration in the liver. The rat right atrium contains about 80 fg angiotensinogen mRNA per g total RNA, while the liver contains 1200 fg angiotensinogen mRNA per μg total RNA. If this is translated into absolute production rates, the heart synthesizes about 1000 to 10,000 times less angiotensinogen than the liver [18].

Experiments with isolated perfused limbs and hearts have provided a good deal of information. The basal level of angiotensin production is very low. The lower limbs produce about 5 fmol/hour, and the cardiac production is undetectable. In contrast, the plasma produces about 1000 times as much angiotensin. Perfusion with exogenous renin causes a temporary increase in angiotensin production. The maximum for the rat heart is 10^4 fmol/min, while angiotensin generation in the isolated limb system is increased 1000 fold, together with a 10 vasoconstriction. The effect of this perfusion was transient, short-lived and could not immediately be repeated. The level of angiotensin formation is correlated with the circulating concentration of angiotensinogen. The results for experiments with isolated kidneys are in agreement. The isolated perfused kidney spontaneously produces little angiotensin. The amount decreases with time, while that of renin increases. Perfusion with exogenous angiotensinogen results in a considerable increase in angiotensin production, vasoconstriction and reduced renin secretion. Perfusion with angiotensinogen re-establishes feedback control of angiotensin production on the system itself [4].

The third major protein component of the renin-angiotensin system is converting enzyme. This is both an enzyme circulating in the plasma and a component of the membranes of endothelial cells and other types of cells. The production of angiotensin II in isolated organ experiments can always be blocked by inhibitors of this enzyme. These pharmacological experiments have shown the specificity of angiotensin II production. They also show that the tissue concentration – probably the endothelium – of the enzyme is able to generate angiotensin II from angiotensin I regardless of the circulating concentration of converting enzyme, while stripping the endothelium from isolated vessels blocks the conversion of angiotensin I to angiotensin II [19]. However, exogenous converting enzyme increases the angiotensin II production of the isolated, perfused kidney system, and in the whole animal, the pulmonary capillary network, which has the highest converting enzyme concentration, can transform all the angiotensin I passing through it into angiotensin II in a single passage.

The present state of our knowledge of the plasma and tissue renin-angiotensin systems can be summarized as follows:
- Active renin is secreted almost entirely by the kidney.
- The liver is the main source of angiotensinogen, but small amounts may also be produced by other tissues.
- Renin, like angiotensinogen, diffuses freely in the interstitial fluid.
- 20% of the renin-substrate reaction occurs in the plasma and 80% in the interstitial fluid.
- The two compartments are not independent.

- Converting enzyme is synthesized and expressed in the endothelium of all tissues.
- Protein and peptides are constantly being exchanged between the two compartments.
- Tissues contain angiotensin II receptors, and the angiotensin II-receptor interaction occurs at the interstitial fluid-cell interface.

Signal transduction of angiotensin II: phosphoinositol pathway

The interaction between type I receptors and angiotensin II leads to activation of the phosphoinositol pathway (PIP) [20] in all target cells [21, 22], including the smooth muscle cells, mesangial cells [23], aldosterone-secreting adrenal cortex cells [24], hepatocytes [25] and cardiocytes.

In the smooth muscle cells, other receptors, including the endothelin, a_1-adrenergic, vasopressin Vl [26], muscarinic acetylcholine, thrombin and thromboxane receptors, are coupled to the activation of the PIP. Their activation on smooth muscle cells leads to an increase in free intracellular calcium and contraction mediated by activation of the PIP.

In addition to these hormonal signals, the PIP in smooth muscle cells can also be activated by an increase in transversal tension [36], and hence cell deformation by stretching. Thus vasomotility can be activated both hormonally and mechanically.

Activation of the PIP involves a cascade of membrane and cytosolic events [27]. The phosphatidylinositols are hydrophobic lipid molecules present in the membrane. Phospholipase C is a membrane protein, as are the Gq proteins, and the receptors (with seven trans-membrane domains). The Gq proteins that bind the receptors to phospholipase C are less well known than the $G_{i,s}$ proteins that bind to the receptors for adenylate cyclase. Nevertheless, the Gq proteins linking the receptor to phospholipase C also seem to be composed of three sub-units (a, β and g), and the a_q sub-unit seems to be specific for this binding. The interaction between angiotensin II and its receptor produces an allosteric change in the conformation of the molecule, which, via an activating G protein (GTP-dependent protein), leads to activation of protein kinase C [28]. In the presence of ATP, this enzyme then cleaves phosphoinositol diphosphate (PIP_2] into inositol triphosphate (IP_3] and diacylglycerol [29]. The hydrophobic lipid, diacylglycerol, remains with the membrane, but the sugar IP_3 is hydrophilic and becomes dissolved in the cytoplasm before being bound by specific receptors on the sarcoplasmic reticulum and the calciosomes [30]. Binding of IP_3 to its sarcoplasmic receptor causes the calcium channels to open on these storage sites, allowing calcium release as a function of the concentration gradient. This results in an abrupt rise in free intracellular calcium [6, 45] and the first component of contraction. During this peak there is also a transient hyperpolarisation of the cell membrane, quickly followed by depolarization and sodium entry

[31–33], leading to the entry of large amounts of calcium from the extra-cellular environment via the calcium channels, and the maintenance of a high concentration of free intracellular calcium [34].

The lipid diacylglycerol that remains attached to the membrane activates protein kinase C. This soluble cytosolic protein is normally inactive because of its allosteric- conformation; one domain, the pseudo-substrate [28], perma-nently inhibits its active site. The second domain is the diacylglycerol binding site, while the third domain is the catalytic sub-unit and includes the kinase active site. When the membrane contains diacylglycerol, the protein kinase C moves to the peri-membrane cytoplasm and binds, via domain 2 to diacyl-glycerol to become activated.

Protein kinase C acts on many systems implicated in the processes of cell differentiation and proliferation. One of the effectors, the sodium-proton exchanger, has recently been cloned. This exchanger, as its name implies, exchanges one sodium ion for one (intracellular) hydrogen ion. When the exchanger is phosphorylated by protein kinase C it becomes more active, pumping out more hydrogen ions, and hence increasing the intracellular pH. This change in intracellular pH is necessary for increased genetic expression and the triggering of the phenomena involved in cell proliferation. The role of protein kinase C in influencing the proliferation phenomena has been studied during cancerous proliferation, in which the PIP is implicated. There is clearly a direct link between activation of the contractility and trophic capacity of smooth muscle cells in response to activation of the PIP.

Reduction of free intracellular calcium: the guanylate cyclases

The cGMP pathway act in the opposite sense to the PIP in the smooth muscle cell [35]. Its activation leads to a drop in free intracellular calcium, and hence to relaxation.

This pathway has three main elements, the guanylate cyclase that is respon-sible for formation of the second messenger, cyclic GMP, adenylate cyclase, that produces cAMP from ATP, and G-kinase [36] the inactive cytosolic protein that is activated by cAMP and cGMP [37] in smooth muscle cells. The substrates for G-kinase are not clearly defined; it indirectly activates the membrane Ca^{++}-dependent ATPase [38] and cytosolic Na^+/Ca^{++} exchange [39]. It may also act on the phospholambans, which are proteins that are also involved in intracellular calcium transport.

G-kinase is particularly tissue-specific. It is mostly found in blood vessel walls [40], making the action of activators of the cGMP pathway very specific. G-kinase has been purified from pulmonary tissue and cloned. It has two isoforms [41]. Studies with anti-G-kinase antibodies show that it is present only in vascular tissue, so that in the heart, only the coronary vessels are immuno-labelled [40].

G-kinase is inactive in the absence of cGMP. Its two-chain structure is similar to that of other kinases, with an inhibitory pseudo-substrate domain that is bound to the active site to inhibit the enzyme in the absence of cGMP, a high-affinity cGMP-binding site and a catalytic domain. The cGMP binds to the G-kinase and changes its allosteric conformation so that the inhibitory domain no longer blocks the catalytic domain.

As its name implies, cGMP is a cyclic nucleotide formed from GTP. One of its main properties, other than binding to G-kinase, is that it can be secreted from the cell. This egression of cGMP is active and can occur against a concentration gradient [42]. It seems to act as a powerful feedback regulator to block the accumulation of cGMP in cells in response to activation of guanylate cyclase. cGMP is rapidly broken down within the cell by phosphodiesterases of varying specificities. Phosphodiesterases I and III seem to be mainly involved in the breakdown of cGMP, while phosphodiesterase II is the main enzyme breaking down cAMP. Phosphodiesterase III seems to be absent from the endothelium [43], and cyclic GMP egression is probably the main metabolism pathway in the endothelial cells.

The enzymes responsible for producing cGMP are the guanylate cyclases. There are two main types: the soluble and the particulate or membrane guanylate cyclases (biologically active ANF receptors) [44]. The soluble guanylate cyclase and two types of particulate guanylate cyclases have been clone. The particulate guanylate cyclases are transmembrane proteins having four domains: an extracellular ANF-binding domain, a short hydrophobic anchoring segment within the plasma membrane, and two intracellular segments. The first of these is the ATP-binding site (by homology with tyrosine kinase) and the second is the guanylate cyclase activity (by homology with the soluble guanylate cyclase) [45]. The ATP-binding site does not seem to have any kinase activity, but the binding of ATP appears to alter the allosteric conformation of the molecule so as to amplify its guanylate cyclase activity.

The physiological activators of particulate guanylate cyclases are the atrial natriuretic factors (ANF and BNF), while soluble guanylate cyclase is activated by nitric oxide.

Activation of the cAMP pathway also leads to smooth muscle cell relaxation, although the calcium concentration in the cardiac muscle cell increases. This is probably due to the presence of G-kinase in the smooth muscle cells. The adenylate cyclase activators, such as β sympathetic stimulation, or prostacyclin, are vasodilators. They also cause an increase in intracellular cAMP (second messenger) concentration. The cAMP probably binds to the G-kinase in the smooth muscle cell, thereby inducing vasodilation. Although cAMP is bound to G-kinase much less tightly than is cGMP, the intracellular concentration of cAMP is 100 times higher than that of cGMP [37].

Intracellular interaction

The actions of the phosphoinositol and guanylate cyclase pathways within the cell are antagonistic. Hence, activation of the PIP results in a drop in the activity of the cGMP pathway [46], while activation of the cGMP system decreases the effects of the PIP on free intracellular calcium concentration.

These interactions have recently been analysed. Activation of the guanylate cyclase system activates the G-kinase, which then phosphorylates G protein binding the receptor and phospholipase C, leading to uncoupling of the receptor from phospholipase C. This cGMP- dependent uncoupling may be completely inhibited by GTPg$_s$, which is an irreversible activator of G protein binding. Thus, activation of the cGMP system not only directly reduces the free intracellular calcium concentration, but also inhibits the response of the PIP to its agonists.

Conversely, activation of the PIP reduces the intracellular concentration of cGMP [47]. The phosphodiesterase activity responsible for breaking down cyclic nucleotides is partially dependent on calcium and calmodulin. Under these conditions, activation of the PIP leads to an increase in phosphodiesterase activity, and hence to an increase in the rate of cyclic nucleotide destruction. In addition, the angiotenin II receptor is negatively coupled to adenylate cyclase. Interaction of angiotensin II with its receptor activates a G protein that inhibits adenylate cyclase.

Regulation of the balance between the two signalling systems

Although the way in which these two pathways are integrated to produce the overall regulation of vascular contractility is complex, it may be simplified for clarity. However, the more the system is simplified, the greater the chance that it will be incomplete. We have seen that there are two hormonal and mechanical activators of the two pathways within the smooth muscle cell. We must therefore describe the role of the endothelium in the regulation of vascular motricity [48].

The endothelial cell has also the two pathways, one for metabolising phosphoinositols [49] and the second for cGMP (SO) and cAMP. While the concentration of G-kinase in the endothelial cell is very low, there are ANF-sensitive particulate guanylate cyclases that can generate cGMP and export it into the extracellular medium. Thus, the cGMP measured in the plasma after stimulation with ANF is mainly of endothelial origin.

The endothelium produces a factor that relaxes the underlying smooth muscle cells, endothelial relaxing factor (EDRF) [51, 52]. This is probably nitric oxide (NO) [53–55]. It also produces a factor that causes the smooth muscle cells to contract, endothelin, whose physiological and pathological roles have not yet to be determined. We shall be mainly concerned with EDRF; as it is the physiological activator of soluble smooth muscle guanylate cyclase.

Furchgott first showed that the endothelium had a vasodilatory action. In the absence of the endothelium, acetylcholine is essentially a vasoconstrictor, while in the presence of the endothelium it is a powerful vasodilator. This phenomenon has since been demonstrated for several hormonal products, such as the kinins, thrombin, vasopressin, endothelin, etc. Most important, it has been shown that the increase in flow [52] increases the shear stress (frictional forces) on the endothelial cell and thus increase EDRF production. The major role of NO has recently been demonstrated by Moncada and co-workers. The endothelial cell produces NO from L-arginine. The NADPH and Ca^{++}-dependent enzyme NO-synthase cleaves the arginine into citrulline and NO. The natural substrate L-arginine may be competitively blocked by pseudo-substrates such as L-monomethyl arginine or L-nitro-arginine, which take the place of arginine and prevent NO production. Removal of the endothelium, which results in a significant drop in the cGMP concentration in the arterial media, was used to demonstrate an endothelium-dependent vasodilatory tone. It has recently been shown that acute in perfusion with L-NMMA (which blocks NO production) completely blocks the vasodilatory response to acetylcholine, and causes a spontaneous increase in the arterial pressure and induces vasoconstriction under normal conditions. Similarly, chronic administration of L-NAME lead to a chronic dose-dependant increase in blood pressure, and a chronic decrease in cyclic GMP content [56]. Thus the chronic vasodilation is dependent on NO production by the endothelium. This has been demonstrated in several organs of both animals and man, but particularly the kidney. NO secretion thus depends on the presence of arginine and the synthase enzyme activity. This enzyme activity is regulated by the endothelial PIP via the Ca^{++} calmoduline pathway.

Hence, the hormonal and/or mechanical signals that activate the PIP in the endothelial cells [57] increase the secretion of NO and induce relaxation of the underlying smooth muscle cells. Blood velocity [58, 59] is the mechanical signal that increases the concentration of intracellular free calcium in the endothelium leading to dilation which tends to normalize shear stress.

Similarly, hormonal signals such as acetylcholine (muscarinic receptors), bradykinin, ADP, and S-hydroxytryptamine all increase the intracellular concentrations of IP_3 and free calcium by

binding to their endothelial receptors. A hormone or a peptide whose action in linked to activation of phospholipase C may thus be either vasodilatory, if its receptors are on the endothelial cells, or constrictor if its receptors are on the smooth muscle cells, or both. The dominance of one or other form of total contractile response will depend on the number of receptors on one or other of the cell types and on the pharmacological dose used.

The presence of biologically active receptors for angiotensin II on endothelial cells remains to be demonstrated, although there have been occasional reports of paradoxal vasodilatory effects. In contrast, this phenomenon is well known for vasopressin, which may be vasodilatory in certain vascular territories, idem for thrombin and endothelin. Other peptides, such as bradykinin [60, 61], are essentially vasodilators because they mostly act on the endothelium.

In the endothelial cell, as in other cells, activation of the PIP also leads to prostaglandin synthesis [62, 63]. The endothelial cell contains the enzymatic equipment necessary for prostacyclin synthesis (phospholipase A2, cyclo-oxygenase, prostacycline synthase). This endothelial prostaglandin relaxes the underlying smooth muscle cells by activating adenyl cyclase to produce cAMP.

However, the vasodilatory effects of bradykinin are completely inhibited by L-NMMA [64–66] and unaffected by indomethacin, which inhibits prosta-glandin synthesis. Thus, activation of NO production plays a key role as compared to PGI_2 production, at least under the experimental conditions tested, in endothelial dependant vasodilatation.

Thus, while there is clearly tonic vasoconstrictor activity that depends directly on the activation of the smooth muscle cell PIP, there is also a permanent vasodilatory tone that depends on the guanylate cyclase system within the smooth muscle cell and on the PIP within the endothelium. Thus vascular contractility is the dynamic algebraic sum of these effects over time and as an adaptive response to changes in the environment and tissue oxygen consumption. In addition to the hormonal signals influencing the two path-ways, there are mechanical signals that contribute to this dynamic equilib-rium. Angiotensin II, a sympathetic stimulation, and increased parietal ten-sion (transverse Laplace forces) are major contributors to vasocontriction tone. ANF, NO production, B sympathetic activation, prostacyclin and in-creased blood velocity all contribute to the vasodilation. Inhibition of either vasoconstriction or vasodilation leads to immediate changes in vasocontractil-ity, depending on how they influence the smooth muscle cell.

Relationship between vasocontractility and vasotrophicity

The mechanical and hormonal signals that induce contractile changes also influence the trophic alterations in smooth muscle cells via the actions of their intracellular messengers. These effects have been studied on cell cultures, and in vivo, particularly for angiotensin II.

In vitro [67–71] angiotensin II alone will increase protein synthesis in cultured smooth muscle cells, stopping short of a total effect at cell multiplica-tion (mitosis). This trophic effect of angiotensin II on cells in culture leads to increased expression of the pro-oncogenes C-Fos and C-Myc, whose products interfere with the nucleus. It also leads to production of growth factors, particularly PDGF, by muscle cells, and as mentioned above, to an increase in intracellular pH. All these trophic effects depend on activation of the PIP, and particularly on protein kinase C.

Other vasoactive hormones, such as endothelin, a adrenergic 23 stimula-tion and bradykinin, are reported to have analogous effects [72]. When these hormones act alone, they behave as hypertrophic factors for smooth muscle cells in culture, when they act synergistically with other growth factors or mechanical factors they increase the proliferative response capacity of smooth

Table 1

Mechanical stimuli	Signal transduction	Trophic effects		
		Smooth muscle growth	Elastin biosynthesis	Collagen biosynthesis
Tensil stress (pressure and dimensions)	PIP	+	−	+
Shear stress and rate (velocity and dimensions)	cyclic GMP	−	+(?)	−

muscle cells. For example, PDGF induces proliferation, addition of angiotensin II has an additive effect, the protein-synthesis stimulating effect facilitates the proliferative effect of the growth factor. These synergistic phenomena are extremely important and probably play a major role in the trophic response in vivo, resulting in proliferation of smooth muscle cells. The very large number of angiotensin II type II receptors present during fetal development is also a strong indication of the possible trophic action of angiotensin II [73].

In vivo, in arterial hypertension the synergy between hormonal factors such as angiotensin II and mechanical ones like increased pressure result in an increase in transversal stress according to the Laplace law ($r = p.r/h$; where r is the stress, p is pressure, r the radius, and h the thickness of the cylinder wall) There are several situations in which the production of angiotensin II is increased and the constriction is unchanged, such as sodium depletion. The trophic capacity of the arterial wall is unchanged in these cases.

The inter-renal aorta coarctation model [74] is also a good example. In the initial phase of this model, the renin-angiotensin system is strongly activated and angiotensin II is produced in all the blood vessels of the animal. However, the increase in arterial pressure only occurs in the sub-strictural segment of the aorta. Here, only the sub-strictural segment thickens, and its incorporation of tritiated thymidine increases, expressing the proto-oncogenes. Therefore, mechanical factors and angiotensin II must act synergistically to bring about major changes in arterial trophicity.

The situation in post-endothelialisation proliferation phenomena is similar [75]. This intimal proliferation is essentially proportional to the production of growth factors, particularly PDGF. But in this situation, when the production of angiotensin II is blocked, there is a lower proliferative response. This suggests synergy with growth factors much like that found in vitro. This effect is also not completely independent of the arterial pressure. It does not require a high angiotensin II concentration.

In contrast, factors that activate the guanylate cyclase system [76] tend to block smooth muscle cell growth, and inhibit their growth in tissue culture.

This depends on both the particulate (ANF) and the soluble forms of guanylate cyclase.In vivo the chronic increase in blood velocity such as in the aorto-caval fistula model, lead to a chronic increase in the arterial wall cyclic GMP content and increase oin arterial dimensions. Conversely the chronic decrease in blood flow lead to a decrease in arterial dimensions and decrease in transversal stress and was associated with a decrease in elastin content [77].

Conclusion

The arterial wall undergoes major phenotypic changes, in arterial hypertension. These changes are regulated by the intracellular balance between the phosphoinositol and guanylate cylcase systems.The net result is an apparent activation of the phosphoinositol pathway in classical model of hypertension whereas the activation of guanylate cyclase system depends on the model used. Nevertheless, chronic complete blockade of NO synthase activity lead also to a new model of hypertension. The relationship between mechanical stimuli, signal transduction and trophic effect could be probably summarized in Table 1.

References

1. Michel JB, De Roux N, Plissonnier D, Anidjar S, Salzmann JL, Levy BI. Pathophysiological role of the vascular smooth muscle cell. J Cardiovasc Pharmacol 1990; 16(suppl. I): 54–511.
2. Campbell DJ. Circulating and tissue angiotensin system. J Clin, Invest 1987; 79: 1–6.
3. Hilger KF, Kuczera M, Wilhalm MJ, et al. Angiotensin formation in the rat hind limb. J Hypertension 1989; 7: 789–98.
4. Misumi J, Gardes J, Gonzales MF, Corvol P, Ménard J. Angiotensinogen's role in angiotensin formation, renin release and I renal hemodynamics in isolated perfused kidney. Am J Physiol 1989; 256: F719-F27.
5. Lentz T, Sealey JE, Lappe RW, et al. Infusion of recombinant human prorenin into rhesus monkeys: effects on hemodynamics, renin-angiotensin-aldosterone axis and plasma testosterone. Am J Hyperten 1990; 3: 257–61.
6. Huang H, Baussant T, Reade R, Michel JB, Corvol P. Measurement of angiotensin II concentration in rat plasma.Physiopathological applications. Clin Exp Hypertens 1989; 11: 1535–48.
7. Campbell DJ. The site of angiotensin production. J Hypertension 1985; 3: 199–207.
8. Admiraal PJJ, Derks FHM, Danser AHJ, Pieterman H, Shalekamp MADH. Metabolism and production of angiotensin I in different vascular beds in patients with hypertension. Hypertension 1990; 15: 44–55.
9. Admiraal PJJ, Derkx FHM, Danser AHJ, Pieterman H, Schalekamp MADH. De novo production of angiotensin I by the affected and unaffected kidney in subjects with renal artery stenosis; role of circulating and non-circulating renin. Hypertension 1990; 16: 555–63.
10. Danser AHJ, Sassen LMA, Admiraal PJJ, Derkx FHM, Verdouw PD, Schalekamp MADH. Regional production of angiotensins I and II. Contribution of vascular kidney – derived renin. J Hypertens 1991; 9(Suppl.6): S234–S5.

11. Admiraal PJJ, Derkx FHM, Schalekamp MADH. Angiotensin II production in different vascular beds in hypertensive subjects. J Hypertens 9(Suppl. 6): S208-S9.
12. Danser AHJ, Koning MMG, Admiraal PPJ, Derkx FHM, Verdouw PD, Schakelamp MADH. Metabolism of angiotensin I by different tissues in the intact animal. Am J Physiol 1992; 263: H418-H28.
13. Danser AHJ, Koning MMG, Admiraal PJJ, et al. Production of angiotensins I and II at tissues sites in the intact pig. Am J Physiol 1992; 263: H429-H37.
14. Reade R, Michel JB, Carelli C, Huang H, Baussant T, Corvol P. Immunisation du rat spontanément hypertendu contre l'angiotensine I. Arch Mal Coeur Vaiss 1989; 82: 1323-8.
15. Michel JB, Guettier C, Reade R, Sayah S, Menard J, Corvol P Immunological approach to the blockade of the renin-angiotensin system. Am Heart J 1989; 117: 756-67.
16. Michel JB, Sayah S, Nussberger J. et al. Physiological and murine renin in spontaneously hypertensive and normotensive ras. Circulation 1990; 81: 1899-910.
17. Ellison KE, Ingelfinger JR, Pivor M, Dzau V. Androgen regulation of rat renal angiotensinogen messenger RNA expression. J Clin Invest 1989; 83: 1941-5.
18. Lindpaintner K, Jin M, Niedermaier N, Wilhelm M J, Ganten D. Cardiac angiotensinogen and its local activation in the isolated perfused beating heart. Circ Res 1990; 67: 564-73.
19. Gohlke P, Bunning P, Unger T. Distribution and metabolism of angiotensin I and II in the blood vessel wall. Hypertension 1992; 20: 151-7.
20. Berridge MJ. Inositol triphosphate and diacylglycerol: two interacting second messengers. Ann Rev Biochem 1987; 56: 159-93.
21. Alexander RW, Brock TA, Gimbrone MA, Rittenhouse SE. Angiotensin increases inositol triphosphate and calcium in vascular smooth muscle. Hypertension 1985; 7: 447-51.
22. Smith JB. Angiotensin receptor signalising in cultured vascular smooth muscle cells. Am J Physiol 1986; 250: F759-F69.
23. Hassid A, Pidikiti N, Gamero D. Effects of vasoactive peptides on cytosolic calcium in cultured mesangial cell. Am J Physiol 1986a; 251: F1018-F28.
24. Capponi AM, Rossier M, Lang U, Lew PD, Valloton MB. Comparison of the signal transduction mechanisms for angiotensin II in adrenal zona glomerulosa and vascular smooth muscle cells. J Hypertens 1986, 4(Suppl. 6): S419 S20.
25. Manger JP, Claret M, Pietry F, Hilly M. Hormonal regulation of inositol 1,4,5 triphosphate receptor in rat liver. J Biol Chem 1989; 264: 8821-6.
26. Capponi AM, Lew PD, Walloton MB. Cytosolic free calcium levels in monolayers of cultured rat aortic smooth muscle cells: effects of angiotensin II and vasopressin. J Biol Chem 1985; 260: 7836-42.
27. Marx JL. Polyphosphoinositide research updated. Science 1987; 235: 974-6.
28. Hardie G. Pseudosubstrate turn off proteinkinase. Nature 1988; 335: 592-3.
29. Griendling KK, Rittenhouse SE, Brock TA, et al. Sustained diacylglycerol formation from inositol phospholipids in angiotensin II stimulated smooth muscle cells. J Biol Chem 1986; 261: 5901-6.
30. Guillemette G, Balla T, Bankal AJ, Spat A, Catt KJ. Intracellular receptors for inositol 1,4,5-triphosphate in angiotensin II target tissues. J Biol Chem 1987; 262: 1010-5.
31. Somlyo AP. Excitation contraction coupling and the ultrastructure of smooth muscle. Circ Res 1985; 57: 497-507.
32. Hamon G Worcel M. Electrophysiological study of the action of angiotensin II on the rat myometrium. Circ Res 1979; 45: 234-43.
33. Hamon G, Moura AM, Papdimitriou A, Worcel M. Effect of angiotensin II on ionic fluxes in rat myometrium. J Pharmacol 1982a; 13: 329-40.
34. Ullian ME, Linas SL. Angiotensin II surface receptor coupling to inositol triphosphate formation in vascular smooth muscle cells. J Bio Chem 1990; 265: 195-200.
35. Murad F. Cyclic guanosine monophosphatase as a mediator of vasodilatation. J Clin Invest 1986; 78: 1-5.

36. Lincoln TM, Johnson RM. Possible role of cyclic GMP dependent protein kinase in vascular smooth muscle function. Dev Cycl Nucleot Prot Phosphor Res 1984; 17: 285–96.

37. Lincoln TM, Cornwell TL, Taylon AE. cGMP-dependent protein kinase mediates the reduction of Ca^{2+} by cAMP in vascular smooth muscle cells. Am J Physiol 1990; 258: C399–C407.

38. Furukawa KI, Ohshima N, Tawada-Iwata Y, Shigekawa M. Cyclic GMP stimulates NA^+/Ca^{++} exchange in vascular smooth muscle cells in primary culture. Biol Chem 1991; 19: 12337–41.

39. Yoshida Y, Sun HT, Cai JQ, Imai S. Cyclic GMP-dependent protein kinase stimulates the plasma membrane Ca^{++} pump ATPase of vascular smooth muscle via phosphorylation of a 240-kDa protein. J Biol Chem 1991; 29: 19819–5.

40. Ecker T, Gobel C, Hullin R, Rettig R, Seith G, Hofmann F. Decreased cardiac concentration of cGMP kinase in hypertensive animals. Circ Res 1989; 65: 1361–9.

41. Wernet W, Flockerzi V, Hofmann F. The cDNA of the two isoforms of bovine cGMP in cultured vascular smooth muscle and endothelial cell. J Biol Chem 1989; 264: 12364–9.

42. Hamet P, Pany S.C, Tremblay J. Atrial natriuretic factor induced egression of cGMP in cultured vascular smooth muscle and endothelial cell. J Biol Chem 1989; 264: 12364–9.

43. Lugnier C, Schini VB. Characterization of cyclic nucleotide phosphodiesterases from cultured bovine aortic endothelial cells. Biochem Pharmacol 1990; 39: 75–84.

44. Michel JIB, Arnal J, F. Le facteur atrial natriurétique: données récentes et perspectives. Arch Mal Coeur 1990; 83: 2111–21.

45. Chang MS, Lowe DG, Lewis M, Hellmiss R, Chen E, Goeddel DV. Differential activation by atrial and brain natriuretic peptides of two different receptor guanylate cyclases. Nature 1989; 341: 68–72.

46. Hirata M, Kohse KP, Chang CH, Ikebe T, Murad F. Mechanism of cyclic GMP inhibition of inositol phosphate formation in rat aorta segments and cultured bovine aortic smooth muscle cells. J Biol Chem 1990; 265: 1268–73.

47. Smith JF, Lincoln TM. Angiotensin decreases cyclic GMP accumulation produced by atrial natriuretic factor. Am J Physiol 1987; 253: C147–C50.

48. Cherry PD, Furchgott RF, Zawadzki JV, Jothianaudau D. Role of endothelial cells in relaxation of isolated arteries by bradykinin. Proc Natl Acad Sci 1982; 79: 2106–10.

49. Lambert TL, Kent RS, Whorton AR. Bradykinin stimulation of inositol polyphosphate production in porcine aortic endothelial cells. J Biol Chem 1986; 261: 15288–93.

50. Van Gett C, Decknyn H, Kienas J, Wittevrongel C, Vermylen J. Guanine nucleotide-dependent inhibition of phospholipase C in human endothelial cells. J Biol Chem 1990; 265: 7920–6.

51. Furchgott RF, Vanhoutte PM. Endothelium-derived relaxing and contracting factors. FASEB J 1989; 3: 2007–18.

52. Griffith TM, Edwards DH, Davies RL, Harrion TJ, Evans RT. EDRF coordinates the behaviour of vascular resistance vessels. Nature 1987; 329: 442–5.

53. Palmer RMJ, Ferrige AG, Moncada S. Nitric oxide accounts for the biological activity of endothelium-derived relaxing factor. Nature 1987; 327: 524–6.

54. Palmer RMJ, Ashton DS, Moncada S. Vascular endothelial cells synthetise nitric oxide from L-arginine. Nature 1988; 333: 664–6.

55. Rees DD, Palmer RMJ, Moncada S. Role of endothelium-derived nitric oxide in the regulation of blood pressure. Proc Natl Acad Sci USA 1989; 86: 3375–18.

56. Arnal JF, Warin L, Michel JB. Determinants of aortic cyclic GMP in hypertension-induced by chronic blockade of NO-synthase. J Clin Invest 1992; 90: 647–52.

57. Schilling WP, Ritchie AK, Navarro LT, Eskin SG. Bradykinin-stimulated calcium influx in cultured bovine aortic endothelial cells. Am J Physiol 1988; 255: H219–H27.

58. Rubanyi GM, Romero JC, Vanhoutte PM. Flow-induced release of endothelial derived relaxing factor. Am Physiol 1986; 250: H1145–H7.

59. Tolins JP, Palmer RMJ, Moncada S, Raij L. Role of endothelim-derived relaxing factor in regulation of renal hemodynamic responses. Am J Physiol 1990; 258: H655–H62.

60. Dixon BS, Breckon R, Fortune J, et al. Effects of kinins on cultured arterial smooth muscle cells. Am J Physiol 1990; 258: C299–C308.
61. Morgan-Boyd R, Stewart JM, Vavrek RJ, Hassid A. Effect of bradykinin and angiotensin II on intracellular Ca^{++} dynamics in endothelial cells. Am J Physiol 1987; 253: C588–C98.
62. Hassid A, Oudinet JP. Relationship between cellular calcium and prostaglandin synthesis in cultured vascular smooth muscle cells. Prostaglandins 1986; 32: 457–78.
63. Furstermann U, Hertting G, Neufang B. The role of endothelial and non endothelial prostaglandins in the relaxation of isolated blood vessels of the rabbit induced by acetylcholine and bradykinin. Br J Pharmacol 1986; 87: 521–32.
64. Aosala K, Gross SS, Griffith OW, Levi R. NG-methyl arginine, an inhibitor of endothelium derived nitric oxide synthesis, is a potent pressor agent in the guinea pig: does nitric oxide regulate blood pressure in vivo. Biochem Biophys Res Commun 1989; 160: 881–6.
65. Whittle BJR, Lopez Belmonte J, Rees DD. Modulation of the vasodepressor actions of acetylcholine, bradykinin, substance P and endothelin in the rat by a specific inhibitor of nitric oxide formation. Br J Pharmacol 1989; 98: 646–52.
66. Moore PK, Al-Swaych OA, Chong NWS, Evans RA, Gibson A. L-NG-nitro artinine, a novel L-arginine-reversible inhibitor of endothelium dependent vasodilatation in vitro. Br J Pharmacol 1990; 99: 408–12.
67. Taubman MB, Berk B, Izumo S, Tsuda T, Alexander RW, Nadal-Ginard B. Angiotensin II induces c-fos mRNA in aortic smooth muscle. J Biol Chem 1989; 264: 526–30.
68. Naftilan AJ, Pratt RC, Dzau VJ. Induction of platelet derived growth factor A-chain and C-myc gene expression by angiotensin II in cultured rat vascular smooth muscle cells. J Clin Invest 1989; 83: 1419–24.
69. Berk BC, Wekshtein V, Gordon HM, Tsuda T. Angiotensin II-stimulated protein synthesis in cultured vascular smooth muscle cells. Hypertension 1989; 13: 305–14.
70. Tsuda T, Griendling KK, Alexander RW. Angiotensin II stimulates vimentin phosphorylation via a Ca^{++}-dependent, protein kinase C-independent mechanism in cultured vascular smooth muscle cells. J Biol Chem 1988; 263: 19758–63.
71. Tsuda T, Alexander RW. Angiotensin II stimulates phosphorylation of nuclear lamins via a protein kinase C-dependent mechanism in cultured vascular smooth muscle cells. J Biol Chem 1990: 265: 1167–70.
72. Downward J, de Gunzburg J, Riehl R, Weinberg RA. P21 ras induced responsiveness of phosphatidyl-inositol turnover to bradykinin is a receptor number effect. Proc Nat Acad Sci USA 1988; 85: 5774–8.
73. Millan MA, Carvallo P, Izumi SI, Zemel S, Catt KJ, Aguilera G. Novel sites of expression of functional angiotensin II receptors in the late gestation fetus. Science 1989; 244: 1340–2.
74. Ollerenshaw JD, Heagerty AM, West KP, Sawles JD. The effects of coarctation, hypertension upon vascular inositol phospholipid hydrolysis in wistar rats. Hypertens 1988; 6: 733–8.
75. Powel JS, Clozel JP, Müller RKM, et al. Inhibitors of angiotensin converting enzyme prevent myointimal proliferation after vascular injury. Science 1989; 245: 186–8.
76. Garg UC, Hassid A. Nitric ox de generating vasodilatators and 8 bromo cyclic GMP inhibit mitogenesis and proliferation of cultured rat vascular smooth muscle cells. J Clin Invest 1989; 83: 1774–7.
77. Languille LB, Bendeck MP, Keeley FW. Adaptations of carotid arteries of young and mature rabbits to reduced carotid blood flow. A J Physiol 1989; 256: H931–H9.

7. Large arteries and epidemiological aspects of hypertension

WILLIAM McFATE SMITH

Introduction

The epidemiological aspects of hypertension most relevant to the large arteries relate to the aging of the vascular system and to factors which predispose to the development of hypertension, which independently and similarly to aging, alter the structure and function of the large arteries. Hypertension in the elderly, particularly systolic hypertension, and the associated vascular risks, and the implications of age for therapeutic interventions on elevated blood pressure, are paramount considerations relative to changes in the structure and function of large arteries [1, 2].

Pathophysiology

The large arteries of the circulatory system have viscoelastic properties, compliance or distensibility, that permit them to modulate the wide fluctuations in pressure generated by the heart, and to facilitate continuous flow through the capillary bed. The media of the arteries is the primary determinant of these physical properties. O'Rourke points out that the elastic fibers bear the generated tension at low distending pressures, while the less stretchable collagen fibers do so predominantly at high pressures, resulting in a nonlinear behavior of arterial wall compliance [3]. The viscoelastic 'reservoir function' of arteries is compromised during aging as they stiffen, dilate, lengthen and their walls thicken.. Hypertension accelerates this process, which has been attributed to cyclic stress acting over many decades [4–7].

Studies of subjects from a community with a low prevalence of atherosclerosis, demonstrate the increase in pulse wave velocity (PWV) with age (Figure 1) [5]. It was also shown in a community with a high dietary intake of salt and a high prevalence of hypertension, that PWV was elevated at any given age compared to normotensives from a community of lower salt intake [8]. In a separate study PWV declined in subjects who voluntarily reduced their salt intake [9]. Levenson et al. have also demonstrated significant decreases

M. E. Safar and M. F. O'Rourke (eds.), The arterial system in hypertension. pp. 107–118.
© 1993 *Kluwer Academic Publishers. Printed in the Netherlands.*

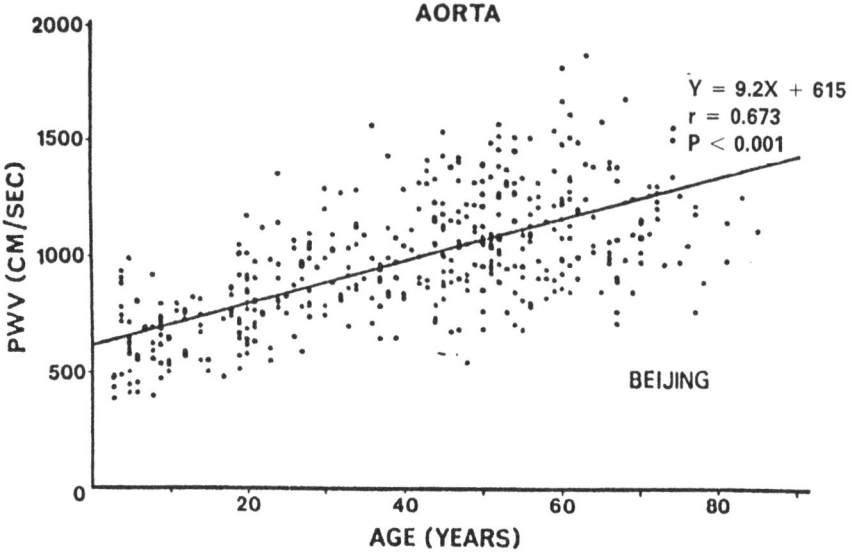

Figure 1. Plot showing relation between aortic pulse wave velocity and age in a group of 480 normal subjects from a community with low prevalence of atherosclerosis. From Avolio et al. [8].

in arterial compliance in the forearm preparation brought about by sodium intake or saline infusion [10].

Loss in aortic compliance, whether due to hypertension or aging, leads to increased impedance to cardiac ejection, usually associated with an increased PWV, early return of the reflected wave, and augmentation of systolic pressure [11]. This contributes to the disproportionate rise of systolic blood pressure with age, and the increasing prevalence of predominantly or isolated systolic hypertension (ISH) in the elderly. ISH developing in previously normotensive individuals, may be the example par excellence of the consequence of altered structure of the large arteries, wherein the elastic fibers of the media have deteriorated and been replaced by less distensible collagen and connective tissue [3]. As noted above, this process apparently proceeds independent of atherosclerosis, and although experimental studies suggest that early diffuse atherosclerosis may be associated with reduced compliance of the carotid artery, the direct application of such studies to human subjects is unclear [12]. ISH may also occur in persons with pre-existent diastolic hypertension whose diastolic pressure declined with age, while systolic pressure level persisted or increased [13]. The prognosis in such cases of 'burned-out' hypertension, may differ from primary ISH.

Diastolic hypertension in the elderly for the most part represents essential hypertension that developed in a younger person and persisted, with or without therapy, among survivors to an older age [1]. The pathophysiology of hypertension in the elderly, as in younger persons, is a consequence of the interaction of multiple pressor mechanisms, with increased total peripheral resistance being the most consistent physiologic change in elderly hypertensives. Age tends to influence these mechanisms in a graded way. Once again, the effects most recognized as being related to aging are the gradual and progressive loss of distensibility of the aorta and large arteries described above, and the reduced effectiveness of baroreceptor reflexes [3, 14, 15].

Prevalence

Estimates of prevalence of hypertension vary not only by the cutpoints chosen to define it, but for any given cutpoint, on the procedures for determining it. Accordingly, due to the biologic variability of blood pressure within individuals, from moment to moment as well as from time to time, predominantly due to environmental influences, the more measures made the more valid the estimate of the true blood pressure. The average of several determinations on each of several occasions is preferable to a single determination on one occasion. Prevalence of hypertension is generally over estimated in population surveys [16]. What is clear is that whatever cutpoint is selected, no matter the procedures used, average diastolic blood pressure (DBP) rises in early adult life and levels off after age 50 or 60 years, while average systolic pressure (SBP) tends to rise linearly with age throughout adult life, with no apparent leveling off [13, 17–19] Figure 2. The prevalence of hypertension therefore rises with age and as conventionally defined is at least two-fold higher in the population over age sixty-five compared to the overall rate. In the United States, where greater than 140/90 mmHg. is the conventional definition for hypertension, over half of all persons over age 65 are hypertensives. Based on the Health and Nutritional Examination Survey (HANES II), 64% of those 65–74 years old are hypertensives; for African-Americans the value is 76% [18]. In the Systolic Hypertension in the Elderly Program pilot study, where diagnosis was based on the average of two determinations on each of two occasions, 75 percent of the population surveyed for eligibility were hypertensive. Numerous studies have demonstrated a steep curvilinear rise in the prevalence of systolic hypertension (Figure 3). The prevalence of isolated systolic hypertension varied from 8% of those age 60–69, to 22% of those 80 years or over, and was higher in blacks than whites, and in women than men (Table 1) [19]. Similar age distributions of hypertension have been observed in autopsy studies [20].

Risk of vascular complications

High blood pressure, particularly high systolic pressure, has been established by prospective epidemiological studies to be a major risk factor for cardiovas-

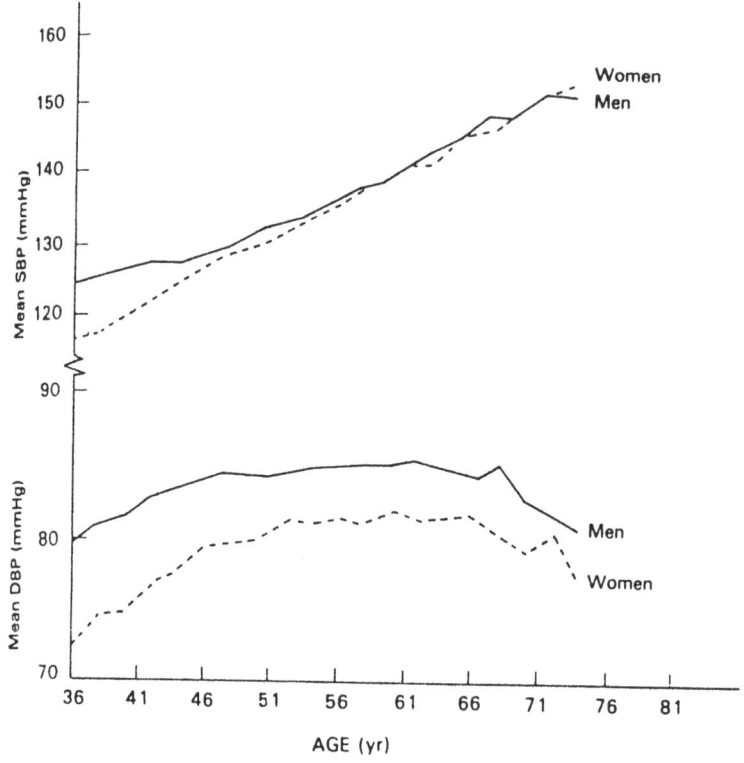

Figure 2. Influence of aging on systolic and diastolic blood pressure in men and women in the Framingham Heart Study – a 24 year cohort. From Kannel et al. [13].

cular complications and total mortality [21–26]. In the elderly, elevated systolic blood pressure is the single greatest risk factor other than age itself. In the Framingham Heart Study, a curvilinear increase in age-adjusted rates of cardiovascular disease and mortality based on systolic pressure was observed (Figure 4). Systolic pressure elevations were more predictive of cardiovascular complications than diastolic pressure, and remained so after adjustment for altered aortic distensibility [13]. In four elderly populations under prospective study in the United States, total mortality rate after five years was predicted by systolic but not diastolic pressure [27]. And although diastolic pressure persists as an independent risk factor in the elderly, ISH, defined as SBP $\geq$ 160 mmHg., and DBP < 90 mmHg, is associated with a three to five fold excess risk for vascular complications. Other studies confirm that total mortality, myocardial infarction, and stroke occur three to five times more commonly in hypertensives based on systolic pressure levels [22–25].

In the Chicago Stroke Study stroke mortality was two and one-half times

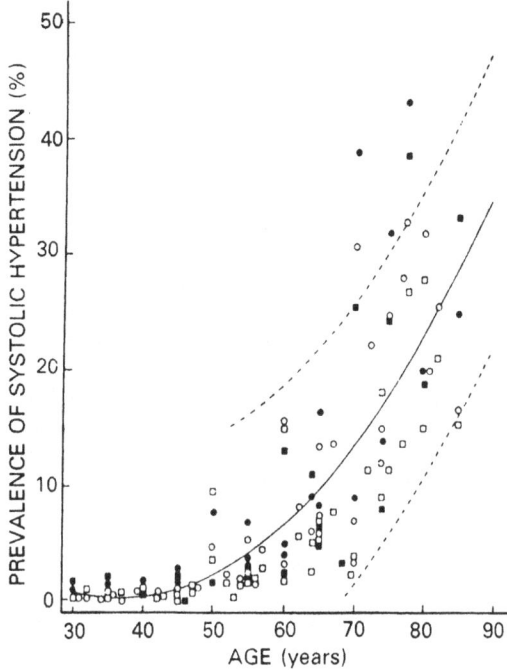

Figure 3. Prevalence of isolated systolic hypertension by the midpoint of the age classes reported in various studies. The 95% confidence interval for the prediction of individual points is presented for the age range 50–90 years. □, white males; ■, black males; ○, white females; ●, black females. Staessen J. [16].

Table 1. Prevalence of ISH in SHEP pilot study

	Age 60–69 years	Age 70–79 years	Age 80+ years
Female			
White	8%	15%	24%
Nonwhite	10%	13%	21%
Male			
White	7%	12%	16%
Nonwhite	8%	9%	19%
Total	8%	13%	22%

ISH = Isolated Systolic Hypertension.
SHEP = Systolic Hypertension in the Elderly Program.

higher in those with systolic hypertension than in normotensive individuals [23]. Colandrea and colleagues followed 72 matched pairs of elderly people (with and without ISH) for five years, observing death, stroke, and myocardial infarction three to five times more frequently in those with ISH [22]. During 6.4 years of follow-up of residents in a white upper middle-class suburb of San Diego California, Garland and coworkers observed in those

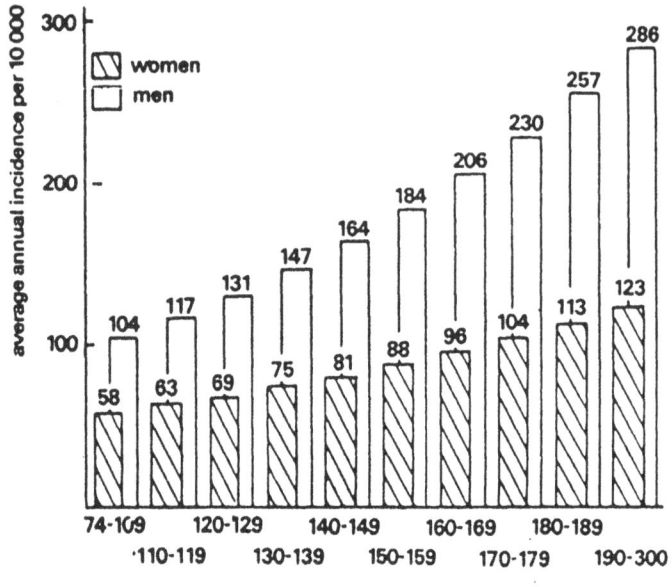

Figure 4. Age-adjusted mortality according to systolic blood pressure at each biennial examination: men and women 45–74. (Framingham Study, 18-year follow-up. From Framingham Monograph, 1974, U.S. Department of Commerce, National Technical Information Service, Springfield, V.A.).

with ISH, an excess risk of death of 50% in both men and women, with a relative risk for stroke of 4.0 in men [24]. Pulse pressure also predicts excess risk but not necessarily independently, being highly correlated with the level of systolic pressure [28, 29].

In accordance with the theory that cyclic stress leads to the structural changes in the media of arteries, one might expect such changes, and subsequent vascular complications, to be associated with and perhaps predicted by pulse pressure, the pulsatile component of blood pressure. This was examined in a population of over 27,000 men and women age 40–69 years, over a mean follow-up period of 9.5 years [30]. Because pulse pressure and mean arterial pressure are so highly correlated, a principal component analysis was performed from which two independent parameters were derived, a steady and pulsatile component index. The steady component of blood pressure, but not the pulsatile, was a strong risk factor for cardiovascular death in both sexes. The authors suggest the pulsatile component index may have some predictive power in older women. In the Framingham Heart Study mean pressure was a better predictor than pulse pressure for CHD in men, the reverse being true for women. However, systolic pressure was the best predictor for both sexes [31].

If as proposed by Simon et al. [32], changes in the vasculature are primary in the development of ISH, (with little or no increase in cardiac output) a view not universally supported clinically or experimentally [33, 34] but supported by computer simulation studies of the arterial system [35]; given the degree of understanding that exists of the pathophysiology of ISH, the identification of predictors or risk factors for ISH through prospective epidemiological study might be expected to provide insights as to etiology. Such studies suggest but do not establish the determinants of ISH. The Framingham Heart Study, employed Cox proportional hazard model regression analyses to assess multiple baseline variables as potential predictors of the occurrence of ISH [29]. The factors included age, sex, four components of blood pressure (systolic and diastolic blood pressure, pulse pressure, and mean arterial pressure), weight, serum cholesterol and uric acid levels, cigarette smoking, heart rate, glucose intolerance, and hematocrit. Age, sex, the four components of blood pressure and increased relative weight in women were the significant independent predictors, the most powerful being the prior levels of the systolic component of blood pressure. While the authors speculate this is consistent with the theory that increased blood pressure is part of the pathophysiologic process leading to an arterial system with reduced elasticity and distensibility, there remains a cart/horse problem for those whose systolic pressure appears to rise coincident with diminishing compliance, or fails to rise in the presence of increasing stiffness. Despite the present understanding of the pathophysiology of age associated elevated systolic pressure, and some knowledge of risk factors for ISH, why some individuals and not others develop it, remains unknown.

Therapeutic considerations

The advisability and merit of treating hypertension in the elderly is thoroughly established. Major randomized clinical trials that included subjects aged 60 or older provided evidence of benefit from treatment equal to that for younger subjects with diastolic hypertension, at least up to age 80 years [36–40]. Moreover, because of the higher rate of events in the elderly, the same relative reduction in complications compared to control groups, results in greater absolute reduction in the number of cardiovascular events in elderly compared with younger people. The older subjects in these trials for the most part had combined systolic (sometimes predominantly) and diastolic hypertension. This was particularly true in the European Working Party on Hypertension in the Elderly trial, and in the recently reported Swedish Trial in Old Patients [39, 41]. The effectiveness of pharmacologic therapy was also demonstrated to be true for ISH in the Systolic Hypertension in the Elderly Program (SHEP) study [42]. The average blood pressure of the 4736 participants in the SHEP trial was 170/77 mmHg. Their average age was 71.6 years, with 13.7% 80 years of age or over. Over one-half were women and 13.9%

Table 2. 5-year cumulative stroke rates for SHEP age, race-sex, and baseline systolic blood pressure subgroups

Variable	Active	Placebo
	M (SE)	M (SE)
Age (years)		
60–69	4.1 (0.7)	5.4 (0.8)+
70–79	5.6 (0.8)	9.0 (1.1)+
80+	7.7 (1.7)	14.4 (2.4)
Race-sex		
White men	5.2 (0.9)	8.7 (1.2)
White women	5.1 (0.8)	6.9 (0.9)+
Black men	9.6 (0.3)	12.3 (0.5)+
Black women	4.0 (1.5)	11.3 (2.5)
Baseline SBP (mmHg)		
160–169	4.2 (0.6)	7.3 (0.9)
170–179	6.0 (1.2)	9.7 (1.3)
180+	7.8 (1.5)	9.0 (1.8)

+ = Difference not statistically significant.
SHEP is Systolic Hypertension in the Elderly Program.

were African-American. Therapy consisting primarily of chlorthalidone 12.5 to 25 mg per day for an average period of 4.5 years, resulted in a reduction of stroke incidence of 36%, of coronary heart disease events (non fatal myocardial infarction and CHD death) of 27%, and of all major cardiovascular events by 32%; all highly significant results. Reduction in stroke incidence was seen in all age and race-sex subgroups including those age 80 and over (Table 2). The reduction in coronary disease incidence is consistent with predictions based on prospective epidemiological studies [43], and is concordant with the Swedish study referred to above and to the Medical Research Council study (MRC). The MRC Treatment Trial of Hypertension in Older Patients used stroke, coronary heart disease, and total mortality as the endpoints in a study which included many with ISH [44]. In this placebo controlled trial, the drug regimens hydrochlorothiazide 25 mg plus amiloride 5 mg daily, and atenolol 50 mg daily, were compared. A 19% reduction in CHD events was reported (159 placebo versus 128 active treatment, $p = 0.08$) The reduction in the CHD rate was seen in the diuretic treated group (12.7 placebo versus 7.7 diuretic, 39% reduction); with no difference between the rate for atenolol and its placebo (12.8 versus 12.7). It is a reasonable inference from the SHEP study, supported by the MRC and the Swedish studies, that middle-aged as well as older people with ISH, and people with less severe ISH, particularly if other risk factors are present, would benefit from such therapy [45] (Table 3). A further reasonable inference is that people with predominantly systolic hypertension will benefit similarly.

The results of these studies should not have been entirely unexpected

Table 3. Reduction of events in active vs placebo groups

	SHEP	MRC	STOP-H
Events	%	%	%
Stroke*	36	25	47
Coronary heart disease*	27	19	28
Cardiovascular*	32	17	40
Total mortality	13	3	43

* =Fatal and nonfatal.
SHEP = Systolic Hypertension in the Elderly Program.
MRC = Medical Research Council trial of treatment of hypertension in older adults.
STOP-H = Swedish Trial in Old Patients with Hypertension.

given the generally excessive intake of dietary salt in western societies, knowledge that sodium intake increases arterial stiffness and systolic blood pressure, particularly in older subjects, and the previously demonstrated effectiveness of diuretics in systolic hypertension [10, 46–48]. Even if the treatment effect of diuretics were only empirical, these findings would be of great significance because of the traditional wisdom that the structural pathology of the large vessels (arteriosclerosis) considered to be responsible for the elevated systolic pressure, would be unresponsive to pharmacologic therapy and such treatment might even be harmful if flow to critical organs were reduced. However, current knowledge of the functional as well as structural factors determining arterial stiffness, suggests that vasodilating drugs, which in addition to lowering peripheral resistance, reduce arterial impedance, constitute a rational approach meriting special consideration. The ability of nitroglycerin, angiotensin converting enzyme (ACE) inhibitors, and calcium antagonists, to alter the vasomotor tone of small and medium-sized arteries such that they become less stiff as they dilate, thereby selectively lowering aortic systolic pressure over and above that of peripheral systolic pressure, suggests a therapeutic strategy of great functional significance [3, 49–53].

Ace inhibitors are effective, beyond that predicted by plasma renin levels, in lowering both systolic and diastolic blood pressure in the elderly, and have been shown to selectively lower systolic pressure more effectively than beta-blockers [54–56]. Calcium channel blockers are also an effective class of antihypertensive agents for the elderly, and like ACE inhibitors have the important functional capability of reducing characteristic aortic impedance [57, 58]. However, their effect on morbidity and mortality has not been established by clinical trial, hence any advantage over diuretic agents remains theoretical. Long-term morbidity and mortality studies comparing the major classes of antihypertensive agents, particularly those capable of dilating small and medium-sized arteries, remains an urgent priority.

References

1. Smith WM. Hypertension in the Elderly. In: Parmley W, Chatterjee K, editors. Cardiology, New York: JB Lippincott Company, 1991; Vol 2, Chap 26: 1–8.
2. Smith WM. Epidemiology of hypertension in older patients. Am J Med 1989(Suppl 3B); 85: 2–6.
3. O'Rourke MF. Arterial stiffness, systolic blood pressure and logical treatment of arterial hypertension. Hypertension 1990; 15: 339–47.
4. O'Rourke MF. Arterial Function in Health and Disease. Edinburgh: Churchill, 1982: 27.
5. Aviolo AP, Deng FQ, Li WQ, et al. Effects of aging on arterial distensibility in populations with high and low prevalence of hypertension: Comparison between urban and rural communities in China. Circulation 1985; 71: 202–10.
6. Sandor B. Fundamentals of Cyclic Stress and Strain, Madison: University of Wisconsin, 1972: 3.
7. O'Rourke MF. Pulsatile arterial hemodynamics in hypertension. Aust NZ J Med 1976; 6(Suppl II): 40–8.
8. Avolio AP, Chen SG, Wang RP, Zhang CL, Li MF, O'Rourke MF. Effects of aging on changing arterial compliance and left ventricular load in a northern Chinese urban community. Circulation 1983; 68: 50–8.
9. Avolio AP, Clyde KM, Beard TC, Cooke HM, Ho KKL, O'Rourke MF. Improved arterial distensibility in normotensive subjects on a low salt diet. Arteriosclerosis 1986; 6: 166–9.
10. Levenson J, Simon AC, Maarek BE, Gitelman GJ, Fiessinger JN, Safar ME. Regional compliance of brachial artery and saline infusion in patients with arteriosclerosis obliterans. Arteriosclerosis 1985; 5: 80–6.
11. O'Rourke MF, Blasek JV, Morreels CL, Kroveta LJ. Pressure wave transmission along the human aorta: changes with age and in arterial degenerative disease. Circ Res 1968; 23: 567–79.
12. Farrar DJ, Bond MG, Riley WA, Sawyer JK. Anatomic Correlates of aortic pulse wave velocity and carotid artery elasticity during atherosclerosis progression and regression in monkeys. Circulation 1991; 83: 1754–63.
13. Kannel WB, Wolf PA, McGee DL, Dawber TR, McNamara P, Castelli W. Systolic blood pressure, arterial rigidity, and risks of stroke: The Framingham Study. J Am Med Assoc 1981; 245: 1225–9.
14. Abboud FM, Houston JH. The effects of aging and degeneration vascular diseases on the measurement of arterial rigidity in man. J Clin Invest 1961; 40: 933–9.
15. Gribbin B, Pickering TG, Sleight P, Peto R. Effect of age and high blood pressure on baroceptor sensitivity in man. Circ Res 1971; 29: 424–31.
16. Staessen J, Amery A, Fagard R: Isolated systolic hypertension in the elderly. J Hypertens 1990; 8: 393–405.
17. Wing S, Aubert RE, Hansen JP, Hames CG, Slome C, Tyroler HA: Isolated systolic hypertension in Evans County. I. Prevalence and screening considerations. J Chronic Dis 1982; 35: 735–42.
18. National Health and Nutritional Examination Survey II: 1976–80: Blood pressure levels in persons 18–74 years of age. (Series 11, No. 234] Hyattsville Maryland: National Center of Health Statistics, 1982.
19. Smith WM, Bagniewska A, Furberg CD, Kuller L, Perry HM, Schnaper H. Blood pressure characteristics of a population aged 60–90 years: SHEP. (abstr). J. Hypertens 1986; 4(Suppl): S564.
20. Kuramoto K, Matsushita S, Kuwajima I. The pathogenic role and treatment of elderly hypertension. Jpn Circ J 1981; 45: 833–43.
21. Kannel WB, Gordon T: Evaluation of cardiovascular risk in the elderly: The Framingham Study. Bull NY Acad Med 54: 573, 1978.
22. Colandrea MA, Friedman GD, Nichaman MZ, Lind CN. Systolic hypertension in the elderly: an epidemiologic assessment. Circulation 1970; 41: 239–45.

23. Shekelle RB, Ostfeld AM, Klawans HF Jr. Hypertension and risk of stroke in an elderly population. Stroke 1974; 5: 71–5.

24. Garland C, Barrett-Conner E, Suarez, Criqui MH. Isolated systolic hypertension and mortality after age 60 years: a prospective population-based study. Am J Epidemiol 1983; 118: 365–76.

25. Abernathy J, Borhani NO, Hawkins CM, et al. Systolic blood pressure as an independent predictor of mortality in the Hypertension Detection and Followup Program. Am J Prev Med 1986; 2: 123–32.

26. Rutan GH, Kuller LH, Neaton JD, Wentworth DN, McDonald RH, Smith WM. Mortality associated with diastolic hypertension and isolated systolic hypertension among men screened for the Multiple Fisk Factor Intervention Trial. Circulation 1988; 77: 505–14.

27. Taylor JO, Cornoni-Huntley J, Curb JD, et al. Blood pressure and mortality risk in the elderly. Am J Epidemiol 1991; 134: 489–501.

28. Siegel D, Kuller L, Lazarus NB, et al. Predictors of cardiovascular events and mortality in the Systolic Hypertension in the Elderly Program Pilot Project. Am J Epidemiol 1987; 126: 385–99.

29. Wilking SV, Belanger A, Kannel WB, D'Agostina RB, Steel K. Determinants of isolated systolic hypertension. J Am Med Assoc 1988; 260: 3451–5.

30. Darne B, Girerd X, Safar M, Cambien F, Guize L. Pulsatile versus steady component of blood pressure: a cross-sectional analysis and a prospective analysis on cardiovascular mortality. Hypertension 1989; 13: 392–400.

31. Kannel WB, Gordon T, Schwartz MJ. Systolic versus diastolic blood pressure and risk of coronary heart disease: The Framingham Study. Am J Cardiol 1971; 27 335–46.

32. Simon AC, Safar ME, Levenson JA, Kheder AM, Levy BI. Hemodynamic mechanisms and therapeutic approach to systolic hypertension. J Cardiovasc Pharmacol 1985; S22–S7.

33. Randall OS, Van den Bos GC, Sipkema P, Westerhof N Systemic compliance: does it play a role in the genesis of essential hypertension? Cardiovasc Res 1984; 18: 455–62.

34. Pasierski TP, Pearson AC, Labovitz AJ. Pathophysiology of isolated systolic hypertension in elderly patients: Doppler echocardiographic insights. Am Heart J 1991; 122: 528–34.

35. Berger DS, Li JK. Concurrent compliance reduction and increased peripheral resistance in the manifestation of isolated systolic hypertension. Am J Cardiol 1990; 65: 67–71.

36. Hypertension Detection and follow-up cooperative group: five year findings of the Hypertension Detection and Followup Program. J Am Med Assoc 1979; 242: 2562–72.

37. Veterans Administration Cooperative Group: Effects of treatment in hypertension. II. Results in patients with diastolic blood pressure averaging 90 through 114 mmHg. J Am Med Assoc 1970; 213: 1143–1152.

38. Management Committee of the Australian Therapeutic Trial in Mild Hypertension: treatment of mild hypertension in the elderly. Med J Aust 1981; 2: 398–402.

39. Amery A, Birkenhager W, Brixko P, et al. Mortality and morbidity results from the European Working Party on High Blood Pressure in the Elderly Trial. Lancet 1985; 2: 1349–54.

40. Coope J, Warrender TS. Randomized trial of treatment of hypertension in elderly patients in primary care. Br Med J 1986; 293: 1145–51.

41. Dahlof B, Lindholm LH, Hansson L, Schersten B, Ekbom B, Wester PO. Morbidity.and mortality in the Swedish Trial in Old Patients with Hypertension (STOP-Hypertension). Lancet 1991; 338: 1281–5.

42. SHEP Cooperative Research Group. Prevention of stroke by antihypertensive drug treatment in older persons with isolated systolic hypertension: Final results of the Systolic Hypertension in the Elderly Program SHEP) J Am Med Assoc 1991; 265: 3255–64.

43. MacMahon S, Peto R, Cutler J, et al. Blood pressure, stroke, and coronary heart disease: Part 1, Prolonged differences in blood pressure: Prospective observational studies corrected for the regression dilution bias. Lancet 1990; 335; 765–74.

44. MRC Working Party. Medical research council trial of treatment of hypertension in older adults: principal results. J Am Med Assoc 1992; 304: 405–12.

45. The Systolic Hypertension in the Elderly Program Cooperative Research Group: Implications of the Systolic Hypertension in the Elderly Program. Hypertension 1993; 21: 1–9.

46. Myers JB, Morgan TO. The effect of sodium intake on the blood pressure related to age and sex. Clin Exp Hypertens 1983; 5: 99–106.

47. Vardan S, Mookherjee S, Warner R, Smulyan H. Systolic hypertension in the elderly. Hemodynamic response to long-term thiazide diuretic therapy and its side effects. J Am Med Assoc 1983; 250: 2807–13.

48. Smith WM, Feigal DW, Furberg CD, et al. Use of diuretics in treatment of hypertension in the elderly. Drugs 1986; 31(Suppl 40: 154–64.

49. Bouthier JD, Safar ME, Benetos A, Simon AC, Levenson JA, Hugues CM. Haemodynamic effects of vasodilating drugs on the common carotid and brachial circulation of patients with essential hypertension. Br J Clin Pharmacol 1987; 21: 137–44.

50. Safar ME, Toto-Moukouo JJ, Bouthier JD et al. Arterial dynamics, cardiac hypertrophy and antihypertensive treatment. Circulation 1987; 75:(Suppl I): 156–61.

51. Safar ME, Laurent S, Bouthier JA, London GM. Comparative effects of captopril and isosorbide dinitrate on the arterial wall of hypertensive human brachial arteries. J Cardiovasc Pharmacol 1986; 8: 1257–61.

52. Yaginuma T, Avolio A, O'Rourke M, et al. Effect of glyceryl trinitrate on peripheral arteries alters left ventricular hydrolic load in man. Cardiovasc Res 1986; 20: 153–60.

53. Latson TW, Hunter WC, Katoh N, Sagawa K. Effect of nitroglycerin on aortic impedance, diameter, and pulse wave velocity. Circ Res 1988; 62: 884–90.

54. Schnaper HW, Stein G, Schoenberger JA, et al. Comparison of enalapril and thiazide diuretics in the elderly hypertensive patient. Gerontology 1987; 33(Suppl 1]: 24–35.

55. Asmar RG, Pannier BM, Santoni JP, Safar ME. Angiotensin converting enzyme inhibition decreases systolic blood pressure more than diastolic pressure as shown by ambulatory blood pressure monitoring. J Hypertens 1988; 6(Suppl 3): S-79-S-84.

56. Gabriel MA, Moncloa F, Walker JF, Gomez HS. Enalapril versus beta-blockers: Differential effect on systolic blood pressure (abstr). Clin Pharm Ther 1986; 39: 194.

57. Leehey DJ, Hartman E. Comparison of diltiazem and hydrochlorothiazide for treatment of patients 60 years of age or older with systemic hypertension. Am J Cardiol 1988; 62: 1218–23.

58. Levinson JA, Safar ME, Simon AC, Bouthier JA, Griener L. Central and arterial hemodynamic effects of nifedipine [20 mg] in mild-to-moderate hypertension. Hypertension 1983; 5(Suppl V): V57–V60.

8. Non-invasive study of the local mechanical arterial characteristics in humans

ARNOLD P.G. HOEKS

Introduction

Various relationships are suggested in the literature to qualify the elastic behavior of (a segment of) an artery as a function of measurable parameters. The expressions, given below, demonstrate the resemblance and clarifies how a given quantity relates to another one [1, 2]:

Distensibility Coefficient	$DC = \dfrac{2\Delta d/d}{\Delta p}$	$[Pa^{-1}]$
Compliance Coefficient	$CC = \dfrac{\pi d \Delta d}{2\Delta p}$	$[m^2/Pa]$
Pulse wave velocity	$p_v = \sqrt{1/\rho DC}$	$[m/s]$
Elastic (Peterson) modulus	$E_P = \dfrac{d\Delta p}{\Delta d} = \dfrac{1}{2DC}$	$[Pa]$
Young's modulus	$E = \dfrac{\rho p_v^2 d}{h} = \dfrac{d/h}{DC}$	$[Pa]$

In the expressions above d and h are the end-diastolic diameter and wall thickness, respectively, Δd is the change in diameter from diastole to systole, Δp is the pulse pressure (systolic minus diastolic pressure), and ρ is the density of blood. Thereby it is assumed that DC is a constant over the actual blood pressure range for the in vivo conditions considered. The pulse wave velocity can be assessed by computing the foot to foot delay between the pressure waves measured simultaneously at 2 sites with a known distance [3]. In non-invasive applications the velocity waveforms, obtained with ultra-sound Doppler equipment, rather than the pressure waveforms are used. The main attraction of this method is that only one parameter has to be measured. On the other hand two measurement systems have to be operated simultaneously. Because of time resolution problems the distance between the sites of measurement should be quite long. Therefore, the pulse wave velocity provides an estimate for the elastic behavior averaged over the segment considered. Non-invasive assessment of the local elastic behavior is

M. E. Safar and M. F. O'Rourke (eds.), The arterial system in hypertension. pp. 119–134.
© 1993 *Kluwer Academic Publishers. Printed in the Netherlands.*

generally based on the measurement with ultrasound echo techniques of the (change in) diameter over a cardiac cycle. The basic concepts of the latter approach and the associated resolution problems will be discussed in the next sections.

Ultrasound techniques

The ultrasound reflection technique is based on the emission of a short acoustic pulse with a high emission frequency and the subsequent reception of the echoes reflected by acoustic interfaces, i.e., boundaries of regions with a different acoustic impedance [4]. The time of flight Δt between emission and the reception of a particular echo corresponds to the distance s between the ultrasound probe and the structure: $\Delta t = 2sc$, where c is the (assumed) speed of sound in the tissue between probe and reflector (for most tissues, except for bone, the sound speed is on the order of 1500 m/s). The factor 2 is due to the round-trip distance (the same distance has to be covered twice). The amplitude of the received echo depends on the local change in acoustic impedance, the orientation of the boundary with respect to the direction of sound propagation, the dimension of the boundary layer, and the distance between probe and boundary. The echo will be maximal if the boundary is perpendicular to the direction of propagation and its size is large with respect to the wavelength λ of the ultrasound in the medium ($\lambda = cf_e$ with f_e the emission frequency). If its size is small (e.g., red blood cells) the ultrasound will be scattered in all directions rather than reflected in a particular direction and only a fraction of the scattered ultrasound energy will arrive at the transducer. That is why the echogenicity of blood is far lower than that of the echo walls. While the ultrasound travels through a medium it is attenuated due to partial reflection and scattering, and due to absorption. Absorption depends on tissue composition and increases with the emission frequency. Therefore, a high emission frequency (up to 10 MHz) can only be used for the investigation of superficial structures, while for the interrogation of, for example, cardiac behavior an emission frequency of 3.5 or 5 MHz is used.

The spatial resolution of an ultrasound system depends on the local width of the ultrasound beam (lateral resolution) and the length of the signal originating from a single reflector (axial resolution). The dimension of the transducer (converting the electric emission signal into an acoustic signal and the received signal back to an electric signal) is on the order of 20 to 40 wavelengths. At an emission frequency of, for example, 5 MHz (corresponding wavelength 300 μm) the diameter of the transducer will be on the order of 10 mm. The local width of the ultrasound beam can be reduced by focussing techniques. The axial resolution is mainly governed by the bandwidth of the transducer, i.e., the range of frequencies the transducer responds to. The larger this frequency range the shorter the received pulse will be if the transducer is activated by a very short electric pulse. The bandwidth of the commonly used transducers is related to its center frequency: the higher the center frequency the larger the bandwidth will be. The gradual improving quality of ultrasound echo systems over time can be mainly attributed to the improvement of the bandwidth center frequency ratio. As for the lateral resolution the attainable axial resolution gets better with an increasing frequency the transducer is tuned to (emission frequency). Since higher frequencies are more strongly attenuated than low frequencies the bandwidth of the received signal (and, therefore, the axial resolution) goes down as the round trip distance increases.

The received signal is amplified, where the amplification gradually increases with depth to compensate for the increasing attenuation in the tissues. In the most simple approach the amplified radio-frequency (RF) signal is rectified and the amplitude (envelope of the RF-signal) as function of depth is displayed (A-mode). Moving structures are visualized by emitting repetitively short bursts in the same direction and displaying the A-mode signals along each other (motion mode or M-mode) with the observed amplitude presented in shades of grey (brightness mode or B-mode). A two-dimensional scan (2D-echo) is obtained by sweeping the ultrasound beam (this can be achieved mechanically or electronically) and putting the envelope as function of depth in B-mode in a corresponding direction and/or position on a screen. If only the direction of the transducer is changed from line to line a sector image is obtained. Displacing the beam in a lateral direction (linear array transducer) gives a rectangular scan format. The attainable image rate goes down with the repetition frequency of the emitted pulses (PRF: pulse repetition frequency) and the number of lines per image. For superficial applications the PRF can be made quite high but for the observation of deeper lying structures a lower PRF has to be used (the echo of these structures should be received before another pulse is emitted). Even then the image rate is generally high enough to give a real-time impression.

Pulse echo systems, operating in M-mode, can also be used for the measurement of the velocity of structures and scatterers as function of time. Only a short segment of the received RF-signal at a preselected delay with respect to emission, corresponding to a given depth, is analyzed. Thereby each emission-reception sequence results in a point of the Doppler signal originating from the selected depth: the Doppler signal is sampled by the PRF. Since in Doppler operation the transducer is activated by a series of pulses rather than a single pulse the sensitive region along the beam (sample volume) is longer than in echo applications.

As mentioned above ultrasound echo techniques can be used to establish the diastolic diameter of a blood vessel and its change as function of time. Before these techniques are discussed in detail a short overview of the history of non-invasive examination of vessel dimensions will be given.

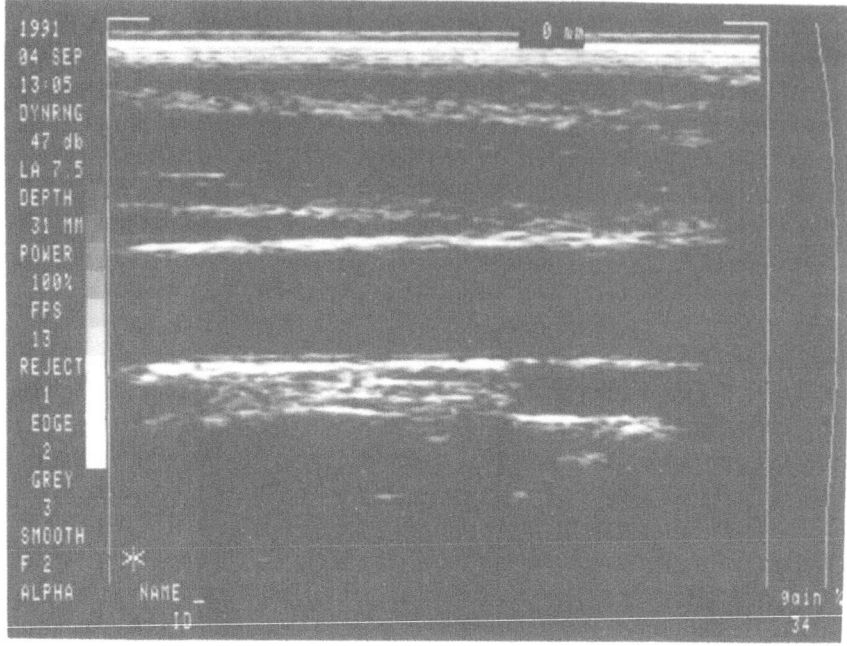

Figure 1. Two-dimensional image (B-mode) of the common carotid artery of a young healthy volunteer, obtained with a 7.5 MHz linear array scanner (ATL Ultramark V). Only where the beam is normal to the wall the intima (and media) can be distinguished.

Historic overview

In a simplified approach an arterial wall is composed of three layers: the adventitia, media and intima. The echogenicity of the adventitia, as compared with the surrounding tissue it is embedded in, is relatively high while that of the media is quite low and of the intima is somewhere in between. For almost all echo-systems the amplitude of the signal returned by blood is too low to be detected and the lumen appears as a black region. The intima is only visible as a separate layer (the media appears as a relative dark line) with a high resolution system if the ultrasound beam is aimed perpendicular to the wall and through the center of the vessel. Figure 1 gives an example of a two-dimensional B-mode image of the common carotid artery of a young, presumably healthy, volunteer. The image is obtained with a 7.5 MHz linear array scanner. The large echoes from the adventitia of the anterior wall tend to obscure the weaker signal from the closely spaced intima. Only at the posterior wall and at those sites where the beam is normal to the wall the intima (and the media) can be observed. Wall thickness measurements are commonly made at the posterior wall.

Arndt [5] was the first to recognize that the (change) in distance between the reflections of the anterior and posterior adventitia along the beam could be used for non-invasive measurement of the artery diameter as function of time. Since he used the crossing of the leading edge of the received signal in A-mode (amplitude tracking) the internal diameter of the artery was overestimated. Moreover, the echogenicity depends on the distance between transducer and the wall and varies with the phase of the cardiac cycle. Therefore, also the change in diameter (and the relative change in diameter) was overestimated.

Because of the gradual improvement of image quality the (change in) location of the walls became also visible on an M-mode display. The measurement of the lumen diameter in diastole and systole can then be made directly from the screen [6, 7]. This is an off-line, time consuming procedure and does not result in a distension waveform.

Because of the problems encountered with A-mode analysis Hokanson switched to the phase of the RF-signal [8, 9]. At the beginning of a measurement short windows are positioned at both walls and the positions of a zero-crossing within these observation windows over time are used as a measure for the distance between the probe and the wall. Thereby, the position of the window is adjusted according to the measured displacement of the wall (zero-crossing tracking). The distance between the selected zero-crossings at both walls represents the diameter as function of time. Since the points of reference can be chosen independent of the local amplitude this method of measurement is far more accurate. Later developments along this line are mainly aimed at the improvement of the detection and processing method [10–14].

Since velocity integrated over time gives displacement the Doppler approach can be employed as well to assess motion. Under the assumption that both walls move with the same speed in opposite directions simple CW-Doppler systems can be used to detect vessel wall motion [15]. However, in practice the walls do not move with the same speed. Moreover, CW-Doppler does not provide information about the initial artery diameter. Pulsed Doppler in combination with a 2D-echo system allows for the simultaneous detection of initial diameter and wall motion. In an early development [16] both sample volumes coinciding with the walls were fixed in depth but later on [17] these sample volumes were allowed to track the moving position of the wall (Doppler tracking). For a long sample volume (long emitted pulse) the initial diameter measurement is rather inaccurate.

The axial resolution is limited by the bandwidth of the transducer in combination with the emitter/receiver characteristics. Operating an ultrasound system in echo mode will give, therefore, the best results for diameter measurements. The change in the location of a zero-crossing can be used to detect displacement (change in position). As will be discussed later this approach is sensitive to phase interference of echo signals returned by closely spaced reflectors. This can be reduced by considering the average behavior of a segment of the RF-signal, as is done in the Doppler approach. A similar

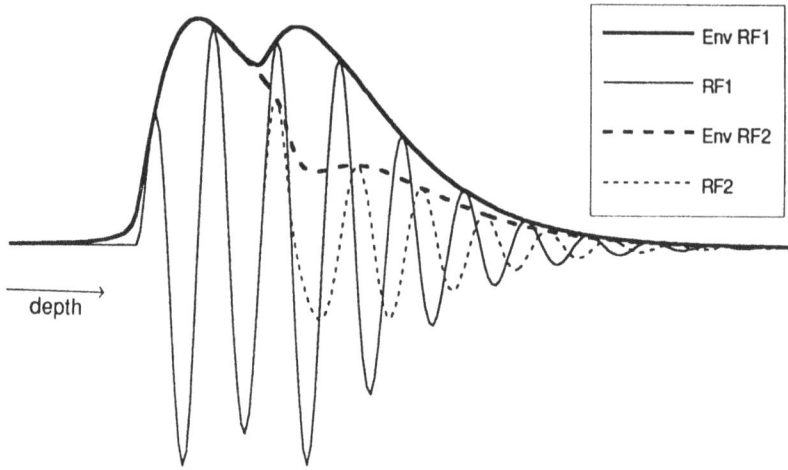

Figure 2. RF-signals and their envelopes based on the superposition of two echo signals with an amplitude ratio of 2, shifted over 2 (situation 1) and 2.5 (situation 2) periods, respectively. An additional shift in phase of 0.5 periods has a great impact on the shape of the envelope.

result can be obtained by cross-correlating [18] the RF-signals within a short segment of two subsequent lines (RF-correlation tracking).

Methods

Amplitude tracking

Generally speaking the acoustic boundaries are not always distinct, do not have the same size, and are not perpendicular oriented with respect to the ultrasound beam. Moreover, the boundaries can be closely spaced, e.g., layers of the arterial wall, causing interaction of the echo signals. To illustrate this effect let us consider an artificial echo signal of the form:

$$d \exp(-d/\lambda) \sin(2\pi d/\lambda)$$

where the distance d is expressed in units of the wavelength λ of the ultrasound in the medium. After one period from the beginning the wave-shape reaches its maximum value and subsequently decays exponentially to zero. The width of the envelope at half its maximum value is about two periods corresponding to a fractional bandwidth (bandwidth divided by center frequency) of the RF-signal of 0.5. This simple example does not take into account the effect of frequency dependent attenuation as function of depth. Figure 2 depicts the superposition of 2 echoes of the above form where the second echo has an amplitude of half the first one. In situation 1 the second echo is shifted in phase over two periods while in situation 2 the shift is 2.5 periods (an additional shift of only half a period). Comparing the envelopes of the signals received in both situations it is noted that due to the interaction of both echoes in situation 1 the interference is constructive (the amplitude is enhanced), while in situation 2 the interference is destructive (the signals tend to cancel). This phase dependent interference is the origin of the speckle pattern in B-mode images especially at sites with diffuse reflectors or scatterers. The speckle size at a larger distance from the transducer is on the order of the local resolution of the ultrasound system. Close to the transducer the ultrasound beam is very inhomogeneous leading to a smaller speckle size and rapidly changing amplitudes with small changes in the distance between reflectors.

Returning to Figure 2 it can be seen that the shape of the trailing part of the signal received dramatically changes with the spacing of the reflectors. Let us suppose this signal is originating from the anterior wall of a blood vessel and that the envelope is used to detect the position of the wall lumen interface using an (arbitrary) threshold level (amplitude tracking). The leading part of the signal is useless for this purpose because it may be clogged by signals originating from other structures the vessel is embedded in. Applying a threshold at the trailing part, e.g., at half the maximum value, will make the result very sensitive to reflector interspacing. A change in interspacing of half a period will result in a change in the detected position of *two* periods, corresponding to an error of one wavelength. Let us consider a system operating at an emission frequency of 5 MHz, corresponding to a wavelength of 300 μm, applied to a vessel with a relative distension of 10%. In a first order approximation the relative change in wall thickness will be on the same order, i.e., the boundaries of a wall with a thickness of 1 mm will move 100 μm with respect to each other. Because of the round trip effect this will induce a change in phase difference of 2/3 of a period. It is therefore quite likely that at some phase of the cardiac cycle phase interference will lead to an overestimation or underestimation of the position of the wall lumen interface. The posterior wall does not cause problems because there the leading part of the signal can be and should be used for position tracking. Therefore, in this example the anticipated error, mainly originating from the anterior wall, will be on the order of half a wavelength (150 μm for a 5 MHz system) which is far too large to follow accurately the change in artery diameter as function of time. The error can only be reduced by employing an ultrasound system with a far better resolution (higher emission frequency, larger bandwidth, dedicated signal processing to enhance the resolution) at situations where echo interaction is not likely to occur.

Amplitude tracking, acting on the envelope of the received signal, has the advantage that it can be executed in real-time. Moreover, it does not impose specific restrictions on the repetition frequency of the M-line other than the frequency content of the displacement waveform. It can even be applied to a video image of a sequence of M-lines [6, 7] but it should be noted that the

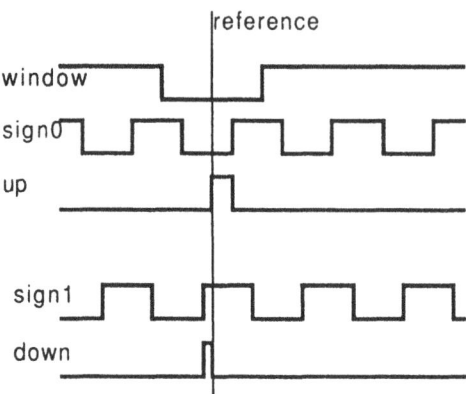

Figure 3. Principle of zero-crossing tracking. For each RF-line the position of the zero-crossing within an observation window is compared with the center of the window. Subsequently, the position of the observation window is moved up (situation 0) or down (situation 1), according to the observed difference in sample points.

presentation of the signal level in shades of grey, due to the compression technique used, changes the relative signal levels. Generally speaking, the diameter of a blood vessel is underestimated by the effective length of the ultrasound pulse used (the response of the anterior wall will trail into the lumen giving a narrower appearance).

Zero-crossing phase tracking

As mentioned above amplitude tracking is quite sensitive to phase interference resulting in a wrong estimation of displacement as function of time. As can be seen from figure 2 the underlying RF-signal is far more stable except for a narrow transition region. The position of a specific zero-crossing within a well-defined echo can then be used as a displacement signal [10–14]. To achieve this the sign of the received RF-signal is sampled at a very high frequency. Within a window (Figure 3) with a length between 0.5 to 1 period of the RF-signal the position of a positive zero-crossing is compared with the middle of the window. Because the position and length of the window (and, therefore, the position of its centre) are expressed in units of the sample clock while the sign is sampled with the same clock any deviation from the center is also given in units of the sample clock. Based on the observed deviation the position of the window is moved up (situation 0 in Figure 3) or moved down (situation 1) to align its center to the positive zero-crossing. The position of the window over subsequent RF-lines in M-mode can, therefore, be used as displacement signal. Its accuracy is completely governed by the frequency of the sample clock. Assuming a frequency of 50 MHz a period of the sample clock will correspond to a depth uncertainty of 15 μm (variance of 19 μm^2). A higher frequency of the sample clock will reduce the error accordingly.

All the processing involved can be executed in real-time, i.e., continuous recordings can be made of the displacement waveform of both walls, and, therefore, of the distension waveform. The only problem is the initial positioning of the sample windows at the reflections of the walls. It is unfeasible to maintain the ultrasound beam at a given direction and, at the same time, adjust the positions of the sample gates. If the investigation is aimed at an artery within a stable structure (e.g., the radial artery) the ultrasound probe can be fixed in a stable support equipped with micromanipulators. The direction and position of the ultrasound beam can then be manually varied until an optimal RF-signal (strong and quite distinct echoes from both walls) is visible on a monitor. Subsequently, the initial positions of the sample gates can be adjusted. While adjusting the gates the tracking algorithm is deactivated but will become active immediately after the control is released. It is preferable to do this in the diastolic phase where the movements of the wall are slow.

Since both windows are positioned at comparable positions of distinct echoes the distance between both minus the length of one window (converted to depth) immediately reflects the diameter of the artery. The accuracy of diameter measurements is fully determined by the resolution of the ultrasound system. The length of the observation window should be long enough to catch a single positive zero-crossing. If occasionally no positive zero-crossing is detected the window will be automatically moved up (or down depending on the preference given) until a zero-crossing is enclosed again. Ambiguity will occur if the window is placed at a transition of echo-signals of different reflectors (see Figure 2). If the interspacing changes during a cardiac cycle, or if the position or angulation of the beam with respect to the arterial walls change, zero-crossings may show up or vanish from the window. The latter situation will change the lock to the nearest zero-crossing causing an incidental error. This may induce a gradual drift in the window position and it is, therefore, necessary to check the position intermittently and, if necessary, to readjust it. At the very moment also systems are available that are able to localize the position of the wall-lumen interface after initial identification of the lumen [10, 13, 19]. From this position both sample volumes move out until they meet a large echo. This procedure is automatically repeated at intervals to ensure that a proper lock position is maintained.

Doppler tracking

The zero-crossing phase tracking technique relies on a lock to a specific feature (a zero-crossing) of the RF-signal received. This works very well if a single distinct reflector is considered. However, if a large number of echo signals interfere the signature of the RF-signal over subsequent lines may change drastically complicating the maintenance of the lock at the pre-

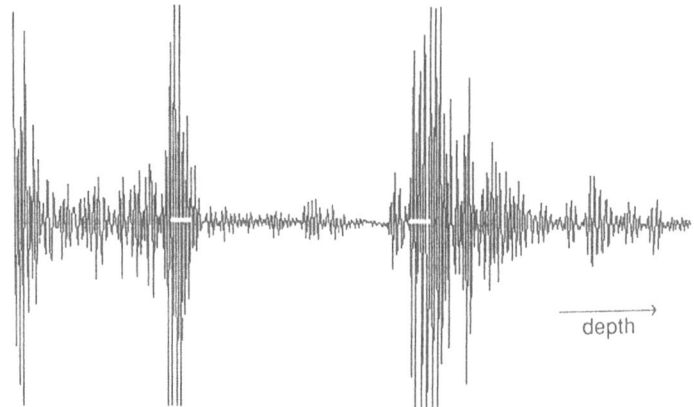

Figure 4. Example of an RF-line covering the common carotid artery. The anterior and posterior wall positions are marked with boxes, where the length of the box indicates the length of the observation window.

defined position. This can be stabilized by considering the phase averaged over a short segment of the RF-signal (a few periods). Conventional pulsed Doppler systems use the (change in) average phase within a specific window over subsequent lines to establish the velocity of the scatterers contributing to that part of the RF-signal. Actually pulsed Doppler systems estimate the mean change in position per RF-line interval. To reduce the variance of the estimate a couple of RF-lines are combined. An integrated change in phase of 2π corresponds to a mean displacement of the RF-signal over one period equivalent to a movement of the reflector over half a wavelength. For large displacements the reflector will partly leave the observation window. There-fore, the position of the observation window is adjusted according to the displacement detected. Again this approach is confronted with the common problem of the initial setting of the observation windows. As stated before, in real-time applications positioning the ultra-sound beam is difficult to combine with the gate adjustment. For the Doppler phase tracking technique [17] this problem is solved by digitizing the received RF-signal at rate of 4 times the carrier frequency and temporarily storing the samples in a buffer memory large enough to hold the original data over a registration interval of a couple of heartbeats. For a 1 MByte memory, configured as 1000 lines of 1000 sample points, a pulse repetition frequency of 250 Hz allows a registration over 4 seconds. After completion of the registration the initial position of the wall-lumen interfaces are identified using the first line stored (Figure 4). From there processing will take care of the detection of movement and readjustment of the sample gates according to the observed displace-ment.

Although in the approach above the phase of the RF-signal, averaged over the sample gate, rather than the instantaneous phase, is considered detection artifacts still occur. These can be effectively reduced by splitting up the sample gate in sub sample volumes, each with a length of one period of the RF-signal. Since all these sub sample volumes should yield the same displacement, comparison of the detector outputs reveals incidental errors which can be compensated for. Another artifact is caused by repositioning of the sample volume(s), where at one side of the sample volume a sample point is removed from the window while at the other end a point is added resulting in a transient. This can be skipped by replacing the computed result around a transient by an extrapolated value. A basic problem is the generation of the conversion clock, synchronous with the emission trigger, and with a frequency of exact four times the emission frequency (most of the echo systems do not have that kind of clock signal readily available). The frequency dependent attenuation will change the spectral distribution of the RF-signal with increasing depth and, therefore, the actual carrier frequency. Henceforth, the true carrier frequency within a given sample window is unknown. The mismatch between actual and assumed carrier frequency will give a scaling error increasing with the discrepancy. However, this error is directly related to the phase of the RF-signal. For a change in phase over one period (displacement over half a wavelength) the net error will be zero.

RF-correlation tracking

Another method to establish a shift in depth of a reflector is based on the evaluation of the cross-correlation function of the RF-signal within an observation window over a pair of subsequent lines [20]. To compute the cross-correlation function the received RF-signal within a window is digitized at a frequency considerably higher than the emission frequency. As for the Doppler method the sample clock should be stable in phase with respect to time of emission. The cross-correlation function can only be calculated for shifts of a multiple of the sample distance. Figure 5 gives an example of the cross-correlation function based on a segment of the signal used in Figure 2 shifted in depth over 1.2 sample points. The horizontal axis gives the lag of the cross-correlation function in units of sample points (the vertical axis is arbitrary). The cross-correlation function exhibits the same periodicity as the RF-signal and its envelope decays faster for systems with a high (axial) resolution, giving a more pronounced peak. The location of the first positive peak of the cross-correlation function (somewhere between 1 and 2 sample points) can only be resolved with an accuracy of the sample distance. A higher sample frequency will improve the accuracy but will make computation more time consuming (a given window will contain more samples and more points of the cross-correlation function have to be computed). However, interpolation techniques can be employed to establish the peak location in between sample points. Since the frequency characteristics of the RFsignal are roughly known it is also possible to develop an alternative method to

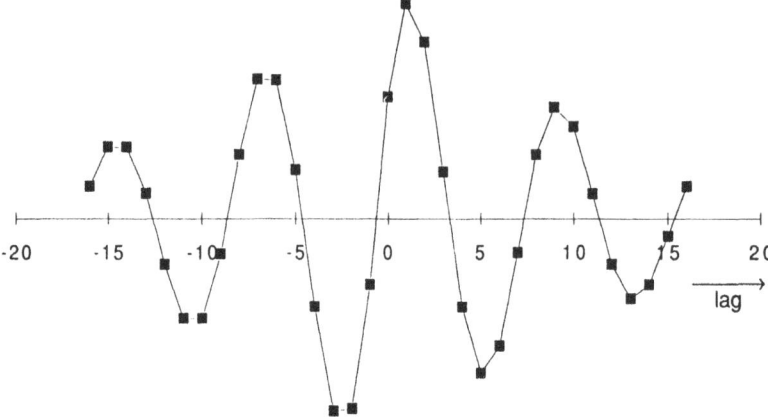

Figure 5. Cross-correlation function of a segment of the signal used in Figure 2 (length 4 periods) shifted over 1.2 sample points in between two observations. Here, the function is evaluated over a larger lag (from −16 to +16 sample points, equivalent to 2 periods) than necessary.

estimate straightforward the peak location accurately without interpolation [18, 21]. Its accuracy improves with the length of the observation window and the number of subsequent RF-lines that are combined. As for the Doppler method the position of the observation window should be shifted if the observed integrated displacement is more than one sample point distance (tracking).

The RF-correlation method is insensitive for phase interference of RF-signals returned by closely spaced reflectors. However, the positive peak of the cross-correlation function will be less pronounced if the phase interference changes strongly from line to line. Since the output of the RF-correlator is presented in (a fraction of) sample points rather than a fraction of an RF-period, as with the Doppler method, the sample frequency can be chosen freely provided it is higher than twice the maximum frequency of the RF-signal. The method can be employed in real-time, with the problem of initial setting of the observation windows, or applied to temporarily stored data.

Discussion

One should distinguish distance resolution and the accuracy in the measured change in distance. The distance resolution heavily depends on the axial resolution of the echo systems used. The higher the bandwidth of the ultra-sound system (this is commonly associated with a higher emission frequency) the better the axial resolution will be. Its theoretical lower limit is $\lambda/2$ in tissue if the fractional bandwidth equals 2. Most systems have a poorer ratio of bandwidth and center frequency and the pulse, received from a single target, will contain several periods. Wide band echo systems, operating at 5 MHz, may achieve an axial resolution on the order of 200 to 400 μm, while a 10 MHz system exhibits a resolution which is twice as good. Of course, these data are given under the assumption that the position of the wall lumen interface can be identified correctly. In a real-time application, without an automatic identification algorithm, the resolution obtained will be worse. Considering an artery with an initial diameter of 6 mm, for a high quality echo system the anticipated relative error in the estimated diameter will be on the order of 2 to 4%. Probably in the future this error can be further reduced by dedicated post-processing of the received signal aimed at the enhancement of the RF-bandwidth [22, 23]. This is of special interest for wall thickness measurements.

All the tracking algorithms (amplitude, zero-crossing, Doppler, RF-correlation) measure movements of the anterior and posterior wall separately. The distension waveform, i.e., the change in diameter as function of time, is obtained by subtracting the posterior displacement waveform from the anterior waveform. This approach makes the result theoretically insensitive for a change in mean position of the artery along the ultrasound beam caused by probe movements and/or shift in vessel position. However, a change in relative position will also affect the local RF-phase interference and, henceforth, the accuracy of displacement detection. Systems relying on the instantaneous phase of the RF-signal (zero-crossing tracking) will be more vulnerable for these artifacts than other ones considering the behavior of the average phase over a short segment of the RF-signal. Unfortunately it is quite difficult to develop a phantom simulating the reflection and scattering behavior of (curved) vessel walls. That is why most of the evaluation studies are carried out with a single reflector, giving better results than can be obtained in an in vivo situation. The quoted theoretical and experimental errors are, therefore, pertaining to the theoretical lower limits. An estimated error of 10 μm at a peak-to-peak excursion of 500 μm gives a relative error of 2%, which is smaller than the anticipated relative error in the diameter measurement. In practical applications the fractional error in the observed distension may be higher, but that is difficult to establish since no objective reference method is available. Reproducibility measurements do not only reflect instrumentation errors but also physiological variations during the measurement.

The processing algorithms automatically compensate for simultaneous displacements of both arterial walls along the ultrasound beam. However, there is no method available to correct for movements of an artery perpendicular to the line of observation due to an unstable probe position and/or movements of the artery itself. Systems with a high lateral resolution (having a narrow ultrasound beam) are more susceptible for this type of artifact. Figure 6, left panel, depicts the situation of an artery observed with a narrow beam. If the artery apparently moves sideways (without changing its diameter) the

narrow beam   broad beam

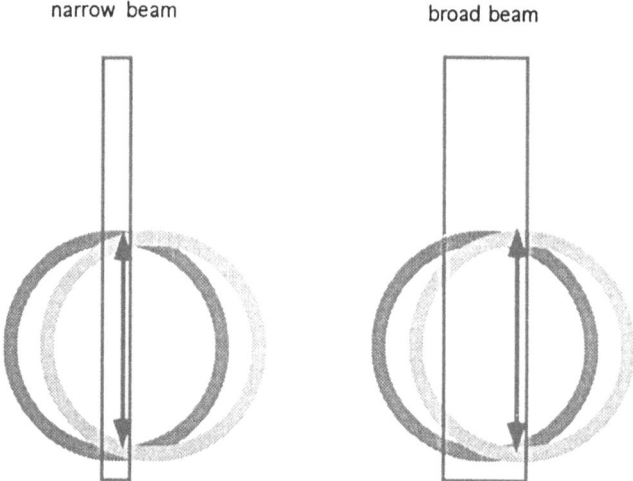

Figure 6. The diameter of an artery, moving in a lateral direction, will be underestimated if the movement is more than half the local beamwidth. For a narrow beam (left) this condition is more critical than for a wide beam (right).

artery will be observed along another line of view. Since the strongest reflections are obtained from the vessel wall segments that are oriented more perpendicular to the beam the line of view will not be the center line of the beam. Yet the diameter will be underestimated and the measured change in diameter will exhibit a negative deflection. For the same apparent lateral displacement a wide beam (Figure 6, right panel) will still allow correct radial measurements. The results are only valid for a lateral motion of the artery of less than half the local beam width. The reflections will be less distinct since also segments of the artery wall at an oblique angle will contribute to the RF-signal, although to a lower extent. To reduce lateral motion artifacts, measurements with a narrow beam should only be performed with stabilized probes (mounted in a holder) on arteries embedded in rigid structures, preventing lateral motion [24].

The measured values of the diameter and (peak-to-peak) distension are used to quantify the mechanical behavior of the arterial wall. Thereby, the observed peak-to-peak distension should be related to the local pulse pressure obtained simultaneously. In practice simultaneous non-invasive pulse pressure measurement is difficult to accomplish. In most cases the local pulse pressure is substituted by a pulse pressure measured as close as possible to the location of interest, e.g., for the radial artery the pulse pressure in the finger tip. But even over this short distance the pulse pressure may change considerably due to pulse wave reflections, generally leading to overestimation of the pulse pressure. As mentioned before the method based on pulse wave velocity avoids the problem of blood pressure measurement simultaneous with the diameter assessment. Presently attempts are made to assess local pulse wave velocity in combination with distension measurement. This approach is based on a single probe double beam configuration, enabling the simultaneous measurement of distension waveforms at two sites at a known distance. However, it is presently still problematic to measure accurately the time shift over a short distance (on the order of a few centimeter) without averaging over a long series of cardiac cycles [25, 26].

Conclusion

Ultrasound techniques provide a means to assess non-invasively the (change in) diameter of peripheral arteries under physiological conditions without introducing any obstruction for the local motion pattern. The (local) spatial resolution of the ultrasound system (beamwidth, RF-bandwidth) has an important effect on the accuracy of the measurement. A change in wall position can be detected with a far higher accuracy than the axial resolution if the RF-signal, rather than its envelope, is considered. Thereby, the processing algorithm locks onto a specific feature of the RF-signal returned by the wall, e.g., a zero-crossing (zero-crossing tracking), the phase of the RF-signal averaged over a short window (Doppler-tracking), or the signal pattern within the observation window (RF-correlation tracking). In real-time applications it may be difficult to identify the correct position of the wall-lumen interface. However, long recordings can be made, provided that the artery does not move in a lateral direction with respect to the beam. On the other hand a frozen image of the RF-signal allows a more careful selection of the wall echo. This requires temporary storage of the RF-signal over a large number of subsequent lines. However, the size of the memory will limit the length of a recording and, therefore, the number of cardiac cycles that can be considered within a single registration. It appears that for all the algorithms based on processing of the RF-signal the anticipated error in the relative distension is dominated by the relative error in the diameter measurement. Further technological research is required to improve the axial resolution, to achieve automatic and accurate identification of the position of the vessel wall lumen boundaries, and to eliminate the problem of local blood pressure registration.

References

1. Silver FH, Christiansen DL, Buntin CM. Mechanical properties of the aorta: a review. Critical Reviews Biomed Eng 1989; 17: 323–58.
2. O'Rourke M. Arterial stiffness, systolic blood pressure and logical treatment of arterial hypertension. Hypertension 1990; 15: 339–47.
3. Lehmann ED, Gosling RG, Fatemi-Langroudi B, Taylor MG. Non-invasive Doppler ultra-

sound technique for the in vivo assessment of aortic compliance. J Biomed Eng 1992; 14: 250–6.

4. Wells PNT. Physical principles of ultrasonic diagnosis. London: Academic Press, 1969.

5. Arndt JO. Über die Mechanik der intakten A. Carotis Communis des Menschen unter verschiedenen Kreislaufbedingungen. Archiv für Kreislaufforschung, 1986; 59: 153–97

6. Blankenhorn DH, Chin HP, Conover DJ, Nessim SA. Ultrasound observation on pulsation in human carotid artery lesions. Ultrasound Med Biol 1988; 14: 583–7.

7. Buntin CH, Silver FH. Noninvasive assessment of mechanical properties of peripheral arteries. Annals of Biomed Eng 1990; 18: 549–66.

8. Hokanson DE, Mozersky DJ, Sumner DS, Strandness DE. A phase locked echo-tracking system for recording arterial diameter changes in vivo. J Appl Phys, 1972; 32: 728–33.

9. Mozersky DJ, Sumner DS, Hokanson DE, Strandness DE. Transcutaneous measurement of the elastic properties of the human femoral artery. Circulation, 1972; 46: 948–55.

10. Gennser G, Lindström K, Dahl P, et al. A dual high-resolution 2-dimensional ultrasound for measuring target movements. Ultrasound Med Biol 1981; 7: 71–5.

11. Groves DH, Powalowski T, White DN. A digital technique for tracking moving interfaces. Ultrasound Med Biol 1982; 8: 185–90.

12. Imura T, Yamamoto K, Kanamori K, Mikami T, Yasuda H. Non-invasive ultrasonic measurement of the elastic properties of the human abdominal aorta. Cardiovasc Res 1986; 20: 208–14.

13. Lindstrom K, Gennser G, Sindberg Eriksen P, Benthin M, Dahl P. An improved echo-tracker for studies on pulse wave in the fetal aorta. In: Rolfe P, editor. Fetal Physiological Measurements 1987; 217–26.

14. Powalowski T, Pensko B. A noninvasive ultrasonic method for the elasticity evaluation of the carotid arteries and its application in the diagnosis of the cerebro-vascular system. Arch Acoustics 1988; 13: 109–26

15. Olsen CF. Doppler ultrasound: A technique for obtaining arterial wall motion parameters. IEEE Trans Sonics Ultrasonics 1977; SU-24: 354–8

16. Hoeks APG, Ruissen CJ, Hick P, Reneman RS. Transcutaneous detection of relative changes in artery diameter. Ultrasound Med Biol 1985; 11: 51–9.

17. Hoeks APG, Brands PJ, Smeets FAM, Reneman RS. Assessment of the distensibility of superficial arteries. Ultrasound Med Biol 1990; 16: 121–8.

18. de Jong PGM, Arts T, Hoeks APG, Reneman RS. Determination of tissue motion velocity by correlation interpolation of pulsed ultrasonic signals. Ultrasonic Imaging 1990; 12: 84–98.

19. Länne T, Stale H, Bengtsson H, et al. Noninvasive measurement of diameter changes in the distal abdominal aorta in man. Ultrasound Med Biol 1992; 18: 451–7.

20. Bonnefous O, Pesqué P. Time domain formulation of pulse-Doppler ultrasound and blood velocity estimation by cross correlation. Ultrasonic Imaging 1986; 8: 73–85.

21. de Jong PGM, Arts T, Hoeks APG, Reneman RS. Experimental evaluation of the correlation interpolation technique to measure regional tissue velocity. Ultrasonic Imaging 1991; 13: 145–61.

22. Eriksen M. Non-invasive measurement of arterial diameters in humans using ultrasound echoes with prefiltered waveforms. Med & Biol Eng & Comput 1987; 25: 189–94.

23. Martin C, Meister JJ, Arditi M, Farine PA. A novel homomorphic processing of ultrasonic echoes for layer thickness measurement. IEEE Trans Signal Proc 1992; 40: 1819–25.

24. Tardy Y, Meister JJ, Perret F, Brunner HR, Arditi M. Non-invasive estimate of the mechanical properties of peripheral arteries from ultrasonic and plethysmographic measurements. Clin Phys Physiol Meas 1991; 12: 39–54.

25. Benthin M, Dahl P, Ruzicka R, Lindström K. Calculation of pulse wave velocity using cross-correlation – effects of reflexes in the arterial tree. Ultrasound Med Biol 1991; 17: 461–9.

26. Struijk PC, Wladimiroff JW, Hop WCJ, Simonazzi E. Pulse pressure assessment in the human fetal descending aorta. Ultrasound Med Biol 1992; 18: 39–43.

9. Geometry and stiffness of the arterial wall in essential hypertension

MICHEL E. SAFAR

Introduction

For many years, large arteries were poorly investigated in hypertension, resulting from two principal reasons. Firstly, the arterial changes were considered to be the simple mechanical consequence of the blood pressure elevation. Consequently, the active intrinsic changes of arterial smooth muscle were considered to be limited to arterioles, with little role of vasomotor tone at the site of large vessels [1]. Secondly, the arteries were investigated using complex mathematical models of the circulation, which only pointed to an increased arterial stiffness of the totality of the arterial tree but could not take into account the heterogeneity of the large vessels of the hypertensive population [2].

In the recent years, the abnormalities of the arterial system in hypertensive subjects were reinvestigated on the basis of two dominant findings. Firstly, hypertension is now considered as a risk factor favouring the arterial complications in several circulations, principally those related to the brain, the heart and the kidney [3]. Secondly, following anti-hypertensive drug treatment, a striking dissociation was observed between the blood pressure reduction and the decrease in morbidity related to arterial changes. Indeed, anti hypertensive therapy decreased the incidence of congestive heart failure and cerebrovascular accidents but did not change substantially the frequency of ischemic heart disease [4]. Such results strongly suggested that active changes of the hypertensive arterial wall were involved following anti-hypertensive therapy and could be the purpose of specific clinical and experimental investigations.

For an adequate study of hypertensive large arteries in vivo, it is important to recognize that the large arteries have two different and inter-related functions, the conduit fonction and the buffering function. The former relates to mean blood flow, which is largelly preserved in hypertension. The latter relates to phasic flow. Indeed any large artery is able to dampen the cyclic flow coming from the heart into a steady flow at the peripheral level, due to its visco-elastic properties. The last years, a particular attempt has been paid

M. E. Safar and M. F. O'Rourke (eds.), The arterial system in hypertension. pp. 135–153.
© 1993 *Kluwer Academic Publishers. Printed in the Netherlands.*

to evaluate the visco-elastic properties of such arteries using non-invasive techniques [5].

The purpose of the present review was to describe these new methologies and to apply them to the hypertensive large arteries in humans, taking into account the large heterogeneity of the various arterial vessels. In this paper, three abnormalities relative to the hypertensive large arteries will be analyzed in detail: (i) pulse pressure is increased in hypertension, (ii) pressure wave reflections are also enhanced, and (iii) there are striking alterations of the geometry and of the function of the arterial system in hypertensive subjects.

Increased pulsatile component of blood pressure in hvpertension

Basic concepts

Human data on arterial pressure are usually obtained from indirect non-invasive measurements. Physicians using these methods have come to think of arterial dynamics exclusively in terms of level of peak-systolic and end-diastolic blood pressures. However, these two values represent only the limits between which arterial pressure fluctuates during a cardiac cycle (Figure 1). Subsequently, from the simple determination of systolic and diastolic blood pressure, no available information is obtained on the shape of the pressure wave itself (2). Nevertheless, from basic physiology, the arterial system may be divided into two distinct and separate functions. The first is the conduit function, the purpose of which is to deliver blood at high pressure to body tissues. The second is to smooth the pulsations caused by intermittent cardiac ejection. From these simple definitions, it is clear that the arterial system behaves both as a conduit and a cushion. Consequently, it is important to evaluate these two functions separately from the analysis of the cyclic characteristics of the blood pressure curve. Such an analysis may be of particular relevance in the case of hypertension.

It is well accepted from the use of Fourier's analysis that an oscillatory phenomenon as the blood pressure curve may be decomposed into a mean value plus a number of sine waves of increasing frequency (2). The harmonic zero reflects the mean value, which represents a sine wave with an infinite period. The first harmonic reflects the heart rate f, and higher harmonics have a frequency of $2f$, $3f$, etc. As shown extensively by digital computers, in the cardiovascular system, about 20 harmonics are sufficient for an adequate reconstruction of the blood pressure curve. Under that condition, a correct description of the curve does not exclusively consider systolic and diastolic pressure, but rather considers the mean pressure and the oscillation around the mean. Mean pressure (often calculated as diastolic pressure plus one-third pulse pressure) is related to steady flow, whereas the oscillation (often

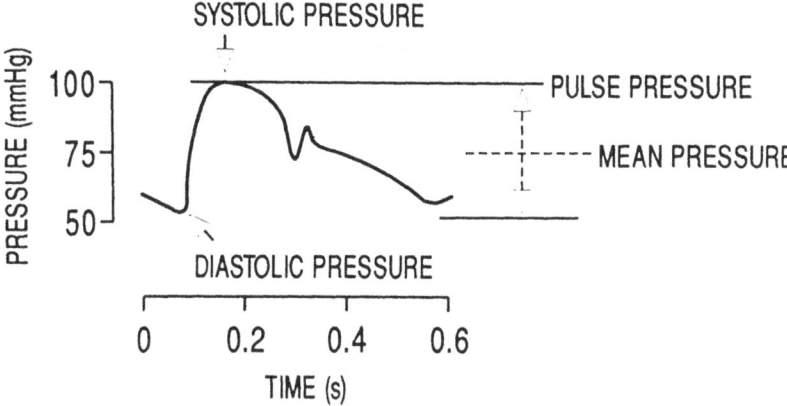

Figure 1. Mean arterial pressure versus pulse pressure.

described as pulse pressure, the difference between systolic and diastolic pressure) is related to pulsatile flow (2) (Figure 1).

Since mean arterial pressure equals the product of cardiac output multiplied by vascular resistance, increased mean arterial pressure (i.e. the classical pattern of hypertension in experimental studies) indicates that, for a given input flow, the elevation of the mean value of pressure is due to an increase in vascular resistance, i.e. to a reduction in the calibre of small arteries (1). However, in hypertension, fluctuations of blood pressure around the mean are also altered, leading to an increase in pulse pressure. In the arterial system, mean arterial pressure and pulse pressure are not completly independent variables: the higher the mean pressure, the higher the fluctuation around the mean. However, it is a common finding that, for a given mean arterial pressure, different values of pulse pressure may be observed, either from one subject to another or in the same subjects investigated beat by beat. This simple observation means that pulse pressure is influenced by haemodynamic mechanisms different from those of mean arterial pressure.

Hemodynamic factors governing pulse pressure

Analytical studies of arterial function consider that the magnitude of pulse pressure is determined by the interaction of an incident pressure wave generated by left ventricular ejection, and one or more reflected waves generated by the arterial system [2]. The magnitude of the incident wave depends on the pattern of left ventricular ejection and arterial stiffness. The magnitude of the reflected waves depends on the value of reflection coefficients but also on the timing and intensity of wave reflection and propagation properties of the arterial system. During systole, the rise in the incident pressure wave up to the time of peak velocity depends on the peak ejection velocity (which in turn is influenced by cardiac performance) and on aortic wave velocity which

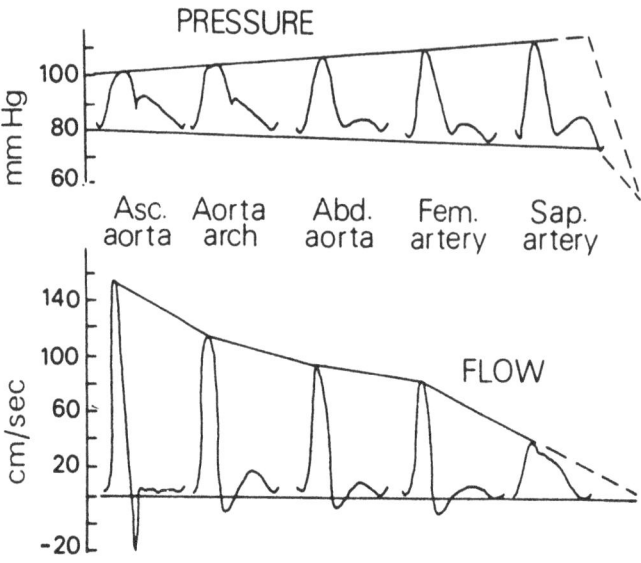

Figure 2. Pulse pressure increases from central to peripheral arteries [2].

depends principally on the viscoelastic properties of the proximal aorta, as described below. However, ventricular ejection and large artery elasticity influence the level of pulse pressure predominantly at the early phase of systole. In the latter phase, wave reflections are also responsible for a further sudden rise in arterial pressure [2].

Reflected waves participate to the increase in pulse pressure through at least two different mechanisms: pulse wave velocity and distance between reflection points and the heart [2]. On one hand, pulse wave velocity increases from the central to peripheral arteries, i.e. towards arteries of lesser cross-sectional area. On the other hand, reflection points are not normally close to the heart since their principal sites are at the origin of resistant arterioles. For that reason, reflected waves generated within the arterial system are responsible for the greater amplitude of pulse pressure in peripheral than in central arteries, with greater systolic pressure in the brachial artery than in the ascending aorta and lower diastolic pressure (Figure 2). Nevertheless, with age, this hemodynamic pattern is attenuated: pulse pressure tends to be similar in all parts of the arterial tree due to the increased speed of wave velocity with age, with a more rapid increase in pulse pressure with age in the thoracic aorta than in peripheral arteries [2]. Interestingly, due to the more important summation of incident and reflected waves with age, the reflected wave returns during the systolic component of the blood pressure curve in the older population whereas it returns during the diastolic component in the younger one [2], causing striking differences in the shape of the bood pressure curve for the same mean arterial pressure.

APPLANATION TONOMETRY

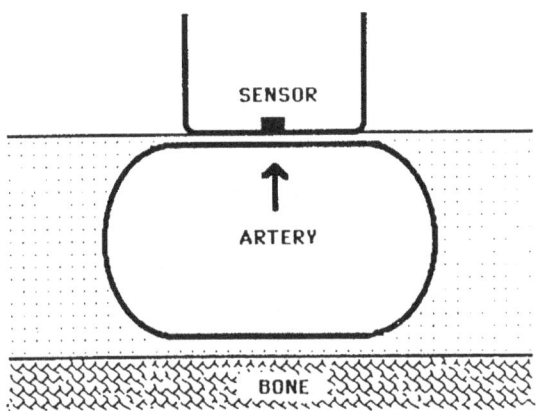

Fig. 3. The principle of applanation tonometry [6].

Non-invasive evaluation of systolic-diastolic vanations of blood pressure in hypertension

To improve the accuracy of nominvasive recording of the arterial pressure wave contour, applanation tonometry may be used, with a pencil-type probe incorporating a high-fidelity strain gauge transducer (Millar instruments Inc, Houston, Tx) [6] (Figure 3). In principle, flattening (applanation) ot a curved surface of pressure-containing structure under the detecting device allows direct measurement of the pressure within. The use and accuracy of the method were tested on the exposed canine femoral artery and percutaneously on the human radial artery [6]. In dogs, waveforms recorded from the exposed artery were virtually identical to direct intraarterial recordings. Analysis of the modulus, percentage of power, and cumulative percentage of power content for each harmonic of the pressure wave showed good correlation between direct and indirect recordings. In humans undergoing catheterization, blood pressure was measured simultaneously by two methods: invasively, at the site of the aortic aortic arch, and non invasively, at the site of the common carotid artery. A significant positive correlation ($r = 0.92$) was observed [7] with a slope equal to 1.05 and an intercept which was not significantly different from zero (0.4 mmHg). In another study in 105 subjects, brachial pulse pressure was measured by conventional sphygmomanometry and radial pulse pressure by applanation tonometry. The two parameters were strongly correlated: $r = 0.97$; slope: 0.98. intercept: 1.4 mmHg [8]. Because the tonometer transducer is small relative to the size of the artery, the positioning of the transducer over the site of the artery is

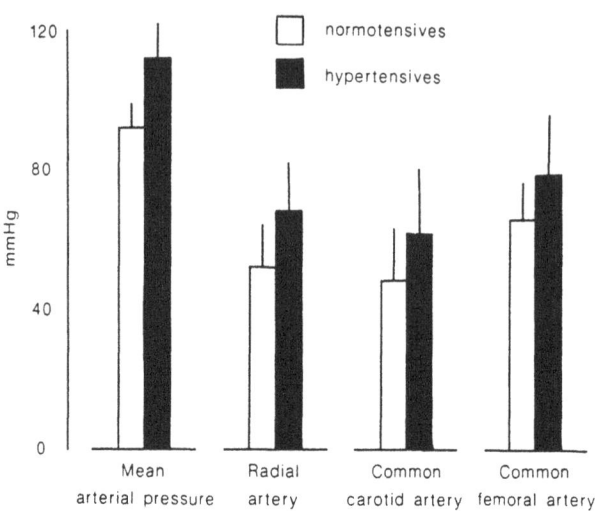

Fig. 4. Pulse pressure in various segments of the arterial tree in humans (personnal data) [8, 11].

quite important to consider in clinical investigation [6]. Firstly, movement of the transducer introduced by the operator's hand or movement of the subject may cause artifacts. This can easily be prevented by the use of a stereotaxic system to fixe the probe, the operator being relaxed and comfortable. Secondly, the hold-down force should be optimized to achieve adequate applanation but to avoid excessive hold-down force. It was found that excessive force leads to two characteristic changes. It is initially accompanied by a gradual increase in the pressure levels recorded in late diastole with a distortion of the diastolic part of the wave shape (often seen as a sharp negative deflection before the succeding systolic upstroke). The change in the value of systolic pressure recorded at this stage is usually minimal. In some cases further increase in hold-down force was accompanied by inversion of the systolic peak. The third source of artifact was found to be due to the angulation between the probe and the vessel. This particularly affects the systolic part of the pressure wave. The probe should ideally be kept close to perpendicular to the vessel axis. In that conditions, intra and inter observer variability of the measurements is below 10%.

The methodology has been applied to subjects with hypertension, either in sustained essential hypertension of the middle age [7] or in end stage renal disease [8]. In both cases, carotid pulse pressure was found to be lower than radial or femoral pulse pressure (Figure 4). The finding was observed to be of same magnitude in normotensive and in hypertensive subjects. However, with age, there is a tendancy for pulse wave velocity to be the same in all

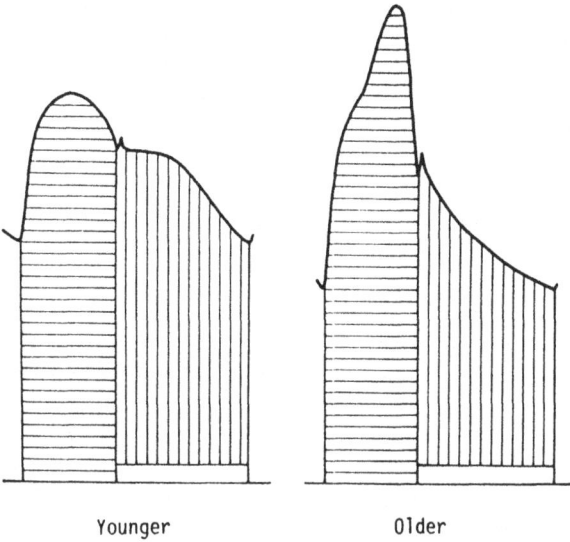

Younger   Older

Fig. 5. Modifications in the shape of the blood pressure curve with age: wave reflections return in diastole in younger subjects and in systole in older subjects [12]. Mean arterial is the same for the two curves.

parts of the arterial tree. Subsequently, pulse pressure is nearly the same in the thoracic aorta and in peripheral arteries, with a higher amplitude in older than in younger subjects [7].

Increased wave reflections in hypertension

As we have seen in the previous paragraph, the intensity of reflected wave depends not only on the rigidity of the arterial wall but also on the site of the reflection points along the arterial tree. The reflected wave will be more pronounced not only if pulse wave velocity is increased (i.e. the aotic wall is more rigid) but also if the reflection points are nearer the heart, leading to a summation between the incident and the reflected waves and therefore to a higher pulse pressure and systolic peak [2]. In normal conditions, reflection points are principally observed at the narrowing of small resistant vessels, thus favoring a return of reflection waves during diastole [2, 9]. However, with aging and hypertension, pulse wave velocity increases markedly and additionnal reflecting points operate closer to the heart, causing a return of reflected waves during systole and the apparition of a late systolic peak [2, 5, 9] (Figure 5). Strong evidence for the role of reflection points to maintain elevated blood pressure results from the increased systolic pressure observed in subjects with coarctation of the aorta [2] or with traumatic amputation of the lower limbs [10]. In both cases, reflection points nearer

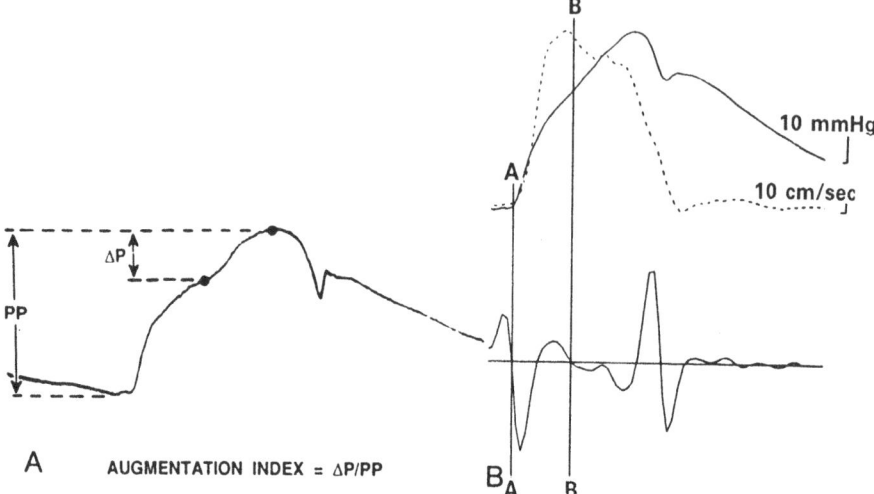

Fig. 6. Wave reflections: definition of the augmentation index [6, 8, 11, 12] see text in A. Difficulties to evaluate the index are noticed in B and detailed in reference 2.

the heart cause a summation of forward and backward waves with a higher systolic peak related to the presence of coarctation or to the amputation of arterial segments. Another example is given by the observation that increased wave reflections are particularly noticed in subjects with reduced height. Indeed, in these subjects, the reduced length of the vasculature contributes to favour reflection sites nearer the heart [11].

For the clinical investigation of wave reflection, it is important to recall that the aortic or central artery pulse pressure (PP) waveforms in man have been well characterized previously on the basis of impedance spectrum [2, 12]. The pressure curve is generally shown to manifest an inflection point which divides the pressure wave into an early and mid-to-late systolic peak (Figure 6). The mild to late systolic peak is taken to be the result of the reflected wave returning from peripheral site (s) and causing an increase of the pulse pressure and systolic blood pressure [2, 12]. As shown in Figure 6, the ΔP to PP ratio defines an augmentation index [12]. Furthermore the time from the foot of the pressure wave to the foot of late systolic peak has been interpreted to represent the travel time of the pulse wave to peripheral reflecting site (s) and its return [2, 12]. Study of the relationship between the aortic pressure waveform and aortic input impedance has shown that a larger secondary rise of PP is associated with an enhanced oscillatory impedance spectrum due to differences in the magnitude of wave reflections and/or interaction of reflection for different sites [2, 12].

Most of the non invasives studies of wave reflections in the literature have been focused on the relationship of the augmentation index with age (Figure 6) [6]. Indeed, the calculation of this index indicates that wave reflections in

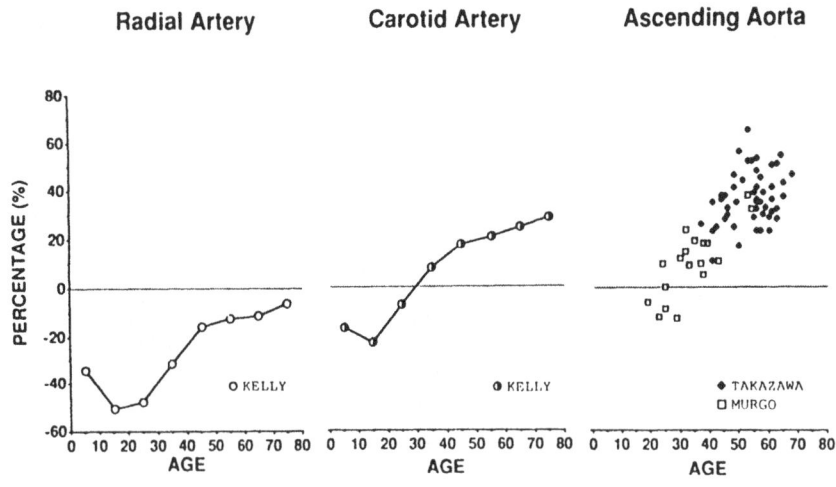

Fig. 7. Increase in augmentation index with age in the literature [6].

Table 1. Carotid pulse wave analysis in control subjects and in hypertensive **patients** with end-stage renal disease (ESRD) [8, 11]

	Control subjects	ESRD patients
Radial artery PP (mmHg)	60.7 ± 16.1	73.7 ± 22.0****
Carotid artery PP (mmHg)	57.3 ± 19.6	73.2 ± 25.7****
Carotid PP/Radial PP (ratio)	0.93 ± 0.14	0.99 ± 0.15**
Augmentation index (mmHg)	7.5 ± 10.5	19.0 ± 15.2****
Augmentation index (%)	9.8 ± 15.6	23.2 ± 15.0****
Heart period (ms)	909 ± 149	840 ± 145***
Aortic PWV (cm/s)	930 ± 196	1035 ± 238***

Values are mean ± SD.
PP, pulse pressure; PWV, pulse wave velocity.
*P < 0.05; **P < 0.02; ***P < 0.01; ****P < 0.001.

the thoracic aorta increase markedly with age (Figure 7). Howewer, this mechanism is amplified in the hypertensive population, in which, at any given value of age, wave reflections are more important than in the normotensive population. Table 1 shows an example of increased wave reflections in hypertensive subjects with end-stage renal disease and undergoing hemodialysis [8]. Similar findings may be observed in essential hypertension.

The importance of wave reflections in hypertension was indirectly shown by the administration of nitrates [13–15]. Indeed, with these agents, later reflection waves may be obtained even without changes in pulse wave velocity when the distance between the heart and the reflection points is increased by drug effects. Early work by Taylor [16] showed that an increase in the arterial cross-sectional area at peripheral bifurcations could theoretically

144   *Michel E. Safar*

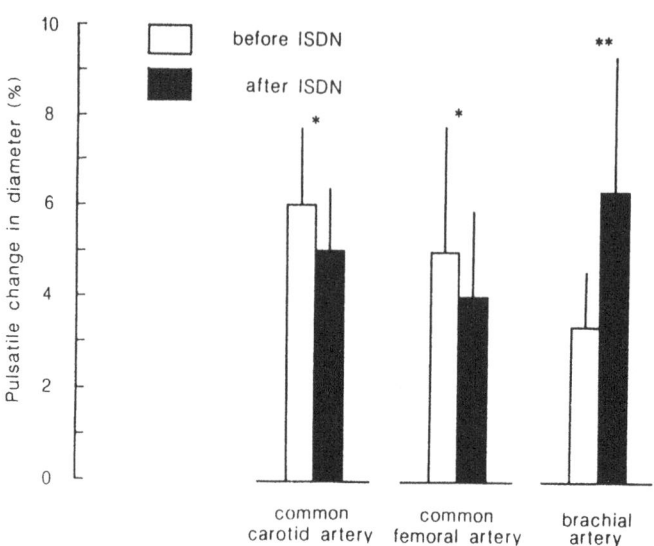

Hypertensive subjects

Fig. 8. Effect of isosorbid dinitrate (ISDN) on the pulsatile change in diameter of various arteries [19].

produce this type of alteration in peripheral reflection patterns. These geometrical modifications might per se reduce the intensity of reflections at the bifurcations so that the total reflections will begin more exclusively at vascular terminations, thus helping to decrease pulse pressure [13–15]. This mechanism has been shown to operate with nitrates, which reduce the amplitude of peripheral vascular reflections and delay the return of these reflections to the aortic root, without any substantial change in ventricular ejection and vascular resistance [13–15]. In normotensive and hypertensive subjects, nitrates dilate much more peripheral muscular arteries than the thoracic aorta [15] (Figure 8), a finding which agrees with the mathematical model described by Taylor.

Geometrical changes of the large arteries in hypertension

In the past years, available non-invasive methods using echography and pulsed Doppler velocimetry have been described to determine the caliber of large arteries, such as in the central aorta, the brachial and the common carotid arteries [17, 18]. Nevertheless, the resolution of the methods was relatively poor. More recently, several devices have been described to measure arterial diameter and wall motion transcutaneously by tracking the echo signals from both the anterior and the posterior walls [19–22]. Earlier instruments used an amplitude tracking method which had several drawbacks

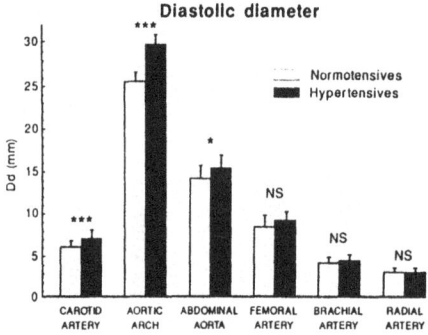

Fig. 9. Diastolic diameter (*Dd*) in various arteries of normotensive and hypertensive subjects [24].

[23]. Surimposed echoes from the tissue surrounding the artery as well as imperfect alignment of the ultrasonic beam perpendicular to the arterial wall caused major unpredictable changes in the amplitude of the echo waveform. New instruments are characterized by sufficient linearity, dynamic range and tracking speed, even when the signal to noise ratio of the original signal is not high.

Nowadays, the vessel wall displacements of peripheral arteries may be measured using very original procedures. The Walltrack system (Maastricht, The Netherlands) [20] was developed in order to measure wall motion of large arteries, such as the brachial and the common carotid arteries, after echographic localisation. Due to the accurate determination of the doppler frequency (phase locked echo-tracking), no stereotaxic apparatus was necessary for obtaining reliable measurements. The Diarad system [21] was developed in order to obtain the pressure-diameter curve of the radial artery by coupling the measurement of systolic-diastolic variations of arterial diameter to those of digital blood pressure, using the advantage of two technical characteristics. First, a pulsed Doppler system coupled to the echo-tracking system allows the localization of this medium-size artery to be done more easily than with a mode echography. Second, the 10 MHz probe and the 11 mm focal length offer a high spatial resolution and an excellent reproducibility for measuring internal diameter and pulsatile changes of the radial artery, provided a stereotaxis apparatus was used. Methodological aspects have been described previously in detail for each of these devices [20, 21]. Inter and intra-observer reproducibility is below 10%.

Figure 9 shows the values of diastolic diameter in various central and peripheral arteries [24]. Whereas the diastolic diameter of the hypertensive carotid artery and of the aorta was increased, no significant change was observed at the site of the brachial, the radial and the femoral arteries, indicating that these latter arteries respond actively to the increase in blood pressure, so that an active constrictive response masked the passive distension

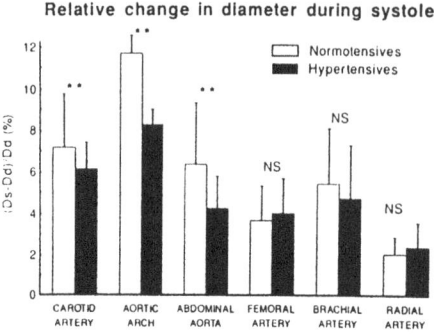

Fig. 10. Pulsatile chance in arterial diameter [$(Ds\text{-}Dd)/Dd$] in various arteries of normotensive and hypertensive subjects [24].

due to the elevated blood pressure. Figure 10 shows the values of the pulsatile changes in diameter (24). Pulsatile changes are maintained within the normal range in peripheral arteries (radial, brachial and femoral arteries) whereas there is a significant reduction at site of the aorta and the carotid artery. Since the pulsatile changes of blood pressure were increased in the latter (see Figure 4), the weight of evidence suggests that the central aorta and the carotid artery responded actively to the increased mechanical signal: a decrease in the pulsatile change of diameter is observed despite the increase in pulsatile pressure.

Finally, these findings strongly suggest that the arteries respond very actively to the long term elevations of blood pressure and that these changes differ in the elastic and the muscular arteries. These observations are corroborated when the role of age is taken into account [24]. Whereas the mechanical properties of the carotid artery and the aorta decrease with age (Figure 11), no comparable relationship may be observed for the radial (Figure 12), the brachial and the femoral arteries. These findings clearly indicate that the visco-elastic properties of the arteries differ greatly in the central and the peripheral compartments of the arterial tree with different changes according to the aging process.

Arterial compliance and distensibility in hypertension

The elastic properties that are characteristic of a particular material are usually expressed in terms of stress/strain ratio, or modulus of elasticity [2]. Young's modulus, for example, is the ratio of a tensile stress to the resulting elongation. Measuring Young's modulus of elasticity is a relatively simple procedure in a purely elastic body where strain is linearly proportional to stress. A plot of stress versus strain is then a straight line, and its slope is Young's modulus. The walls of blood vessels, however, like many other

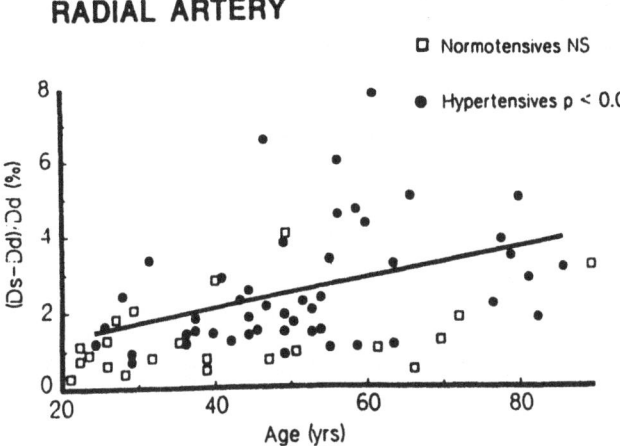

RADIAL ARTERY

Fig. 11. Pulsatile change of arterial diameter [$(Ds - Dd)/Dd$] of the carotid artery: relationship with age [24].

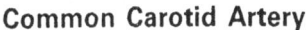

Common Carotid Artery

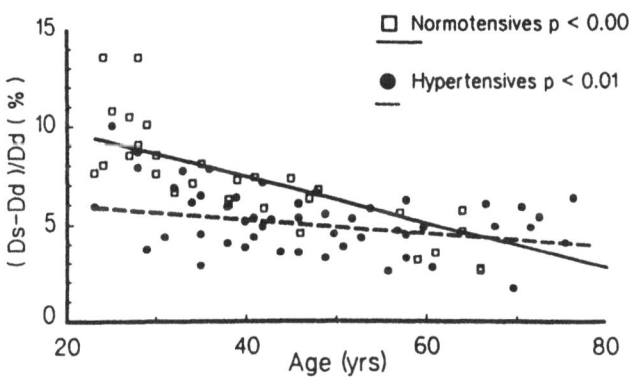

Fig. 12. Pulsatile change of arterial diameter [$(Ds\text{-}Dd)/Dd$] of the radial artery: relationship with age [24].

nonhomogeneous materials, exhibit a curvilinear stress-train relationship. The elastic modulus varies with the degree of extension, becoming greater as length increases. Under such conditions it is advantagenous to define the elastic modulus at a particular length as the tangent to the stress-strain curve at that point. Nevertheless, since wall thickness is often unknown during experiments in vivo, several approximations values have been proposed to evaluate arterial elasticity.

Table 2. Carotid artery versus femoral artery arterial parameters in a population of mixed normotensive and hypertensive subjects [7] (see Table 1 for abbreviations)

	Carotid	Femoral	p
Mean blood pressure	112 ± 2	108 ± 2	NS
Pulse pressure (mmHg) tonometry)	52.7 ± 2.2	62.5 ± 2.5	0.0001
Diastolic arterial diameter (mm)	6.79 ± 0.10	9.14 ± 0.19	0.0001
Ds − Dd (um)	406 ± 16	314 ± 15	0.0001
(Ds − Dd)/Dd(%)	6.07 ± 0.28	3.47 ± 0.18	0.0001
Distensibility coefficient (KPa 10^{-3}3)	21.6 ± 1.75	9.36 ± 0.58	0.0001
Cross-sectional compliance (m² kPa^{-1} 10^{-7})	7.42 ± 0.46	6.20 ± 0.28	0.05

± 1 SEM

The distension of an artery (change in diameter) during a cardiac cycle depends on the elastic characteristics of the vessel wall (and the surrounding tissues) and the local pulse pressure according to a curvilinear relationship [2]. The slope of this relationship can be expressed by the compliance C, defined as: $C = dV/dP$, were dV represents systolic-diastolic changes of the volume of an arterial segment and dP the pulse pressure (systolic minus diastolic blood pressure). Subsequently, compliance during the cardiac cycle decreases with pressure and comparison between normotensive and hypertensive subjects requires an evaluation of compliance for the same pressure. Assuming that the increase in volume is only caused by the distension of the artery (and not by elongation), the cross sectionnal compliance CC (compliance per unit of length) can be also expressed as: $CC = dA/dP$, where A is the arterial cross-sectional area. To consider the effect of the distension on the stretching of the arterial wall, a distensibility coefficient DC (distensibility per unit of length) may be defined as $DC = dA/A/dP$. Therefore, the quantity DC represents the strain of the arterial wall for a given pulse pressure and pertains to the mechanical loading of the artery during a cardiac cycle. As for compliance, distensibility during the cardiac cycle decreases with pressure and comparison between normotensive and hypertensive subjects requires an evaluation of distensibility for the same pressure. In humans, CC and DC are often calculated from non-simultaneous measurements of pulsatile changes of diameter and pressure on the same (or very near) arterial segments and therefore are presented rather as estimations than as direct measurements.

Table 2 indicate as examples the values of compliance in some segments of the arterial tree [7]. In hypertension, the distensibility of the carotid artery and the aorta are decreased, in agreement with the decreased systemic compliance and distensibility already observed in hypertensive subjects [2, 5, 25]. In contrast nearly normal values are observed for peripheral arteries as the radial artery. Even when the compliance of the radial artery is evaluated for the same pressure in normotensive and hypertensive subjects, compliance was normal or even slightly increased in hypertensives [26]. Such findings again indicate that, in the presence of elevated blood pressure, the mechanism of the compliance alterations differ greatly in the different parts of the arterial tree. However, since the compliance changes predominate largelly in the central arteries and contribute mainly to the decrease in the systemic arterial compliance already observed in hypertension [2, 5, 25], only the changes in the mechanical properties of these arteries will be analyzed extensively in this part of the review.

Theoretically, the passive mechanical properties of the vessel wall, and therefore arterial stiffness, are predominantly influenced by one or several of the structural components of a given artery: endothelium, adventitia or media [27]. Basically, the major contribution of structural factors to the mechanical vessel properties is assumed to arise from the inner intima and the media, which consist mainly of smooth muscle, elastin and collagen. The effects of each of these components, individually and collectively, are expected to determine primarily the mechanical properties of the vessel wall and therefore arterial stiffness and pulse pressure, principally at site of the aorta and of its major branches.

In order to explain the respective role of smooth muscle, elastin and collagen on the mechanical properties of the vessel wall, Burton [28] showed that Young's modulus for non contracting smooth muscle was very low and approximated 6×10^4 dyne/cm^2, making it far more extensible than the vessel wall. On the other hand, Young's modulus of isolated elastic tissues was estimated to be 3×10^6 dynes/cm^2 and that of collagen about to be 10^9 dynes/cm^2, indicating that these two components had the major contribution to the passive mechanical properties of the vessel wall. This assumption was clearly shown in Dobrin's experiments [29] in which human isolated arterial vessels were studied in the presence of elastase and collagenase. With elastase, the pressure-volume relationship of the arterial vessel was shifted toward higher values of arterial diameter and volume, indicating that the loss of elastin influenced greatly the geometry of the vessel without changing its elastic property (i.e. the slope of the curve). On the other hand, with collagenase, the slope of the curve changed greatly, indicating a decreased stiffness of the vessel wall, without substantial change in its geometry. Finally, it appears that the passive visco-elastic properties of the vessel wall are principally determined by the elastic on collagen ratio, a parameter which is greatly influenced both by age and hypertension.

From the macroscopic standpoint, the age changes in the larger arteries appear to support the experimental findings described above. An increase in aortic mass, lumen size and wall thickness has been shown in humans and various other species [27]. These changes are more prominent in the subendothelials layer and the media with an increase in connective tissue content. The most conspicuous changes are elastin fragmentation and calcification and increase in collagen content [27]. Such findings are predominantly responsible for the increased pulse wave velocity with age already reported [2]. Morphological changes of arterial smooth muscle also appear to undergo

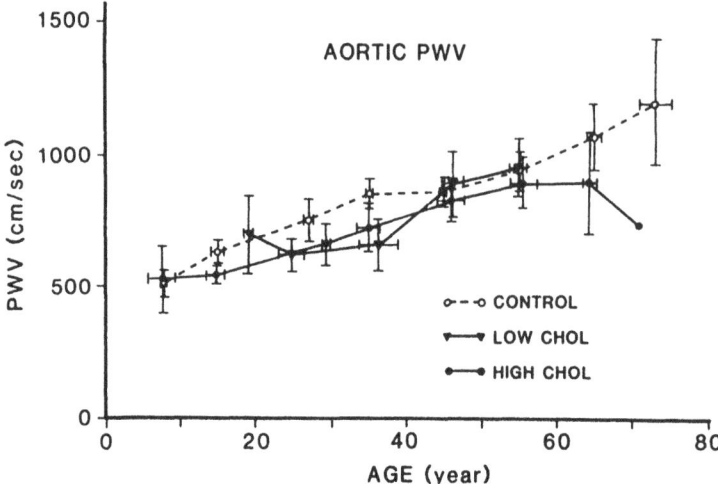

Fig. 13. Relationship of pulse wave velocity (PWV) wlh age. Notice that the relationship is identical whatever the level of total plasma cholesterol (chol) [2]. However, it is well known that, at any given value of age, PWV is higher in hypertensive than in normotensive subjects.

age changes although they have less been extensively studied. The age-related changes in the arterial wall are also accellerated in the presence of hypertension. Indeed, the most common model to account for the overall properties of the vessel wall reflects the role of elastin in low values, of the muscle in intermediate values and of the collagen fibers within the higher values of the distending pressure. Finally, with age and hypertension, the vessel wall is composed of increasing amounts of collagen which plays a dominant role in the mechanical properties of the aorta and its branches and acts as a constraining coat once the strain reaches a given level [30].

Finally, structural factors seem predominant to explain the increased arterial stiffness which occurs with aging and hypertension in the aorta and its major branches. Increased arterial stiffness contributes to accelerate pulse wave velocity (Figure 13) and to produce earlier reflected waves, thus contributing to increase pulse pressure. In this context, changes in arterial smooth muscle tone are probably of lesser influence. Indeed in younger people, the elastic structure of the aorta is predominant whereas, in the older subjects, collagen acts as a constraining coat impeding the muscle to participate to the aortic stiffness changes through constriction and relaxation. Indeed, studies of peripheral arteries in rat and man [31, 32] have shown that, whereas changes in arterial smooth muscle tone may influence substantially arterial stiffness in younger animals, no significant role may be observed in older animals [31]. Nevertheless, such aspects have not yet been fully investigated in the literature, particularly for peripheral arteries. In addition, it is unknown if changes in endothelium function with age and hypertension [31, 33] may also influence arterial compliance and stiffness.

Conclusion

There are important abnormalities of the arterial system in hypertension but they are heterogenenous in nature. Indeed the arterial system may be divided into two compartments: a central compartment involving the aorta and the origin of its major branches, and a peripheral compartment involving the more distal arteries.

In the central compartment, the cross-sectional area is substantially increased, with an increase in pulse wave velocity and a decrease in distensibility. Increased wave reflections predominate in the central thoracic aorta, contributing to increase greatly pulse pressure and to cause a predominant increase in systolic over diastolic blood pressure. All these processes are strongly age dependent and may contribute greatly to the developpment of cardiac hypertrophy [34] and finally to cardiovascular morbidity and mortality. Interestingly, increased pulse pressure has been shown to be an independant cardiovascular risk factor for cardiac death, and not for cerebral death [35].

In the peripheral compartment, the cross-sectional area is poorly modified in hypertensive subjects, with little changes in compliance and distensibility, as observed at the site of the radial artery. The contrast between the dilated central arteries and the unchanged diameter of peripheral arteries may contribute to the changes in the site of the reflection points, making them closer to the heart. These arteries are poorly sensitive to pressure changes (in contrast with central arteries) but respond very rapidly to changes in vasomotor tone, in the same way as resistant arteries [19, 32].

The heterogeneity of the hypertensive arterial system seems largely dependant on the differences in structure of the arterial wall. In the central compartment, the elastin and collagen content predominates on the arterial smooth muscle whereas an opposite pattern is observed for peripheral arteries, leading to different ratios between the distensible (elastin ± smooth muscle) and the non distensible (collagen) material. Whether these changes play a role in the arterial injury observed in hypertensive subjects remain an important question which requires further investigations.

References

1. Folkow B. Physiological aspects of primary hypertension. Physiol Rev 1981; 62: 347–54.
2. Nichols WV, O'Rourke MF. McDonald's blood flow in arteries. Theoretical, experimental and principles. Third Edition. ed. Arnold E, London, Melbourne, Auckland, 1990: 77–142, 216–269, 283–269, 398–437.

3. Kannel WB, Stokes JII. Hypertension as a cardiovascular risk factor. In Bulpitt CJ. editor. Handbook of Hypertension, Vol 6, Epidemiology of Hypertension. Amsterdam: Elsevier Science, 1985: 15–209.

4. Thompson SG. An appraisal of the large-scale trials of antihypertensive treatment. In: Bulpitt CJ. editor. Handbook of Hypertension, Vol. 6, Epidemiology of hypertension. Amsterdam: Elsevier Science, 1985: 331–43.

5. Safar ME. Pulse pressure in essential hypertension: clinical and therapeutical implications. J Hypertens 1989; 7: 768–76.

6. Kelly R, Hayward C, Ganis J, Daley J, Avolio A, O'Rourke M. Noninvasive determination of age-related changes in the human arterial pulse. Circulation 1989; 80: 1652–9.

7. Benetos A, Laurent S, Hoeks AP, Boutouyrie PH, Safar ME. Arterial alterations with aging and high blood pressure – A noninvasive study of carotid and femoral arteries. Arterioschlerosis and Thrombosis 1993; 13: 90–97.

8. London GM, Marchais SJ, Safar ME, et al. Aortic and large artery compliance in end-stage renal failure. Kidney International, 1990; 37: 137–42.

9. Latham RD. Pulse propagation in the systemic arterial tree. Westerhof N, Gross DR, editors. Plenum Press New York and London, 1989: 49–68.

10. Labouret G, Achimastos A, Benetos A, Safar M, Housset E. L'hypertension artérielle systolique des amputés traumatiques. Press Med. 1983; 211: 1349-54.

11. London GM, Guerin AP, Pannier B, Marchais SJ, Metivier F, Safar ME. Increased systolic pressure in chronic uremia: role of arterial wave reflections. Hypertension 1992; 20: 10–19.

12. Murgo JP, Westerhof N, Giolma JP, Altobelli SA. Aortic input impedance in normal man; relationship to pressure shapes. Circulation 1980; 62: 105–116.

13. Latson TW, Hunter WC, Katoh N, Sagawa K. Effect of nitroglycerin on aortic impedance, diameter and pulse wave velocity. Circ Res 1988; 62: 884–90.

14. Yaginuma T, Avolio AP, O'Rourke MF et al. Effect of glyceryl trinitrate on peripheral arteries alters left ventricular hydraulic load in man. Cardiovasc Res 1986; 201: 153–60.

15. Safar ME. Antihypertensive effects of nitrates in chronic human hypertension. J Applied Cardiol 1990; 5: 69–81.

16. Taylor MG. Wave travel in arteries and the design of the cardiovascular system. In: Attinger EO, editor. Pulsatile Blood Flow. New York, McGraw Hill, 1964: 343–7.

17. Safar ME, Peronneau PA, Levenson JA, Toto-Moukouo JA, Simon A Ch. Pulsed Doppler: Diameter, Blood flow velocity and volumic flow of the brachial artery in Sustained essential hypertension. Circulation 1981; 63: 393–9.

18. Isnard RN, Pannier BM, Laurent S, London GM, Diebold B, Safar ME. Pulsatile diameter and elastic modulus of the aortic arch in essential hypertension: a non-invasive study. J Am Coll Cardiol 1989; 113: 399–405.

19. Laurent S, Arcaro G, Benetos A, Lafleche A, Hoeks A, Safar ME. Mechanism of Nitrate-induced improvement on arterial compliance depends on vascular territory. J Cardiovasc Pharmacol 1992; 19: 641–49.

20. Hoeks APG, Brands PJ, Smeets GAM, Reneman RS. Assessment of the distensibility of superficial arteries. Ultrasound Med Biol 1990; 16: 121–8.

21. Tardy Y, Meister JJ, Perret F, Waeber B, Brunner HR. Assessment of the elastic behaviour of peripheral arteries from a noninvasive measurements of their diameter-pressure curves. Clin Phys Physiol Meas 1991; 12: 39–54.

22. Kawasaki T, Sasayama S, Yagi S, Asakawa T, Hirai T. Noninvasive assessment of the age related changes in stiffness of major branches of the human arteries. Cardiovasc Res 1987; 21: 678–87.

23. Arndt JO, Kober G. Pressure diameter relationship of the intact femoral artery in conscious man. Pfluegers Arch 1970; 318: 130–46.

24. Boutouyrie P, Laurent S, Benetos A, Girerd X, Hoeks A, Safar M. Opposite effects of ageing on distal and proximal large arteries in hypertensives. J Hypertens 1992; 10(Suppl 6): 587–591.

25. Liu Z, Ting C-T, Zhu S, Yin FCP. Aortic compliance in human hypertension. Hypertension 1989; 140: 129–36.
26. Laurent S, Hayoz D, Trazzi S, Boutouyrie P, Waeber B, Omboni S, Brunner H, Marcia G, Safar M. Isobaric compliance of the radial artery is increased in patients with essential hypertension. J of Hypertension 1993; 11: 89–98.
27. Yin FCP. The aging vasculature and its effects on the heart. In Weisfeldt ML, editor. The aging heart (aging Vol 12), New York: Raven Press, 1990: 137–213.
28. Burton AC. Relation of structure to function of tissues of the wall of blood vessels. Physiol Rev 1954; 34: 619–42.
29. Dobrin PB, Baker WH, Gley WC. Elastolytic and collagenolytic studies of arteries: implications for the mechanical properties of aneurysms. Arch Surg 1984; 119: 406–9.
30. Remington JW. The physiology of the aorta and major arteries. In: Handbook of Physiology, Sect. 2, Circulation, Vol 2, American Physiological Society, Washington, D.C., 1963.
31. Benetos A, Beriaziz H, Albaladejo P, Levy BI, Safar ME. Physiological and pharmacological changes in the carotid artery pressure-volume curve in situ in rats. J of Hypertension 1992, 10(Suppl 6): S127–S131.
32. Safar ME, Levy BI, Laurent S, London GM. Hypertension and the arterial system: clinical and therapeutic aspects. J Hypertens 1990; 8 (suppl 7): S113–9.
33. Furchgott RF, Zawadzki JV. The obligatory role of endothelial cells on the relaxation of arterial smooth muscle cells by acetylcholine. Nature (London) 1980; 288: 373–6.
34. Safar ME, Toto-Moukouo JJ, Bouthier JA, et al. Arterial dynamics, cardiac hypertrophy, and antihypertensive treatment. Circulation 1987; 75 (suppl 1): 156–61.
35. Darne B, Girerd X, Safar ME, Cambien F, Guize L. Pulsatile versus steady component of blood pressure,: A cross-sectional analysis and a prospective analysis on cardiovascular mortality. Hypertension 1989; 13: 392–400.

10. Arterial system, left ventricular structure and function

RENÉ GOURGON and ALAIN COHEN-SOLAL

Introduction

In systemic hypertension, the left ventricle (LV) is both [1] a culprit participating in the pathogenesis of hypertension and a victim, cardiac and coronary complications being the most frequent and severe among those of the disease.

For several years, the deleterious and "independent" prognostic signification of LV hypertrophy (LVH) has been unanimously recognized and improvements of Doppler-echocardiography have allowed easier evaluation of changes in mass (m), geometry and function of the LV.

The aim of this chapter is not to review all the aspects of the LV in hypertension (some remarkable general reviews are available [2–4]), but to briefly address:

– the relations between the physical properties of the arterial system (AS) and LV systolic load;
– the modifications of mass, geometry and function of the LV observed in hypertension, more heterogeneous than previously described. As after myocardial infarction, "remodeling" has gained a important role besides classical hypertrophy [5–8];
– the main implications, especially the therapeutic and prognostic ones, resulting from these changes of the LV and the AS.

Systolic load of the left ventricle and arterial impedance

The simplistic assimilation of hypertension to a LV pressure overload and of aortic pressure (AoP) to the systolic load of the LV has led to a double misunderstanding because:

– the LV pump participates in the genesis of hypertension;
– aortic pressure does not represent the systolic load of the LV pump or muscle.

M. E. Safar and M. F. O'Rourke (eds.), The arterial system in hypertension. pp. 155–179.
© 1993 *Kluwer Academic Publishers. Printed in the Netherlands.*

LV pump participates to the establishment and persistance of hypertension

Whatever the "primum movens" of hypertension, modifications of the LV and especially exaggeration of the ejection function of the LV pump are required for the initial establishment of sustained hypertension. Generally, in hypertension, cardiac output (CO) is preserved and aortic pressures are increased: less so diastolic arterial pressure (DAP) than mean aortic pressure; but mainly systolic arterial pressure (SAP), end-systolic aortic pressures (ESP), pulse pressure and mean pressure during ejection. This results, as with aging, in the fact that the pulsatile stroke work of the LV is increased compared to the continuous stroke work (evaluated by the simple product of mean AoP by CO). Specificity of this observation is illustrated by the result of the use of vasoactive drugs in normal and hypertensive subjects [9]. In the former, the SWp/SWm ratio (SWp: pulsatile stroke work; SWm: continuous stroke work) is not modified by perfusion of angiotensin, a reduction of cardiac output being observed simultaneously to the increase of AoP. In the latter, after perfusion of sodium nitroprusside, SWp and SWm decrease simultaneously, but the SWp/SWm ratio remains higher, at identical AoP, than in normals. The sole alteration of the transfer function of the arterial system, observed with aging and in hypertension, if not accompanied by a simultaneous improvement of the ability of the LV to match it, would not be sufficient to determine all the hemodynamic modifications observed in systemic hypertension [9–12]. Thus, systemic hypertension is characterized by structural and functional modifications of both the arterial system and the LV, the adaptative or primary parts of these modifications being probably different, depending on the situation. The delay of reinstallation of hypertension after cessation of a prolonged treatment also illustrates the physiopathologic role of the overall cardiac and arterial systems.

Aortic or left ventricular systolic pressures do not represent the systolic load of the left ventricle

Systolic load of the left ventricle in fact depends, for one part, on the intrinsic properties of the LV, and for another part, on the physical properties of the arterial system, at best represented by its entry or input hydraulic impedance [9, 11, 13].

The terms of preload, afterload and total load, are clearly defined for the study of the contraction of an *isolated papillary muscle*:
- preload is the force passively exerced on the ventricular muscle which, as a function of its distensibility, determines its initial length before contraction;
- afterload is the additional force imposed to the muscle all along the shortening period;
- total performed force is the sum of preload and afterload. It is constant (contraction is called isotonic) all along the experimental contraction and,

for a definite inotropic state, determines the final length of shortening. At identical final length, corresponding to a definite inotropic state and a total performed force, the part of afterload decreases if preload is increased and reciprocally. In all cases, total performed force is the sum of the two forces imposed to the muscle, independant of its intrinsic properties of distensibility or inotropy.

Thus, the amplitude and the velocity of shortening of the papillary muscle depend on the inotropic state and the loading conditions, both easy to define and settle experimentally, load being constant all along the contraction.

For the *intact LV*, substitution of the term afterload to the one of total systolic load is first of all inappropriate. Mainly, pressures generated during filling and ejection are very different from the experimental loading conditions, especially as independence towards LV and constancy during ejection are concerned [11, 13]. Finally, the LV is both a muscle, characterized by its intrinsic properties of extension and contraction, and a pump which overall performances during filling and ejection (end-diastolic volume, EDV; end-systolic volume, ESV; stroke volume, SV; ejection fraction, EF) depend on:

– the properties of the muscle,
– its mass,
– its geometrical arrangements, and
– the loading and ejection conditions related to the properties of the up-stream venous and downstream arterial systems.

Aortic pressure is not an independent variable, but is determined by the characteristics of both the arterial system and the LV pump

Mean aortic pressure (MAoP) equals the product of total systemic resistance (TSR) (if venous pressures are neglected) by cardiac output. TSR characterize the distal arterial system (but also incorporates blood viscosity) and represent the continuous term of the spectrum (of modulus) of aortic impedance. CO depends on heart rate (HR), contractility, filling and ejection conditions of the LV pump.

Instantaneous aortic pressures generated during ejection depend on the instantaneous output of the LV and the physical properties of the arterial system (characteristic impedance (Zc) – reflected waves), characterized by the different harmonics of the spectrum of modulus [9, 11, 13–15]. The proximal arterial system (AS) represents the interface between LV pump and the distal AS; its characteristics determine the actual opposition to ejection of the LV: Zc represents only 10% of TSR. The parallelism between TSR, which characterize the distal AS, and the properties of the proximal AS, is not necessarily strict, as demonstrated by the study of normal and pathologic subjects and illustrated by the use of vasoactive drugs [9, 16]. Moreover, aortic pressure, because of the instantaneous variations of flow, is not constant during LV ejection, contraction being called auxotonic. Finally, only aortic impedance, even if it does not have the dimension of a force, appears to be, all along ejection, constant and independent of the characteristics of the LV, and thus able to characterize the factors external to the LV and that oppose to its ejection [9, 11–15, 17, 18].

The LV is both a muscle and a pump

If for both, the external part of opposition to ejection is represented by aortic impedance, analysis of the generated "load" is different in each case.

For the LV muscle, assuming the hypothesis of an ellipsoid of revolution, taking into account at every moment instantaneous generated pressures, mass and geometry of the LV pump, calculation of stresses (σ) (forces at midwall) is possible and represents the best approach of the systolic load which thus depends on factors external to the LV: aortic impedance, representing the aortic part of LV load; and factors intrinsic to the LV (mass, geometry, function), which determine (a) for a given aortic impedance, stroke volume and instantaneous output, and (b) for a given aortic pressure, generated stress. Moreover, these latters are not constant during LV contraction and one can calculate maximal, mean and endsystolic stress; their respective physiologic meaning (regulation of the adaptation of mass and geometry to a mechanical overload, determination of the metabolic demand per gram of myocardium; and determination of the end-systolic volume), is certainly not identical.

Analysis of the *LV pump* is carried out by use of pressure – volume relations [9], LV volume and pressure being not independent one of another. Output of the LV pump depends on the aptitude of the LV to face all the external factors that oppose its ejection. Generated pressures depending on the properties of both the LV and the AS, separation of a pressure load imposed by the AS and a volume load imposed by the LV (or even the venous system) is thus also artificial.

Establishment of spectra of aortic impedance comes up again various difficulties

– It is technically difficult, requiring high fidelity measurements – still nowadays invasive – of pressure and flow in the LV or the aortic root (if one neglects the initial difference of driving pressure).
– The spectra of modulus and phase cannot be expressed by a single number; these spectra only offer various numbers representative of the different properties of the AS at different frequencies.
– Finally, if a spectrum of impedance is, at a given instant, independent of LV properties, properties of the proximal AS (including stiffness, diameter...) vary with aortic pressure and thus, even for constant TSR, cardiac output.

The first two reserves lead to the use of simplified indices of aortic impedance more easy to determine, but whose limits have to be known:

- Characteristic impedance neglects the reflected waves, but can be calculated from diameter and stiffness of the initial aorta [20]. It appears to be generally well correlated to Zc, calculated by averaging the high frequency harmonics of the spectrum of modulus.
- The velocity of propagation of the pulsatile wave (Co) can be calculated by non invasive technics in the thoracic aorta (directly or indirectly, from the modulus of elasticity pressure – strain) and for the overall aorta [21]. It measures aortic stiffness, and is the main determinant of Zc and of the delay of return of the reflected waves.
- Ea was defined by Sunagawa and coll. [12] as the effective elastance of the arterial system by the ratio ESP/SV. ESP/SV = (TSR × HR) + Ea'; HR: heart rate (min^{-1}); Ea' = (ESP − MAoP)/SV. End-systolic pressure (ESP), independently of its role in the detemination of ESV, is undoubtly a point particularly representative of the instantaneous aortic pressure. For given cardiac output and stroke volume, ESP depends on MAoP (and thus on TSR) and on the difference ESP − MAoP. This latter is determined by characteristic impedance, amplitude and overlaping (time of return related to arterial stiffness) of the reflected waves. Taking into account SV tends to correct ESP from the part taken by LV pump itself in the determination of ESP. But Ea does not have the physical dimension of an impedance (it also incorporates heart rate) and ESP, isolated, does not give an idea of all the pressures and stress generated by the LV during ejection. A recent experimental and clinical article of Kelly et al. [22], nevertheless, elegantly illustrates the practical interest of this approximated measurement of the aortic part of the systolic load of the LV.

Left ventricle and systemic arterial hypertension*

In systemic hypertension, the structural and functional changes of the LV allow normalization of wall stress, although this latter may also be found less frequently to be decreased or even increased. Theoretically, LV "adaptation" could simply occur by positive inotropic stimulation, but this would increase metabolic demands by gram of myocardium. In all chronic mechanical overload situations, it is admitted that changes in LV mass and geometry occur to normalize wall stress and thus metabolic demands per gram of myocardium. However, nearly all the experimental and clinical studies have stressed the heterogeneity of LV changes in hypertension and suggested that factors, hemodynamic and non-hemodynamic ones, that determine LV mass, geometry and function, are far more complex than initially suspected. We will successively review:
- the more usual ways of evaluating LV function,

---

*In order to avoid the dilemma of a causal interpretation, this chapter is entitled "LV and hypertension" and not "LV of hypertension".

- the main modifications of the LV observed in hypertension and their various determinants,
- some aspects of the functional coupling between the LV and the AS and their possible consequences.

Evaluation of the left ventricle

The left ventricle is both a *pump*, generating pressure and delivering output, and a *muscle*, characterized by its intrinsic properties of contraction, relaxation and extension. Non-invasive isotopic and especially ultrasound techniques have taken precedence over the traditional hemodynamic and angiographic ones. In all cases, a very strict methology has to be required, as well as a critical knowledge of the methods and indices used, in order to avoid incorrect or exaggerated interpretation of the results. If LV wall thickness (h) is not homogeneous, multiplication of the echographic incidences is necessary, but quantification remains difficult. The ratio between septal and posterior wall thicknesses gives a simple but important information on the heterogeneity of the LV.

LV pump and muscle have to be described in quantitative, geometric and functional terms.

- *LV mass* (m), in absolute values or indexed by body surface area, is usually measured by angiography and/or echocardiography; only an increase of m (and not of wall thickness (h)) defines hypertrophy.
- *LV geometry* is generally expressed in terms of m/EDV or h/r ratio (r: LV end-diastolic longitudinal and/or transversal radius). LV geometry is different according to the pathology, aimed, if appropriated, at normalizing stress. An increase of the m/EDV ratio defines concentric remodeling or hypertrophy. One has to remember that because of LV form, maintaining constant the m/EDV ratio implies, in case of dilatation, a progressive wall thickening (4); and that an increase of the m/EDV ratio necessarily implies a concentric remodeling whatever the EDV.
- Objective of the evaluation of *LV function* is two-fold: characterization of the LV both during ejection and filling; and characterization of the properties of the LV chamber from the pressure-volume relations (pump function) and of the LV muscle from the stress-volume relations.

LV performance during ejection, sometimes restrictively called systolic, depends on loading conditions and contractility.

'*Pump function*'' indices measured during ejection: ejection fraction (EF), mean velocity of shortening ($\overline{VCF}$), are negatively related to maximal, mean or end-systolic stress. Among all indices, the most independent from loading conditions and the most representative of the contractile function of the LV pump is the maximal slope of the systolic pressure-volume relation [19] (probably incorrectly considered to be linear) (E max, active maximal elastance). This maximal slope is generally obtained and measured at end-systole according to the relation E max = ESP/(ESV − Vd) (Vd: ordinate at the origin). It necessitates determination of the end-systolic pressures and volumes corrresponding at least to two different levels of pressure, but at constant inotropy and heart rate.

For the evaluation of *LV muscle function*, slopes of the positive $ES\sigma$-ESV or negative $\overline{VCF}$-σ or EF-σ relations (this latter being not entirely indepen-dent of EDV) are generally used, instead of the tridimensional force-velocity-length relation, difficult to establish in man. Another more simple method is to index the actually measured EF by a theoretical EF calculated from stress and a normal regression line of reference defining a corrected EF [23].

LV function during filling (sometimes incorrectly and restrictively called diastolic) results from two successive and entirely different mechanisms:
- *Relaxation*, at end systole, which velocity depends on velocity of deacti-vation (related to inotropy), loading conditions (and thus on pressure, mass and m/EDV) during contraction and relaxation, and electrical and anatomic synchronisation of the LV muscle;
- *Diastole*, period during which LV muscle is passive, at rest, and the pressure-volume relationship exponential. LV chamber distensibility (evaluated by the time constant of this exponential relation kp) increases as intrinsic muscle distensibility is better and/or h/r ratio lower. Measure-ment of mitral velocities by Doppler-echocardiography easily allows ap-preciating filling conditions. But correct analysis of LV filling function can only be realized if are taken into account driving pressure (for evaluating the characteristics of the pump) and geometry of the chamber (for charac-terizing the muscle).

Evaluation of the segmental properties of the LV chamber and muscle is based on the same principles. However, precison is much more difficult and sometimes irrealistic because of difficulties of modelisation, yet debated for a normal and homogeneous ventricle.

LV modifications (and its determinants) in hypertension

Only the changes of the LV directly related to hypertension and without clinical sign of heart failure will be discussed here. Changes secondary to complications of the disease, coronary ones especially, are excluded. Numer-ous haemodynamic, isotopic and echocardiographic studies have generally shown that, in systemic hypertension:
- LV mass is increased in about half of the cases, considering the generally admitted higher echocardiographic limits of respectively 110 and 135 g/m^2 of body surface area in women and men [24];
- m/EDV is almost always more or less markedly increased;
- muscle contractility is normal most of the times, sometimes increased, sometimes decreased and its intrinsic distensibility normal or decreased;
- finally, systolic function of ejection of LV pump is generally increased, filling function altered and overall function preserved.

However, individual responses are heterogeneous, in relation with the variety of factors implicated in the determination of mass, geometry and function of the LV.

Determinants of mass

Main determinants of mass are [25, 26]:
- body surface area (BSA) and weight,
- pressures (the relative roles of rest, ambulatory and exercise pressures will not be discussed here);
- stroke volume (and EDV), positively correlated with m (all factors also well established for the athlete's heart); and
- intrinsic contractility of the muscle, which is negatively correlated with m (an increase of m being able to "compensate" an alteration of the inotropic state).

A specific role of the pulse pressure (and thus of aortic distensibility) has recently been discussed [27, 28]. Another important determinant is aging [5, 21, 22] (which yet per se represents a systolic pressure overload, but conversely, the young are more easily able to increase their LV mass). Blood viscosity, sodium intake and plasma volume, genetic factors (LV hypertrophy appears to be relatively more frequent in women and in blacks) and neuro-hormonal factors, especially the noradrenergic and the renin-angiotensin-aldosterone systems, the parathyroids, various vasoactives peptides and "growth factors", are also involved. The absence of close correlation between LV mass and the various aortic pressures has led to emphasise on the importance of non-hemodynamic factors in the regulation of LV mass and to suggest the role of primary (non adaptative) structural modifications in the establishment of hypertension. Actually, without neglecting the importance of genetic factors (ability to increase LV mass, a real predisposition to hypertension, is not equal in all individuals and increase of mass may precede hypertension), the debate remains open because:
- diversity of the haemodynamic factors alone is sufficient to explain several individual disparities,
- some neurohormonal modifications may perhaps only be mediators in an adaptative genesis which different steps remain largely unknown [29].

In practice, diversity of the factors determining LV mass, if not limiting the epidemiologic value of LV mass, explains that, depending on the reference norms and the characteristics of the populations, prevalence of echographic LV hypertrophy (LVH) in hypertension varies from 25 to 60% in the studies, and should incitate to personalize interpretation of a LV mass.

Increase of m/EDV

Increase of m/EDV is, in hypertension as in aortic stenosis, mandatory to normalization of systolic stress. This increase may theoretically be achieved by wall thickening and reduction of internal diameters, yielding only a mild increase of LV mass. But in clinical pratice, this scheme is not the most frequently observed and its deleterious consequences on LV filling and preservation of stroke volume are obvious. m/EDV is more closely related to the various aortic pressures and physical properties of the arterial system (Zc, Co, Ea) than m [16, 21, 27, 30]. Similarly, in some hypertensions as in hypertrophic cardiomyopathies, an increase of m/EDV appears to be able to compensate for a reduction of the inotropic properties of the LV myocardium. On the other hand, m/EDV is not positively correlated with SV (on the contrary). As for mass, the mechanisms inducing LV geometric changes in hypertension, as well as the relative importance of adaptative processes or primary abnormalities, are still imperfectly known. The close correlation observed between m/EDV and Zc or Co suggests joint structural modifications of both the AS and the LV and/or a causal relationship between the ones and the others. In hypertension, systolic stresses and especially end-systolic stress are generally normal, and changes in LV mass and geometry are said to be appropriate. Nevertheless, situations exist where systolic stress is increased or, on the contrary, reduced. In the first case, LV is insufficiently adapted to generated pressures and/or stroke volume and/or intrinsic properties of its muscle (as in dilated cardiomyopathies). If systolic stress is decreased, it may correspond to an "overcompensation" of hypertension by the LV, or to geometric modifications "compensating" both a mechanical overload and, as in hypertrophic cardiomyopathies, decreased contractility. Evaluation of LV muscle function is necessary in order to make the distinction.

Studies dealing with LV pump and muscle function in hypertension have reported non unequivocal but in general coherent results

LV muscle function in hypertension
In at least 50% of the subjects and sometimes more, depending on the series, except for methodologic differences, LV muscle contractility and intrinsic distensibility are considered normal. In 10 to 25% of the subjects depending on the studies, systolic function of the muscle seems to be altered [16, 31, 32], more frequently in case of associated obesity. This feature generally represents so-called "pathological" LVH as opposed to the excellent functional properties of the "physiological" LVH, e.g. in athletes. Passive distensibility of these pathologic muscles is generally reduced. These functional changes are generally explained by abnormalities of the beta-adrenergic receptors, fiber disarray and mainly fibrosis. It seems now likely that myocytic hypertrophy (actual muscular LV) are under the control of mechanical factors whereas development of interstitial, perivascular and vascular wall collagen fibrosis are under the control of hormonal factors, especially aldosterone [33]. Thus, regulation of connective tissue growth seems to respond to stimuli and pathways different from the ones governing myocytes growth. Conversely, in some subjects, 25% approximately in the series of Lutas and coll. [23] and de Simone and coll. [34], contractile function of LV muscle appears to be increased with even a bimodal distribution of the population. This generally

corresponds to "borderline" or moderate hypertension, characterized by an "hyperdynamic" state associating increased cardiac output and normal or midly reduced systemic vascular resistances. But increased contractile function of LV muscle has also been reported in other forms of hypertension and even in some systolic hypertensions in the elderly. It is not at present demonstrated that the noradrenergic system is the sole implicated nor that this profile always represents an initial stage in the establishment of some hypertensions. An increase of myocardial function seems enable LV to compensate for a quantitative and geometric defect of its adaptation.

LV pump function and hypertension

Maximal active elastance of the LV pump, sometimes only approximated by the simple ESP/ESV ratio, is generally increased in hypertension, even in subjects with altered myocardial contractility [16]. It is related to Ea and m/EDV and reflects the ability of the overall LV pump to maintain normal or even reduced ESV, despite increases in aortic pressures, especially ESP.

LV filling is often and early altered, even before there is increase in LV mass. Relaxation is slowed probably because of the increase in m/EDV reducing the effective load opposing to LV wall at this time. Diastolic distensibility is also reduced by increase of m/EDV and sometimes reduction of intrinsic distensibility of the muscle. This results in
– an increase in LV filling pressures;
– and at identical age and heart rate, an increase of the A/E ratio in the echocardiogram in most of hypertensive subjects; this aspect is unanimously recognized as the earliest indice of the consequences of hypertension on LV.

As in normals, A/E is related to age and SAP, but is independent of LV mass and very rarely found to be related to wall thickness or the h/r ratio. These observations are not easy to explain and should probably bear some relation with the complexity of the mechanisms regulating LV filling [35]. Nevertheless, increase in the atrial contribution of a less compliant LV filling results in left atrial hypertrophy and/or dilatation and explains the poor haemodynamic tolerance of atrial tachycardia or fibrillation during hypertension.

Overall LV pump function is preserved in a very large majority of cases: SV is preserved, stroke work (SW) and power (W) are increased, EF is generally within normal ranges. Table 1 summarizes the main correlations between the characteristics of the LV and the arterial system obtained by our group in 25 normals (N) and 20 subjects with sustained hypertension (HT) (arterial pressure > 160/90 mm Hg); Table 2 the ones between m or m/EDV and the indices of muscle and pump function of the LV.

LV function during exercise has been studied in some cases. A reduced

Table 1. Simple matrix of the correlation between structural and functional LV indices and arterial function indices

r p	MAoP		Co		Ea		TSR		HR		Ea'		SW	
m	0.59	<0.001	0.66	<0.001	0.39	<0.01	0.44	<0.005	–		0.53	<0.001	0.53	<0.001
m/EDV	0.72	<0.001	0.81	<0.001	0.76	<0.001	0.71	<0.001	0.33	<0.05	0.59	<0.001	–	NS
E$_{lv}$	0.46	0.001	0.43	<0.005	0.55	<0.001	0.49	0.001	–		–	NS	–	NS
corrected EF	–	NS	–	NS	–	NS	–	NS	–	NS	–	NS	–	NS
k$_p$	0.63	<0.001	0.56	<0.001	0.65	<0.001	0.57	<0.001	0.28	0.06	0.42	<0.005	–	NS

(n = 45).

Table 2. Simple matrix of the correlations between LV mass and structure and indices of LV muscle and pump function

r ⟍ p	m		m/EDV		EF corrected	
EVG	–		0.59		0.33	
		NS		<0.01		<0.05
k_p	0.40		0.57			
		<0.01		<0.001		
corrected EF	−0.52		–			
		<0.001		NS		

(n = 45).

maximal exercise capacity is generally observed, in part due to the premature stopping of the tests because of an excessive increase in blood pressure and/or an early acceleration of heart rate. In some hypertensive patients with LVH, EF increases less during exercise, the respective role of alteration of systolic and/or diastolic function having been discussed. Association of overweight, important sodium intake or "eccentric" hypertrophy seems to be deleterious. It has recently been demonstrated that physical training may allow a reduction in MAoP after several weeks in some hypertensions; LV mass is not reported to be concomitantly reduced, probably because of the increase in SV, but no deleterious consequence on the LV seems to contra-indicate exercise. It has not been demonstrated that a "supranormal" function of the LV pump observed at rest in some hypertensives may correspond to an abnormal increase of arterial pressure during exercise.

Classification of the LV in hypertension
Classification of the LV in hypertension is made difficult by individual dispar-ities. If the objectives (search of a particular etiological profile, mainly re-finement of the prognostic signification of LVH) are common to the various authors, criteria (m, m/EDV, function, σ . . .) differ. The results of a recent and remarkable Italian and North-American study [5] should, at least at the present state of our knowledge, be use as a framework. It was conducted in 165 untreated hypertensive subjects (arterial pressure always higher than 140/90 mm Hg) and 125 normotensive subjects of identical age, weight, body surface area and sex-ratio. Depending on the distribution of the echocardio-graphic values of m and h/r, compared to the normals, hypertensives were classified in 4 groups:
– In 52% of them, m and h/r were within the limits of the normal subjects. This represents an overall subgroup of intermittent (normal MAoP or moderate hypertensives, which h/r ratio, however, was significantly in-creased compared to normals. ESσ, LV pump and muscle function were on average identical to the ones of the normals.
– 13% had a normal LV mass, but a markedly increased h/r ratio. This.

exclusive "concentric remodeling" of the LV corresponds to more elevated peripheral resistances and lower cardiac output than in the other hypertensives. Observation of decreased ES is compatible with an "overcompensation" of the pressure overload, since it appears yet to be in part "compensated" by the reduced SV and a relative hypovolemia. LV muscle function is on average normal, but when standard deviations are considered, it seems likely that it was depressed in some subjects.

– 8% only of these LV exhibit the traditional pattern of homogeneous concentric LVH, with a joint increase of m and h/r. SAP and DAP are more elevated in this group than in the other hypertensives. ESσ are also lower than normal and seem, because of the apparent normal LV muscle function, to be related to an overcompensation of the LV.

– 27% have a LVH qualified as eccentric by the authors as m is increased and h/r within the extreme limits of the normals. However, h/r ratio is on average statistically higher than in normals. This group has two particular characteristics: (1) more spherical form of the LV, increase in ED diameter and SV suggest the existence of a volume overload associated with hypertension or generating it (calculated TSR are on average normal); and (2) an insufficient hypertrophy is present at least in some subjects.

Indeed, ES stresses are not significantly different, but tend to be more elevated than in normals and the standard deviation is particularly large. Muscle function (expressed in percentage of a theoretical "normal" EF calculated from ESσ) is roughly normal. But it may be overestimated in this group where ED diameter is increased and the amplitude of standard deviation is compatible with the existence of an alteration of myocardial contractility in some subjects and, on the contrary, an increase in others.

These results confirm the heterogeneity of LV mass, geometry and function previously described in hypertension by haemodynamic or echocardiographic studies. The main differences between the other series of the literature and ours [16, 31, 32, 36] may be explained by difference in population (generally, only hypertension with arterial pressure constantly higher than 160/90 mm Hg having been considered).

Two particular clinical forms deserve individualised consideration: assymetrical septal hypertrophy (ASH) and hypertension of the elderly.

– Assymetrical septal hypertrophy (ASH) (septal thickness/posterior wall thickness >1.3) is from far the most frequent of the heterogeneous wall thickening patterns in hypertension. Its prevalence is variously appreciated (from 5 to 55% of hypertensives). Sometimes considered most frequent in borderline hypertension, in hyperdynamic states or in the aged, ASH does not appear to be related to age, sex or clinical characteristics.

– Aging is accompanied, even when DAP is normal, by systolic hypertension and the physiologic changes of the AS and the LV (hypertrophy and concentric remodeling) are close to the ones observed in hypertension.

Therefore, it is not surprising than the association of age with authentic systolo-diastolic hypertension leads to a higher prevalence of concentric LVH

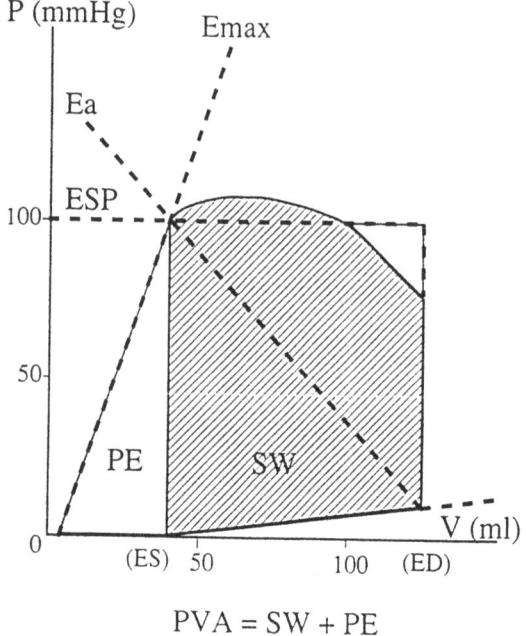

$$PVA = SW + PE$$

Figure 1. Schematic representation of a left ventricular (LV) pressure (P)-volume (V) relation. ED: end-diastole, ES: end-systole, ESP: end-systolic pressure, SW: stroke work, PE: potential energy, PVA: pressure-volume area, Ea: ESP/stroke volume, Emax: LV ma.ximal active elastance.

and filling modifications. It is in the elderly that functional intraventricular obstructions have been described and that the differentiation from authentic hypertrophic cardiomyopathies may be difficult. Nevertheless, overall function of the LV pump remains generally preserved, even in the few subjects in whom alterations of LV muscle properties have been observed.

Ventricular-arterial "coupling" in hypertension

There are several ways of assessing the LV–AS coupling [37], and the various characteristics of an arterial system favouring relatively low systolic arterial pressures and relatively high diastolic arterial pressures in consideration to the aortic pressure have been previously analyzed [38]. Similarly, the main relations between on the one hand m, m/EDV and Emax, and on the other hand various indices of the AS have been discussed in the previous paragraphs. In this chapter, we will only address the "functional" coupling between LV active maximal elastance and arterial effective elastance, evaluated by the Ea/Emax ratio, because of its role in the overall function of the LV, the achievement of a "maximal" stroke work and part of the mechanical efficiency of the LV pump (Figure 1). Actually:
- Ea/ Emax represents a main determinant of EF: Ea/Emax =

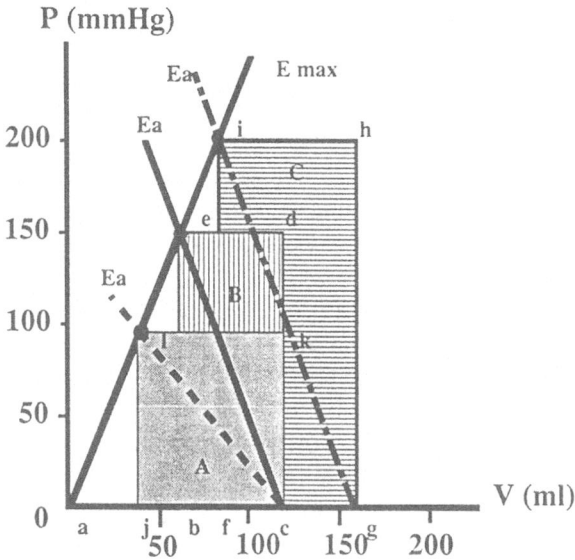

Figure 2. Relations between on one hand Emax, Ea, and the Ea/Emax ratio, and on the other hand SV and ejection fraction (EF), stroke work (Wc) and the Wc/PVA ratio. For given Emax and end-diastolic volume (EDV) of respectively 2.5 mm Hg·ml^{-1} and 120 ml (beat A and B), maximal stroke work is obtained when Ea/Emax =1, but in this case, SV, EF and Wc/PVA decrease. (A) Ea/Emax = 0.50, SV = 80 ml, EF = 0.66, Wc (rectangle jckl) = 8000 mmHg·ml, Ep (triangle ajl) = 2000 mm Hg·ml, Wc/PVA = 0.80. (B) Ea/Emax = 1, SV = 60 ml, EF=0.50, Wc (rectangle bcde) = 9000 mm Hg·ml, Ep (triangle abe) = 4500 mm Hg·ml, Wc/PVA = 0.66. For a given Ea/Emax, SV and Wc increase with EDV but EF and Wc/PVA remain unchanged. (C) Ea/Emax = 1, VS = 80 ml, FE = 0.50, Wc = (rectangle fghi) = 16000 mm Hg·ml, EP (triangle afi) = 8000 mm Hg·ml, Wc/PVA = 0.66.

(ESV − Vd)/SV = EDV/SV − Vd/SV − 1. In the absence of LV dilatation, Vd may be neglected in face of SV and Emax approximated by the sole ratio ESP/ESV. EF is thus directly related to the systolic function of ejection of the LV pump and inversely proportional to the transfer function of the arterial system, illustrating well the importance of the physical properties of the AS in the determination of the overall function of the LV pump.

– Maximal stroke work is the one possibly performed by LV pump for a given value of Emax [39]. It depends on EDV and on the Ea/Emax ratio. For a given EDV, a simple arithmetic calculation demonstrates that maximal work is achieved when Ea = Emax and thus Ea/Emax = 1 (Figure 2).

– Suga et al. [40] have experimentally demonstrated that myocardial VO$_2$ per gram and per beat (m VO$_2$) was proportional to the total pressure-volume area (PVA) (PVA = cardiac stroke work (SW) + potential energy (PE)) under the ESP/ESV relation of the LV (Figure 1). Ordinate at the origin increases with metabolism and inotropy, but the slope remains unchanged. Nozawa et al. [41] have confirmed in situ these results on the dog intact heart. The slope of the mVO_2/SPV relation is identical in case of LVH. Potential modifications of the slope of this relation with inotropy have led to contradictory results [39,42]. The mechanical efficiency of the LV may thus be decomposed into two parts, one corresponding to the SW/SPV ratio, the other depending on the proper energetic demands of basal metabolism and inotropy. Indeed, SW/PVA is inversely related to Ea/Emax.

Thus, for a given Emax, the function of the arterial system, evaluated by Ea, determines the achievement of a SW more or less close to the maximal stroke work, and in part the mechanical efficiency of the myocardium. A normal LV functions with a Ea/Emax ratio close to 0.60 [43], thus relatively far from the maximal possible stroke work, but with an "economic" efficiency SW/PVA of about 0.75. In case of LV failure, the Ea/Emax ratio increases, approaching the maximal possible stroke work [43] but decreasing the SW/PVA ratio. These observations emphasize the two alternative finalities of the behaviour of the LV and the LV· AS couple, achievement of a more important stroke work on one hand or efficiency on the other hand.

This aspect of the ventricular-arterial coupling is illustrated by our data in normals (N) and subjects with sustained hypertension (HT). The clinical characteristics, the techniques used, the measures and calculations performed (except those concerning the functional coupling between the LV and the AS) have been previously reported [16]. By comparison with the EF of the normals ($64 \pm 6\%$), patients with hypertension can be separated in three groups: HT 1 – normal EF (n = 8), HT 2: increased EF ($>70\%$) (n = 5), HT 3: decreased EF ($<57\%$) (50–57 %) (n = 7). SW/ PVA ratio was 0.78 ± 0.05 in normals and 0.78 ± 0.02, 0.88 ± 0.03, 0.70 ± 0.02 respectively in HT 1, 2 and 3.

End-diastolic pressures and volumes of normals, HT and the three sub-groups of HT are represented with the corresponding values of Ea and Elv (Elv = ESP/ESV and approximates Emax if Vd is neglected) in Figures 3, 4. Ea and its various components (TSR, HR, Ea') are increased in HT compared with normals but identical to the three groups of HT. Only hetero-geneity of ESP/ESV differenciates each of the three groups of HT and determines the observed differences in the Ea/Elv, EF and SW/PVA ratio, differences much more important than observed with only aging.

Interpretation of these results should be cautious because of methodologic limits: ESP and ESP/ESV especially are only approximated values of the aortic pressures of ejection and of Emax, respectively; and because of their consequences on the efficiency and the metabolic demands of the myocar-dium remains hypothetical in the absence of concomitant measure of mVO_2 and of the PVA/mVO_2 relation. Nevertheless, they confirm that, regarding the relatively univocal changes of the AS, the LV response in hypertension is heterogeneous in terms of m, m/EDV, systolic function of ejection and

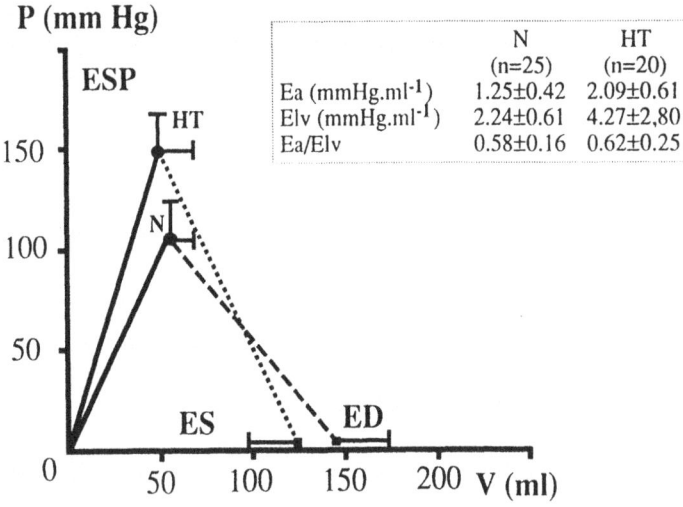

Figure 3. Left ventricular end-diastolic (ED) and end-systolic (ES) pressures (P) and volumes (V) in normals (N) and hypertensives (HT).

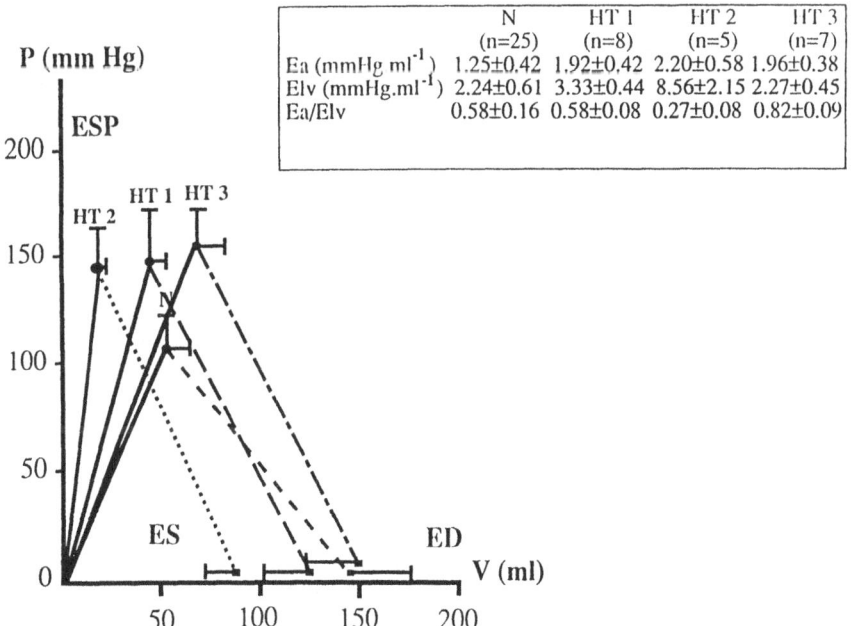

Figure 4. Left ventricular end-diastolic (ED) and end-systolic (ES) pressures (P) and volumes (V) in normals (N) and hypertensives (HT).

also LV–AS coupling. Such an approach is likely to be considered in evaluating and following an hypertension in order to explain the respective prognostic significations of the changes of m, geometry and function of the LV pump and muscle.

Pronostic and therapeutic consequences

Left ventricle and prognosis of hypertension

In hypertension, the "independent" deleterious prognostic signification of electrocardiographic LVH, especially when accompanied by abnormalities of repolarisation, has been recognized for a long time [44] and confirmed [45–47]. More recently, this prognostic signification has been extended to echographic LVH [48, 49]. If LVH may be considered in some cases as a simple marker of the risk of extracardiac complications, associated or resulting myocardial ischemia, heart failure, arrhythmias – statistically and reasonably – promote LVH as an authentical and independent cardiovascular risk factor.

Myocardial ischemia

Even in the absence of coronary atheroma, myocardial ischemia is probably frequent within LV in hypertension. Reasons for myocardial ischemia with angiographically normal coronary arteries are multiple in hypertension (4).

– Metabolic demands may be increased: there is a positive relationship between the overall myocardial metabolic demands in oxygen and LV mass and also a positive relationship between the metabolic demands in oxygen per gram of myocardium and end-systolic stress which may be increased in case of quantitative or geometrically inappropriate LV and/or defect in contractility.

– Reduction of the exchange capacities of the coronary circulation has also been suggested: reduction of capillary density with increase in intercapillary distance, reduction of the area/volume of the hypertrophied cell.

– But reduction in coronary reserve is the main accused. Reasons are numerous: insufficient development, especially in adults, of the coronary circulation, compared to the development of LV mass, with a positive correlation between LV mass and reduction of coronary reserve; increase in systolic stress increasing the level of the plateau of coronary autoregulation; increase in extravascular resistances by increase of diastolic pressures and stress altering subendocardial perfusion; vascular wall thickening and increase in interstitial and perivascular fibrosis; increase in blood viscosity; delay of diastolic perfusion resulting from prolongation of relaxation . . . .

A relation between reduction of coronary reserve and extent of fibrosis has also been established. The role of an abnormality of coronary arterial muscle has been suggested in hypertensives without hypertrophy or proximal coronary artery disease by an abnormal vasoconstrictive response observed after ergonovine infusion. The same group [50] has more recently obtained results compatible with abnormalities of the endothelial function in the coronary circulation in hypertension: acetylcholine (endothelium-dependent vasodilator) reduces arterial diameter and reduces coronary blood flow in 8 hypertensives compared to 6 normal subjects. On the contrary, response to nitroglycerin (endothelium – independent vasodilator) is identical in both groups. Thus, both anatomic distal coronary circulation and "functional" coronary pathologies probably coexist in hypertension, but their evaluation remains difficult and the therapeutic consequences still belong to the research field.

In Practice
As authentical myocardial ischemia with angiographically normal coronary arteries is possible in systemic hypertension, anginal pain, electrocardiographic abnormalities (at rest, exercise or during Holter monitoring) suggesting ischemia and even – at least for some authors – defects in myocardial scintigraphy during exercise or after dipyridamole infusion have a low specificity for the diagnosis of coronary artery stenoses.
– The high prevalence of obliterative coronary atherosclerosis complicating systemic hypertension increases the incidence and severity of myocardial ischemia in hypertension
– A pathogenetic role for ischemia is often suggested in ventricular hyperexcitability and "pathological" LVH, in part mediated by increase in the proportion of non-muscular tissues (fibrosis, necrosis . . .). Moreover, acute myocardial ischemia may result in systolic dysfunction and aggravation of diastolic dysfunction in systemic hypertension.
– Coronary complications are the most frequent and lethal during hypertension, and the particular severity of myocardial infarction has long been recognized. Moreover, recent results suggest an increase in coronary risk in treated hypertensive with coronary insufficiency when DAP is decreased below 85 mm Hg. Risks of an a excessive reduction of DAP may be easily explained: in case of proximal coronary stenosis, coronary driving pressure is lower than central DAP, and reduction in coronary artery reserve increases the critical pressure below which coronary blood flow decreases with pressure.

Left ventricular failure
The risk of left ventricular failure doubles when LVH is present. Alterations in LV filling are early markers of an impact of hypertension on the LV, but isolated, they rarely result in congestive LV failure. However, a poorly distensible LV is particularly sensitive to even mild alterations of the systolic performance, these latter appearing to be constant with time because of the development of a pathological LVH and/or myocardial ischemia. LV failure with normal (or nearly normal) ejection function of the LV pump (mildly or

not dilated LV) is frequent. Alteration of the intrinsic contractility of the muscle with increase in collagen and occurence of fibrosis or low end-systolic stress constitute deleterious markers in the disease.

Ventricular arrhythmias

Since the first observations of Clémenty et al. [51], the high prevalence of ventricular hyperexcitability associated with electric or echographic LVH has been largely confirmed. These ventricular arrhythmias appear to be more frequent and electrically more severe in the elderly or when LV mass, end-systolic stress or EDV are increased. Myocardial ischemia or associated coronary microcirculation abnormalities represent independent risk factors and the role of some treatments, at rest and during exercise, diuretics especially, has also been suggested. However, the real prognostic signification of these ventricular arrhythmias, and especially their relation with potential sudden deaths, remains to be established.

What risks for which left ventricle?

Finally, the present debate is no more to discuss the deleterious signiflcation of LVH but, because of the individual disparities of the LV in hypertension and the necessarily large ranges of "normal" LV mass, to affirm the cardiac and extra-cardiac prognostic signification of some changes of the LV. Existence of concentric LVH has a predictive value of LV failure; coronary complications and an electric or echographic LVH also are independent markers of the risk of occurence of cerebrovascular accidents. Similarly, abnormalities of the optic fundus or proteinuria appear to be more frequent in some concentric LVH. Low end-systolic stress has a deleterious prognostic signification. In the spontaneously hypertensive rat, depression of LV muscle function also appears as the most sensitive of the markers. Finally, Koren et al. [52], with a ten years follow-up, have reported that the highest risk was observed in systemic hypertension with concentric LVH (21% of deaths, 31% of clinical events) and the lowest risk in hypertension with normal LV geometry (no death, only 11% of clinical events), risk being intermediate for patients with concentric remodeling of the LV or so-called eccentric LVH. Further studies are obviously required to more precisely define, in terms of mass, geometry, function (pump-muscle, ejection-filling), the left ventricules at risk and to determine the overall genetic, haemodynamic, neurohormonal factors which give to the changes of the LV, both actor and victim in hypertension, the signification of a marker as well as a risk factor.

Therapeutic consequences

Unlike cerebrovascular complications, cardiac and coronary complications are incompletely prevented by antihypertensive treatments, at least with the traditional ones and within the ranges of follow-up of the large controlled trials. This evidence, the reasons of which are poorly understood and probably not unequivocal, constitutes a current therapeutic challenge for the future.

LVH regression

LVH regression has been for some years a main target of the treatment of systemic hypertension. It has been observed with almost all antihypertensive treatments. LVH regression becomes noticeable within a few weeks, but is prolonged for several months. It is generally associated with a regression of LV filling abnormalities. Systolic function of the LV pump is preserved or even improved. As for valvular cardiopathies, it is however possible that even a complete correction of the mechanical overload may not always and entirely normalize the left ventricle. Slow albeit possible regression of collagen overload [53] however constitutes a good indirect argument in favour of a progressive improvement of cardiac muscle function. Sustained improvement of potential LV failure, arrhythmias and to a lesser extent myocardial ischemia, obviously results from LVH regression. Since the expected variations of LV mass with treatment are generally lower than 15%, a real methodologic problem, due to the imperfection of measurement techniques (ultrasonic especially [54]) and mainly their intra and interindividual reproducibility (requiring a rigorous methodology, which is not always the case) [24] arises. Three points require brief comments:

– Improvement in prognosis by LVH regression by itself has not yet been definitely demonstrated, even if some preliminary results seem to confirm this hypothesis [55, 56].
– All antihypertensive treatments do not have – at identical reduction of mean aortic pressure – the same efficacy on LV mass reduction [57]. But few comparative controlled studies are available and a too simplistic LV mass/MAoP relationship fails to recognise the multifactorial determination of LV mass.
– The cardiac consequences of systemic hypertension correspond to a disease of the overall cardiovascular system. LVH regression should be paralleled by a joint and harmonious improvement of heart and artery remodeling and reparation [52], even if the evolutive modifications of the one and the other are dissociated in time [58].

Finally, LVH probably only represents the most rough expression of the cardiac consequences of systemic hypertension. The exemple of athletes demonstrates that all LVH are not necessarily deleterious and that the adaptative function of LVH may and should be respected. Since now, we can use techniques of exploration allowing us to refine, in terms of mass, geometry and function, the various components of the cardiac consequences of hypertension. The main objective of treatment is obviously to control hypertension, but also to guide and correct the mechanisms that render LVH inadapted or dangerous. It may be possible that improvements in genetics and pharmacology may give us tomorrow the tools for correcting the mismatch in structure and function of the LV – arterial system coupling induced by hypertension or even for preventing its establishment in identified high-risk subjects.

"Logic" of the medical treatment of hypertension [59–60]

A better understanding of the deterrninants of the systolic load of the LV may explain, for a large part, the observed disparities between reductions in AoP and LV mass.

– Antihypertensive treatments that decrease AoP but increase cardiac output do not reasonably have significant effect on LV mass [61, 62]. On the other hand, dietetical actions, by reducing overweight or sodium overload are remarkably effective.

– Exclusive vasodilators of the distal arterial system only very incompletely reduce the real opposition to LV ejection (represented by Zc and the reflected waves) in contrast to vasodilators having simultaneously a direct action on proximal or intermediate arteries which decrease aortic impedance to frequencies requiring the most of LV energy [9, 38]. Some preliminary results suggest that nitrate derivatives (or molsidomine), potent vasodilators of the intermediate arterial and venous systems, would take a role in the treatment of systolic hypertension by selectively reducing impedance to LV ejection [63] and probably also systolic volumes during exercise.

– Drugs that, by reaction, "stimulate" the neurohormonal systems implicated in the genesis of LVH do not produce a complete reduction of LV mass, at least when used alone. On the contrary, those who decrease the activation of these systems and/or have a direct trophic inhibitory action appear to that extent highly more effective. The experimentally deleterious influence on the development of non-muscular tissues of the agents stimulating the renin-angiotensin-aldosterone system does not have received at the present time clinical confirmation.

– Beyond controlling arterial tension levels, taking care of the target organs and especially of the left ventricle are part of the criteria of efficacy of an antihypertensive treatment. Such an attitude probably has a double advantage: the subject being its own control, it tends to "rub" the individual disparities in LV mass determination, and it allows a personalized treatment, eventually modified following the results of each particular case.

Improvement in understanding the physiopathology and the treatment of systemic hypertension, disease of the overall cardiovascular system, should now progress by managing the prevention and the correction of the multifactorial determinants of the arterial disease and aging.

References

1. Tarazi RC. The role of the heart in hypertension. Clin Sci 1982; 63: 347–58.

2. Frohlich ED, Chobanian AV, Devereux RB et al. The Heart in Hypertension. N Engl J Med 1992; 327: 998–1008.
3. Pearson AC, Pasierski T, Labovitz AJ. Left ventricular hypertrophy: diagnosis, prognosis, and management. Am Heart J 1991; 121: 148–57.
4. Strauer BE. Cardiopathie hypertensive. In: Swynghedauw B, ed. Hypertrophie et insuffisance cardiaques. Paris: INSERM, 1990: 479–504.
5. Ganau A, Devereux RB, Roman MJ, et al. Patterns of left ventricular hypertrophy and geometric remodeling in essential hypertension. J Am Coll Cardiol 1992; 19: 1550–8.
6. Gosse P, Dallocchio M. Remodelage ventriculaire gauche dans l'hypertension artérielle. Physiopathologie. Arch Mal Coeur 1991; 84(IV): 69–72.
7. Swynghcdauw B. Remodeling of the heart in response to chronic mechanical overload. Eur. Heart J 1989; 10: 935–43.
8. Weber KT, Anversa P, Armstrong PW, et al. Remodeling and reparation of the cardiovascular system. J Am Coll Cardiol 1992; 20: 3–16.
9. Merillon JP, Fontenier GJ, Lerallut JF, et al. Aortic input impedance in normal man and arterial hypertension: its modification during changes in aortic pressure. Cardiovasc Res 1982; 16: 646–56.
10. Milnor WR. Cardiac dynamics. In: Milnor WR, ed. Hemodynamics. Second Edition. Baltimore: Williams and Wilkins, 1989: 260–93.
11. Nichols WW, O'Rourke MF. Input impedance as ventricular load. In: Nichols WW, O'Rourke MF, ed. McDonald's Blood Flow in Arteries, 3rd Edition, London: Edward Arnold, 1990: 330–42.
12. Sunagawa K, Maughan Wl, Burkhoff D, Sagawa K. Left ventricular interaction with arterial load studied in isolated canine ventricle. Am J Physiol 1983; 245: H773–80.
13. Milnor WR. Arterial impedance as ventricular afterload. Circ Res 1975; 36: 565–70.
14. Merillon JP, Lebras Y, Chastre J, et al. Forward and backward waves in the arterial system, their relationship to pressure waves form. Eur Heart J 1983; 4 (suppl G): 13–20.
15. Simon ACh, O'Rourke M, Levenson J. Arterial distensibility and its effect on wave reflection and cardiac loading in cardiovascular disease. Coronary Artery Dis 1991; 2: 1111–20.
16. Merillon JP, Motte G, Masquet C, Azancot I, Guiomard A, Gourgon R. Relationship between physical properties of the arterial system and left ventricular performance in the course of aging and arterial hypertension. Eur Heart J 1982; 3 (suppl A): 95–102.
17. Levy BI, Safar M. Postcharge ventriculaire et impedance aortique. In: Swynghedauw B, ed. Hypertrophie et insuffisance cardiaques. Paris: INSERM, 1990: 563–72.
18. O'Rourke MF. Part 4: Clinical implications of altered cushioning function. In: O'Rourke MF, ed. Arterial function in health and disease. Edinburgh: Churchill Livingstone, 1982: 185–261.
19. Suga H, Sagawa K. Instantaneous pressure-volume relationships and their ratio in the excised, supported canine left ventricle. Circ Res 1974; 35: 117–26.
20. Merillon JP, Motte G, Fruchaud J, Masquet C, Gourgon R. Evaluation of the elasticity and characteristic impedance of the ascending aorta in man. Cardiovasc Res 1978; 12: 401–6.
21. Dahan M, Paillole C, Ferreira BV, Gourgon R. Doppler echocardiographic study of the consequences of aging and hypertension on the left ventricle and aorta. Eur Heart J 1990; 11 (suppl G): 39–45.
22. Kelly RP, Ting CT, Yang TM, et al. Effective arterial elastance as index of arterial vascular load in humans. Circulation 1992; 86: 513–21.
23. Lutas EM, Devereux RB, Reis G, et al. Increased cardiac performance in mild essential hypertension. Left ventricular mechanics. Hypertension 1985; 7: 979–88.
24. Devereux RB. Evaluation of cardiac structure and function by echocardiography and other non invasive techniques. In: Laragh JH, Brenner BM, ed. Hypertension: Pathophysiology, diagnosis, and management. New York: Raven Press, 1990: 1479–92.
25. Devereux RB, Pickering TG, Alderman MH, Chien S, Borer JS, Laragh JH. Left ventricular

hypertrophy in hypertension. Prevalence and relationship to pathophysiologic variables. Hypertension 1987; 9 (Suppl II): II-53–60.

26. Ganau A, Devereux RB, Pickering TG, et al. Relation of left ventricular hemodynamic load and contractile performance to left ventricular mass in hypertension. Circulation 1990; 81: 25–36.

27. Girerd X, Laurent S, Pannier B, Asmar R, Safar M. Arterial distensibility and left ventricular hypertrophy in patients with sustained essential hypertension. Am Heart J 1991; 122: 1210–4.

28. Pannier B, Brunnel P, El Aroussay W, Lacolley P, Safar M. Pulse pressure and echocardiographic findings in essential hypertension. J Hypertens 1989; 7: 127–32.

29. Swynghedauw B, Moalic JM, Delcayre C. Genèse de l'hypertrophie cardiaque. Induction mécanique et changements transitoires de l'expression de signaux de croissance. Synthèse des protéines, du RNA et du DNA. In: Swynghedauw B, ed. Hypertrophie et insuffisance cardiaques. Paris: INSERM, 1990: 21–66.

30. Bouthier JD, De Luca N, Safar ME, Simon ACh. Cardiac hypertrophy and arterial distensibility in essential hypertension. Am Heart J 1985; 109: 1345–52.

31. Boudoulas H, Mantzouratos D, Sohn YH, Weissler AM. Left ventricular mass and systolic performance in chronic systemic hypertension. Am J Cardiol 1986; 57: 232–7.

32. Takahashi M, Sasayama S, Kawai C, Kotoura H. Contractile performance of the hypertrophied ventricle in patients with systemic hypertension. Circulation 1980; 62: 116–26.

33. Weber KT, Brilla CG. Pathological hypertrophy and cardiac interstitium. Fibrosis and renin-angiotensin-aldosterone system. Circulation 1991; 83: 1849–65.

34. De Simone G, Lorenzo LD, Costantino G, Moccia D, Buonissimo S, Divitis OD. Supernormal contractility in primary hypertension without left ventricular hypertrophy. Hypertension 1988; 11: 457–63.

35. Ollivier JP, Gaillard JH, Quatre JM, Assoun B, Bussy E, Plotton C. Vieillissement naturel, hypertension artérielle et remplissage ventriculaire gauche. Arch Mal Coeur 1990; 83: 1143–7.

36. Gosse P, Roudaut R, Durandet P, Le Herissier A, Dallochio M. Caractéristiques morphologiques et fonctionnelles du coeur dans l'hypertension artérielle non traitée. Arch Mal Coeur 1991; 84: 1033–7.

37. Shroff SG, Weber KT, Janicki JS. Coupling of the left ventricle with the systemic arterial circulation. In: Nichols WW, O'Rourke MF, ed. McDonald's Blood flow in Arteries, 3rd Edition. London: Edward Arnold, 1990: 343–59.

38. O'Rourke ME. Steady and pulsatile energy losses in the systemic circulation under normal conditions and in simulated arterial disease. Cardiovasc Res 1967; 1: 313–26.

39. Nozawa T, Yasumura Y, Futaki S, Tanaka N, Uenishi M, Suga H. Efficiency of energy transfer from pressure-volume area to external mechanical work increases with contractile state and decreases with afterload in the left ventricle of the anesthetized closed-chest dog. Circulation 1988; 77: 1116–24.

40. Suga H, Hayashi T, Shirahata M. Ventricular systolic pressure volume area as predictor of cardiac oxygen consumption. Am J Physiol 1981; 240: H539–44.

41. Nozawa T, Yasamura Y, Futaki S, et al. Relation between oxygen consumption and pressure-volume area of in situ dog heart. Am J Physiol 1987; 253; H31–40.

42. Wolff MR, De Tombe PP, Harasawa Y, et al. Alterations in left ventricular mechanics, energetics, and contractile reserve in experimental hcart failure. Circ Res 1992; 70: 516–29.

43. Asanoi H, Sasayama S, Tomoki K. Ventriculoarterial coupling in normal and failing heart in humans. Circ Res 1989; 65: 483–93.

44. Kannel WB, Gordon T, Offutt D. Left ventricular hypertrophy by electrocardiogram: prevalence, incidence and mortality in the Framingham study. Ann Intern Med 1969; 71: 89–105.

45. Dunn FG, McLenachan J, Isles CG, et al. Left ventricular hypertrophy and mortality in

hypertension: an analysis of data from the Glasgow Blood Pressure Clinic. J Hypertens 1990; 8: 775–82.

46. Girerd X, Darne B, Lang T, Le Heuzey JY, Chretien J, Guize L. Mortalité cardiovasculaire en fonction de l'hypertrophie ventriculaire gauche électrique dans une population d'hommes. Presse Méd 1989; 18: 332–5.

47. Multiple Risk Factor Intervention Trial Research Group. Baseline rest electrocardiographic abnormalities, antihypertensive treatment, and mortality in the multiple risk factor intervention trial. Am J Cardiol 1985; 55: 1–15.

48. Casale PN, Devereux RB, Milner M, et al. Value of echocardiographic measurement of left ventricular mass in predicting cardiovascular morbid events in hypertensive men. Ann Intern Med 1986; 105: 173–8.

49. Levy D, Garrison RJ, Savage DD, Kannel WB, Castelli WP. Prognostic implications of echocardiographically determined left ventricular mass in the Framingham heart study. N Engl J Med 1990; 322: 1561–6.

50. Brush JE, Faxon DP, Salmon S, Jacobs AK, Ryan TJ. Abnormal endothelium-dependent coronary vasomotion in hypertensive patients. J Am Coll Cardiol 1992; 19: 809–15.

51. Clementy J, Levy S, Dallocchio M, Bricaud H. Propriétés électrophysiologiques du coeur dans l'hypertension artérielle. Ann Cardiol Angéiol 1980; 29: 245–9.

52. Koren MJ, Devereux RB, Casale PN, Savage DD, Laragh JH. Relation of left ventricular mass and geometry to morbidity and mortality in uncomplicated essential hypertension. Ann Intern Med 1991; 114: 345–52.

53. Motz W, Strauer BE. Left ventricular function and collagen content after regression of hypertensive hypertrophy. Hypertension 1989; 13: 43–50.

54. Savage DD, Garrison RJ, Kannel WB, Anderson SJ, Feinleib M, Castelli WP. Considerations in the use of echocardiography in epidemiology. The Framingham study. Hypertension 1987; 9 (Suppl II): II-40–44.

55. Koren MJ, Savage DD, Casale PN, al et. Changes in left ventricular mass predict risk in essential hypertension. (abstract). Circulation 1990; 82 (suppl III): III-29.

56. Levy D, Salomon M, Kannel WB, Agostino RB, Belanger AJ. Prognostic Implications of serial changes in QRS voltage in subjects with ECG evidence of left ventricular hypertrophy: the Framingham study. (abstract). Circulation 1991; 84 (suppl II) II-605.

57. Dahlof B, Pennert K, Hansson L. Reversal of left ventricular hypertrophy in hypertensive patients. A metaanalysis of 109 treatment studies. Am J Hypertens 1992; 5: 95–110.

58. Asmar RG, Pannier B, Santoni J Ph, Laurent St, London GM. Reversion of cardiac hypertrophy and reduced arterial compliance after converting enzyme inhibition in essential hypertension. Circulation 1988; 78: 941–50.

59. O'Rourke M. Arterial stiffness, systolic blood pressure and logical treatment of arterial hypertension. Hypertension 1990; 15: 339–47.

60. Safar ME, Toto-Moukouo JJ, Bouthier JA, Asmar RE, Levenson JA, Simon ACh. Arterial dynamics, cardiac hypertrophy and anti-hypertensive treatment. Circulation 1987; 75 (suppl II): II-156–161.

61. Julien J, Dufloux MA, Prasquier R, et al. Effects of captopril and minoxidil on left ventricular hypertrophy in resistant hypertensive patients: a 6 month double-blind comparison. J Am Coll Cardiol 1990; 16: 137–42.

62. Leenen FHH, Tsoporist J. Cardiac volume load as a determinant of the response of cardiac mass to antihypertensive therapy. Eur Heart J 1990; 11: 100–6.

63. Kelly RP, Gibbs HH, O'Rourke MF, et al. Nitroglycerin has more favourable effects on left ventricular afterload than apparent from measurement of pressure in a peripheral artery. Eur Heart J 1990; 11: 138–44.

11. Autonomic nervous system and large conduit arteries

GÉRARD M. LONDON and MICHEL E. SAFAR

Introduction

The vessels have the ability to alter their caliber and to influence the regional vascular resistance and capacitance through the modification of the neuronal discharge or changes in circulating catecholamines. Several in vitro studies demonstrated the extreme diversity of responses in the control of vascular tone of large conduit arteries and smaller resistive vessels [1], resulting from differences in the response to adrenoreceptor stimulation and antagonism between large and small arteries. Firstly, aorta and large conduit arteries which contain highly sensitive vascular smooth muscle cells have an excess of alpha^1-adrenoreceptors, and are quite sensitive to adrenergic stimulation [2, 3]. Second, abrupt decrease in responsiveness to catecholamines occurs close to the roots of many aortic branches, and continue to fall-off as the arteries get smaller and further divide [4]. Finally, the sympathetic control of vascular tone of large arteries is more sensitive to alpha-adrenergic blockade, than that of smaller vessels [5].

Due to the ability of small arteries and arterioles to adapt their myogenic activity to a bewildering variety of regional, local, and systemic factors [1], it is widely conceded that the major circulatory correlates of vascular smooth muscle contraction are to be found in the microvasculature. In contrast with such a diversity and specialization, large conduit arteries were frequently considered as simple conduits. Indeed, there seems to be little evidence in vivo that vasomotor changes in large arteries occur independently of those in the resistive vessels [6]. Nevertheless, caliber changes of the large conduit arteries can occur in two ways: (i) – passively, due to local or systemic changes in transmural pressure, and (ii) – actively, due to changes in vascular smooth muscle contraction. Thus, constriction or dilatation of arterioles distal to the large arteries may modify the geometric and physical characteristics of the conduit vessel through two possible mechanisms. First, arteriolar vasomotion may induce systemic or local blood pressure changes which could passively alter the diameter of the artery and its viscoelastic properties [6]. Secondly, arteriolar constriction or dilatation may modify the arterial wall

M. E. Safar and M. F. O'Rourke (eds.), The arterial system in hypertension. pp. 181–194.
© 1993 *Kluwer Academic Publishers. Printed in the Netherlands.*

smooth muscle tone actively throughout the endothelium-dependent mechanism of 'high-flow dilation' [7, 8]. However, there is evidence that the tone of large arteries may be regulated actively, and studies in isolated vessels, animals and humans suggest that large conduit arteries respond directly to both autonomic reflex and neurohumoral stimulation [9–14]. Nevertheless, during changes in sympathetic activity the alterations in the caliber and viscoelastic properties of conduit arteries depends also on the balance between passive and active forces acting on the vessel wall.

In this report we shall consider the arteries as a target for autonomic control, and the influence of the autonomic nervous system on the control of large arteries function in experimental conditions and in humans will be analyzed.

Basic concepts

Experimental studies in anesthetized animals in vivo or arterial preparations in vitro have indicated that changes produced by catecholamines or autonomic nervous system, affect the dimension as well as the viscoelastic properties of the large conduit arteries [9–14]. The extent of arterial diameter changes depends on the basal diameter, on the structure of their walls, on the resting tone [15–17], on the species [6, 9], on age [13] and the method used [6].

The diameter changes in the large central arteries are small in comparison with changes in medium-sized and small arteries or arterioles [6]. In most physiological conditions the diameter of intrathoracic arteries changes 8% to 18% with each cardiac cycle, whereas the diameter of systemic arteries changes 8% to 10% [18]. In dogs the maximum norepinephrine-induced constriction of the aorta was 6% of the outer diameter [9], while the hemorrhage or lumbar sympathetic stimulation produced a constriction of about 10% [10, 19]. The response of the artery were more pronounced in the rabbits where the range of diameter changes occurred with 6% norepinephrine constriction and 17% phenoxybenzamine dilation [20]. Active changes in the diameter of muscular, medium – sized arteries are greater in magnitude than those in central arteries [6]. The range of diameter changes observed during norepinephrine perfusion vary from 40% [21] in the sheep carotid artery to 55% in the dog iliac artery [22].

The question of the physiological role of the diameter changes observed in central and large arteries is addressed since these diameter changes have little effect on resistance to steady flow [6, 17, 23]. However, due to a complex interaction between active changes in the vascular tone, transmural pressure and, resulting cross-sectional area of arteries, the response of large arteries to reflex stimuli have repercussions on pulsatile arterial hemodynamics and arterial viscoelasticity [6, 23]. Nevertheless, several studies reported conflicting results regarding the effect of vasomotor tone on arterial stiffness

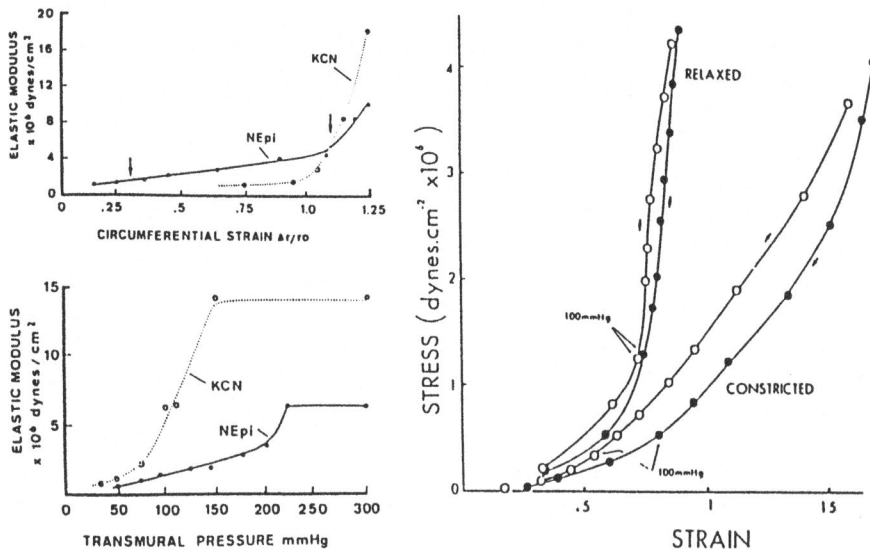

Figure 1. Left panel: Elastic moduli of relaxed and constricted carotid artery as function of strain or pressure (from Dobrin and Rovick [15]). Right panel: Stress-strain relationships of relaxed and constricted carotid artery derived from data of Dobrin and Rovick [15] by Gow [6]. Strain was calculated by using 'unstressed' circumference obtained at pressures of 5 mmHg.(Reproduced with permission of American Physiological Society).

and elastic modulus. Whereas some authors found that stimulation of smooth muscle increases vessel stiffness [24], others reported a decrease [25] or no modification of elastic properties [13]. Whether vasoconstriction increases or decreases the elastic modulus of the arterial walls depends on whether the control and constricted vessels are compared at the same transmural pressure, circumference, strain and stress (Figure 1) [15–17]. This is related to the non-linear behavior of the stress-strain relationship, and the unstressed diameter of the vessel which is different in the constricted and relaxed artery [6, 15, 16].

Smooth muscle cells contraction in the arterial walls is largely in the circumferential direction and has two interrelated consequences: (1) to cause vessel constriction, and (2) to alter vessel resistance to distension [26]. For a constant transmural pressure the constriction reduces the diameter of the arteries and has as a consequence a decrease of the distending force which is the product of transmural pressure and diameter. The principal consequence of these changes are twofold. Firstly, there is an alteration of the strain-stress relationship with a lower stress for a given strain (fractional increase in circumferential length or diameter of the artery) [6]. Secondly, the other consequence of active contraction is the increase resistance of the vessel wall to distension [26]. This second effect is related to decrease in arterial diameter (at any pressure the distending force is lower for smaller diameter) and to the increase in the elastic modulus of contracted muscle (active stiffness)[26]. Indeed adding a viscoelastic element (active muscle) during contraction would increase vessel wall stiffness. Study by Dobrin and Rovick [15] showed that this is the case when the elastic modulus was plotted as a function of strain. However the same study showed that muscle activation decreases the elastic modulus when this was plotted as a function of pressure [15]. Analysing the same data, but calculating the strain from appropriate unstressed circumferences, Gow [6] demonstrated that at most strain and stress values, and at comparable distending pressures, the slope of stress-strain curve is lower, that is, elastic modulus is lower for constricted than for relaxed vessels (Figure 1). This apparent paradox could be explained by the reciprocal variations in active stiffness (contracted muscle) and passive stiffness (connective tissue elements).

During, contraction the elastic modulus of the smooth muscle element increases and the vessel diameter decreases. The decrease in the vessel diameter is accompanied by a retraction of connective tissues and a decrease in the elastic modulus of the collagen and elastic fibers. This decrease in passive stiffness exceeds the increase in active stiffness provided by muscle contraction [26]. The final effects of vasoconstriction of conduit arteries on their distensibility depends on whether the vasomotor changes are exerced against a maintained or increased arterial pressure [6]. When the blood pressure is maintained constant, the vasoconstriction decreases the elastic modulus while the vasodilation increases it. When the vasoconstriction is exerced during an elevation of blood pressure, then two opposing tendencies interact: (i) passive distension of the arteries with a tendency to increase the diameter, and (ii) smooth muscle contraction which increases the resistance of the artery to inflation and limits the diameter increase.

From these considerations it follows that arterial distensibility during sympatho-adrenal vasoconstriction is determined by these two opposing tendencies [6]. On one hand, sympathetic stimulation induces an increase in vasomotor tone of precapillary resistance vessels and an elevation of arterial pressure. This has as a consequence a passive circumferential distension of the conduit arteries and an elevation of the elastic modulus by a tension applied on elastin and collagen fibers. On the other hand, the sympathetic stimulation induces a contraction of smooth muscle cells in the arterial walls, limiting the pressure induced passive distension of the arteries and the rise of the elastic modulus is less. Therefore, the sympathetic stimulation increases the elastic modulus of major systemic arteries, but the active vasoconstriction of these large vessels to some extent offset the pressure induced increase in elastic modulus due to the systemic vasoconstriction of resistance vessels [6]. The alterations of the diameter and elastic modulus of the large arteries during systemic sympatho-adrenal vasoconstriction (and/or vasodilation) influence the opposition of the arterial system to pulsatile flow, expressed as impedance [6, 17, 23]. It has been shown that impedance rises in the systemic circulation during reflex sympathetic stimulation as a result of an active reduction of cross-sectional area [27, 28].

Thus, even if the physiological variations of large arteries diameter are small, they influence arterial distensibility, which is an important determinant of vascular impedance and cardiac afterload. In adapting their geometry and viscoelastic properties to hemodynamic changes of the resistive vessels (or to systemic influences) the large vessels participate to ventricular/vascular coupling and efficient control of the circulation.

Methodological aspects of the study of the autonomic control of conduit arteries in humans

The role of autonomic nervous system on the control of systemic and/or local vascular tone has been investigated for a long time. The respective contribution of beta and alpha receptors and their subclasses were described, in particular on the basis of the administration of selective agonists and antagonists [29, 30]. The forearm vascular circulation was the most widely used model for the studies of the reflex and sympatho-adrenal regulation of the vascular tone [14, 31, 32]. The majority of the studies of forearm circulation used the plethysmography for measuring blood flow and the observed changes in flow could be interpreted solely as due to changes in peripheral resistances, i.e to dilatation or constriction of the small arteries and arterioles [14, 31, 32].

An adequate understanding of hemodynamics in the conduit arteries is impossible without a knowledge of large arteries caliber and its alterations. Indeed, the large arteries have two distinct interrelated functions: (i) to deliver an adequate supply of blood to body tissues (the conduit function characterized be steady flow and steady pressure and their relationship, governed by the Poiseuille's law) and, (ii) to smooth out the pulsations occurring with intermittent ventricular ejection (cushioning function) characterized by oscillatory pressure and flow and their frequency dependent relationships which depends principally on the diameter of the artery and the mechanical properties of the arterial walls [23]. Thus, methods which permit an evaluation of hemodynamics of large conduit arteries in humans should be described in detail.

In recent years new methods using pulsed Doppler flowmetry were introduced in clinical research, which permit measurement of arterial diameter in man [33]. With the pulsed Doppler velocimetry the inner diameter of the brachial artery and superficial straight arteries may be measured in situ. In addition to the sequential determination of the arterial diameter, the pulsed Doppler system allows the blood velocity to be separately and continuously measured, giving indirect information on the instantaneous fluctuations of the vasomotor tone of forearm arterioles [33, 34].

With the older pulsed Doppler systems, the measurements of large artery diameter have two characteristics. Firstly, only mean diameter is measured, secondly the determination can only be performed sequentially. Indeed, the internal diameter is determined from peak velocity profiles obtained by electronically moving a measurement volume across the arterial lumen. It is possible to locate precisely the proximal and the distal wall of the artery corresponding respectively to the first and the last Doppler signals received and to deduce by their interval the internal diameter of the brachial (or other) artery. The methodology has been described and validated elsewhere [33]. As already published the reproducibility of the diameter measurements, determined from sequential recordings during 90 minutes period, approximates 3.1% [33]. The principal limitation of the determination is the resolution of the sample volume size. Indeed, any value of diameter change less than 0.034 cm cannot be detected, and the diameter measurement is overestimated with a maximum of 0.34 mm [33].

Instantaneous values of blood flow velocity may be obtained with the same probe containing two transducers, forming between them an angle of 120 degrees, so that, when Doppler signals recorded by each transducer are equal in absolute value, the ultrasonic incidence with the vessel axis is 60 degrees. The reproducibility of blood velocity measurement is $14 \pm 3\%$ [34]. The pattern of changes in blood flow velocity gives indirect information concerning hemodynamic changes occurring during various physiological manoeuvers. For instance, during mental stress, brachial blood flow velocity increases 2 to 3 times [35]. Since the increase in cardiac output measured simultaneously is small in comparison to the large increase in blood flow velocity, the most likely explanation for the velocity increase is that forearm vascular resistance decreases. This is indirectly evidenced by the significant relationship between brachial blood flow velocity measured with the pulsed Doppler system and the forearm vascular resistances, calculated from simultaneous plethysmographic measurements [36]. In some subjects the magnitude of spontaneous variations of brachial blood flow velocity represent 3 to 6 fold minimum values. Hand exclusion attenuates these spontaneous fluctuations confirming that the cutaneous territory of the hand is principally responsible [35]. Brachial artery diameter changes observed during various physiological and pharmacological conditions do not exceed 15%, representing less than a 32% changes in cross-sectional area [34, 37–39]. Using a cylindrical representation of the artery, it can be assumed that variations of blood velocity account for the main part of the changes in volumic blood flow. Therefore, instantaneous fluctuations of blood flow velocity indicate that the vasomotor tone of arterioles is under permanent adjustment by local and systemic factors. As already mentioned, a flow-dependent mechanism can link changes in large artery caliber to changes in arteriolar vasomotor tone. For a clinical evaluation of this mechanism, flow velocity and arterial diameter may be studied before and after distal wrist occlusion. When the wrist cuff is deflated, reactive hyperemia increases blood velocity up to 8 fold with a parallel increase of arterial diameter of $12 \pm 2\%$. Since myogenic relaxation and the vasodilating effect of recirculating metabolic compounds can be easily excluded, a velocity-dependent mechanism is the most likely explanation for the large artery relaxation [37, 39]. Used in parallel with the measurement of arterial diameters, the determination of arterial pulse wave velocity permit the determination of arterial compliance and to have a deeper insight into the arterial function [23, 40].

More modern echotracking techniques have been developed recently, permitting measurement of the systolic-diastolic variations of arterial diameters with a high degree of resolution and reproducibility. Coupled with the use of applanation tonometry, which allows non-invasive measurement of pulse pressure in peripheral and central arteries, these methods allow direct determination of changes of arterial mechanical properties; their introduction into clinical research will certainly permit a better knowledge of arterial physiology [41, 42].

Response of brachial artery to orthostatic maneuvers

In humans, both lower body negative pressure and passive elevation of the legs with head-down tilt have been used to simulate orthostatic maneuvers.

Lower body negative pressure (LBNP)

Lower body negative pressure (LBNP) decreases the cardiopulmonary blood volume and pressure. According to the degree of negative pressure used the LBNP could realise a conditions of a specific unloading of cardiac mechanoreceptors (from −5 to −20 mmHg) or can mimic a true orthostatic stress (−40 mmHg) [39]. In all circumstances the LBNP is a good circulatory model of the enhancement or stimulation of sympathetic activity.

Anderson and Mark [39] have demonstrated that LBNP caused constriction of the brachial artery and a decrease in brachial artery flow. Because the LBNP induced sympathetic constriction of small resistive vessels the decrease in brachial artery diameter could be secondary to flow-mediated regulation. The absence of reduction in arterial diameter when LBNP was applied after distal circulatory arrest suggested that orthostatic maneuvers influence large artery diameter through primary control of resistance vessels and velocity-mediated regulation. Increase in adrenergic activity with LBNP is not only associated with hemodynamic alterations in large peripheral arteries, but induce also changes in aorta. Thus, Madkour et al. [43] have shown LBNP induces a decrease in aortic compliance in parallel to an increase in plasma norepinephrine and a reduction of systolic blood pressure. The respective role of aortic diameter changes on the compliance changes was not evaluated [43].

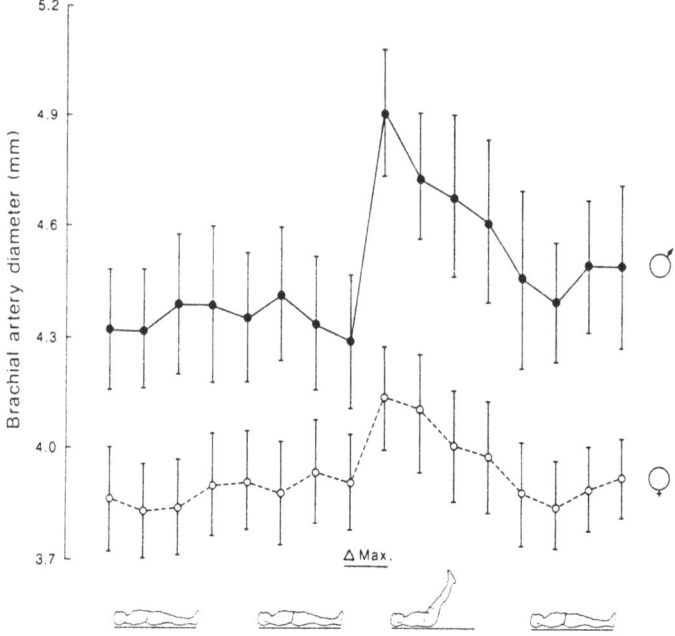

Figure 2. Brachial artery (BA) diameter changes induced by orthostatic maneuvers. Leg raising in supine subjects induce a significant increase in BA diameter [38].

Passive elevation of the legs

A passive elevation of the legs in a recumbent subject is an effective technique that increases venous return, cardiopulmonary blood volume and cardiac filling pressure [44]. Roddie et al. [45] reported that such a leg elevation induced reflex vasodilatation of forearm skeletal muscle arterioles through the stimulation of cardiopulmonary receptors and consequent inhibition of sympathetic vasomotor discharge. In a recent study using a dual crystal pulsed Doppler system, we observed that the passive elevation of the legs in recumbent subjects, besides inducing a decrease in forearm vascular resistances and plasma renin activity also induced an sustained increase in brachial artery diameter and brachial artery flow velocity (Figure 2) [38]. The initial maximum response after leg raising represented an increase of 12.9 ± 1.6% of the baseline brachial artery diameter. Changes in the arterial caliber occurred in the absence of arterial pressure modifications and the arterial relaxation was due to changes in vascular smooth muscle cells activity. Whether the arterial relaxation associated with cardiopulmonary baroreflex stimulation results directly from the inhibition of sympathetic activity remains uncertain. Indeed leg raising induces a reflex vasodilation of forearm skeletal arterioles and a decrease in vascular resistances [38, 44, 45]. Such a decrease in vascular resistances is associated with an increased distal outflow from the brachial artery and an increase in blood velocity [38]. Endothelial cells, when exposed to greater shear stress caused by an increase in blood velocity, induce relaxation of underlying smooth muscle and arterial relaxation [46]. During the initial response to leg raising brachial artery diameter increased together with an increase in blood velocity. Moreover, during this peak response the variations in diameter and velocity were significantly correlated. The higher was the increase in blood velocity, the higher was the increase in arterial diameter. Therefore a velocity-dependent increase in brachial artery diameter, consecutive to reflex vasodilation of forearm resistant vessels could be the initiating mechanism. Nevertheless the increase in arterial caliber observed after leg raising was long-lasting while the increase in blood velocity was observed only during the initial period and the possibility of a direct reflex control of large conduit arteries should be considered [38].

A number of standard techniques were applied to demonstrate the reflex nature of forearm resistance vessels changes in humans during cardiopulmonary receptor stimulation [39, 44, 45]. The use of these techniques to analyse separately the control of conduit arteries and resistive vessels is difficult. Indeed there seems to be little evidence that vasomotor changes in large arteries and microvasculature occur independently of each other [6]. Under that condition, the maneuvers that could block an eventual direct reflex control of large arteries would also block the reflex control of resistance vessels and vice versa.

An exaggerated response of forearm resistance vessels following stimulation of cardiac mechanoreceptors has been observed in human hypertension [47].

Response of small and large arteries to catecholamines

Infusion

One recent study has documented the in situ reactivity of large arteries to infused norepinephrine [34]. Using pulsed Doppler flowmetry, the response of brachial artery diameter/ flow velocity, blood flow and vascular resistances to subpressive dose of norepinephrine was studied in 9 normotensive people and 19 essential hypertensive patients. Brachial artery hemodynamic parameters were studied before and after the administration of placebo (glucose) or increasing doses of norepinephrine (10, 20, and 40 ng/kg/min iv) given in a single blind fashion. While the placebo infusion did not modify the brachial artery flow or diameter, the infusion of norepinephrine was accompanied by a significant decrease in brachial artery diameter, blood velocity, volumic flow and conductance. The changes observed in essential hypertensives were amplified in comparison with those observed in normotensive subjects. The changes in brachial artery diameter occurred in the absence of systemic arterial pressure variations. Change in brachial artery diameter was significantly correlated to change in plasma norepinephrine; the greater the rise in plasma norepinephrine, the greater the decrease in brachial artery diameter. Although the conclusion that the constriction of brachial artery is norepinephrine dependent is logical, norepinephrine induced also a constriction of small arteriolar resistances vessels and this can have direct repercussions on the upstream artery. A myogenic constriction cannot be excluded as a consequence of redistribution of local intravascular pressures. It seems improbable that myogenic response could cause the constriction of the brachial artery since large arteries do not exhibit substantial myogenic response. The changes in flow velocity can also be involved. Nevertheless a flow-dependent endothelial mechanism was unlikely since in response to the largest doses of norepinephrine blood velocity decreased to a smaller extent than the decrease in arterial diameter, and the changes in diameter and blood velocity were not correlated. Furthermore, in hypertensive patients, alpha-1 blockade by Urapidil increased markedly blood flow velocity but did not change brachial artery diameter [48], indicating that diameter changes are not necessarily the consequence of velocity alterations.

The action of epinephrine infusion on brachial artery hemodynamics was evaluated by Anderson and Mark [39]. They measured the brachial artery diameter and flow in 3 subjects before and during a 30-minute infusion of epinephrine at 1.5 microgr/min. Contrasting with the results observed during norepinephrine infusion, epinephrine did not change brachial artery diameter despite an increase in brachial artery blood flow velocity.

Response of brachial artery to cold pressor test

Anderson and Mark measured changes in brachial artery diameter and flow in 15 subjects while a cold pressor test (CPT) was performed in the contralateral arm [39]. CPT reduced the brachial artery diameter from 4.94 ± 0.18 to 4.38 ± 0.18 mm and brachial flow velocity from 10.2 ± 1.4 to 4.7 ± 0.6 cm/sec. This decrease in brachial artery diameter was observed in the presence of a significant increase in arterial pressure, and was therefore related to active smooth muscle contraction. CPT was able to cause brachial artery constriction also after circulatory arrest induced by wrist occlusion. These findings were interpreted by the authors as suggesting a direct sympathetic stimulation with an exclusion of flow-mediated changes. This could suggest a neurogenic sympathetic constriction or a constriction secondary to increases in circulating catecholamines, especially epinephrine. The fact that infusion of epinephrine did not constricted the brachial artery favored the hypothesis of a direct neurogenic effect [39].

Using echotracking systems, other recent studies have demonstrated that during CPT arterial compliance calculated from the systolic-diastolic changes in radial artery diameter and pressure is significantly decreased suggesting that an increase in sympathetic tone and/or circulating catecholamines alter mechanical properties of the arteries by a direct action on the arterial walls [35, 41, 50, 51].

Response of brachial artery to mental stress

Mental stress is a classical maneuver to study vascular responses to sympatho-adrenal stimulation, and to detect pressor hyperresponsivness in hypertensive patients [49].

The effects of mental stress on brachial artery hemodynamics of normotensive and hypertensive patients has been evaluated [35]. A 2 minutes long mental arithmetic stress increased arterial pressure and brachial blood flow velocity. However brachial artery diameter did not change. The absence of increase in brachial artery diameter suggested that some mechanisms such as myogenic or catecholamine-induced vasoconstriction may have offset the increase in large conduit artery diameter which would have been the consequence of: passive arterial-pressure dependent distension; velocity-dependent vasodilation; cholinergic vasodilation [35, 50].

The effects of mental stress (2 min of mental arithmetic) on arterial compliance and systolic-diastolic variations of radial artery diameter was performed in man using echotracking system coupled with Finapres for the simultaneous measurement of blood pressure [51]. During mental stress, mean radial artery diameter did not change in spite of the increase in mean blood pressure. Systolic-diastolic variations in radial artery diameter decreased significantly whereas pulse pressure increased. Arterial compliance, calculated for the instantaneous level of mean blood pressure significantly decreased indicating that increase in sympathetic activity alter viscoelastic properties of the arterial wall through a direct effect on the arterial wall.

References

1. Bevan JA, Bevan RD. Changes in arteries as they get smaller. In: Vanhoutte PM, editor. Vasodilatation: Vascular smooth muscle, Peptides, Autonomic nerves, and Endothelium. New York: Raven Press, 1988: 55–60.
2. Aars H. Diameter and elasticity of the ascending aorta during infusion of noradrenaline. Acta Physiol Scand 1971; 83: 133–8.
3. Cox RH. Effects of norepinephrine on mechanics of arteries in vivo. Am J Physiol 1976; 231: 420–5.
4. Laher I, Bevan JA. Alpha adrenoreceptor number limits response of some rabbit arteries to norepinephrine. J Pharmacol Exp Ther 1985; 233: 290–7.

5. Owen MP, Quinn C, Bevan JA. Phentolamine-resistant neurogenic constriction occurs in small arteries at higher frequencies. Am J Physiol 1985; 249 (Heart Circ Physiol 18]: H404–H14.

6. Gow BS. Circulatory correlates. vascular impedance, resistance, and capacitance. In: Bohr DF et al. editors. The Cardiovascular System, Vol II. Vascular smooth muscle. Baltimore: American Physiological Society (The Williams & Wilkins Company) 1980: 353–408.

7. Furchgott RF, Zawadzki JV, Cherry PD. Role of endothelium in the vasodilator response to acetylcholine. In: Vanhoutte PM, Leusen I, editors. Vasodilation. New York: Raven Press, 1981: 49–66.

8. Pohl U, Holtz J, Busse R, Bassenge E. Crucial role of endothelium in the vasodilator response to increased flow in vivo. Hypertension 1986; 8: 37–44.

9. Barnett GO, Mallos AJ, Shapiro A. Relationship of aortic pressure and diameter in the dog. J Appl Physiol 1961; 16: 545–8.

10. Pieper HP, Paul LT. Responses in aortic smooth muscle studied in intact dogs. Am J Physiol 1969; 217: 154–160.

11. Gero J, Gerova M. Sympathetic regulation of arterial distensibility. Physiol Bohemoslov 1969; 18: 480–1.

12. Gerova M, Gero J. Range of the sympathetic control of the dog femoral artery. Circ Res 1969; 24: 349–59.

13. Pagani M, Mirsky I, Baig H, Manders WY, Kerkhof P, Vatner SF. Effects of age on aortic pressure-diameter and elastic stiffness stress relationships in unanesthetized sheep. Circ Res 1979; 44: 1420–9.

14. Hughes AD, Thom SAM, Martin GN, et al. Size and site-dependent heterogeneity of human vascular responses in vitro. J Hypertens 1988; 6(Suppl 4]: S173–S5.

15. Dobrin PB, Rovick AA. Influence of vascular smooth muscle on contractile mechanics and elasticity of arteries. Am J Physiol 1969; 217: 1644–51.

16. Gow BS. The influence of vascular smooth muscle on the viscoelastic properties of blood vessels. In: Bergel DH, editor. Cardiovascular Fluid Dynamics. New York: Academic Press 1972 Vol II: 65–110.

17. McDonald DA. Blood Flow in Arteries. London: Arnold, 1974.

18. Dobrin PB. Mechanical properties of arteries. Physiol Rev 1978; 58: 397–460.

19. Gerova M, Gero J, Dolezel S, Blazkova-Huzulakova I. Sympathetic control of canine abdominal aorta. Circ Res 1973; 33: 149–52.

20. Aars H. Effects of altered smooth muscle tone on aortic diameter and aortic baroreceptor activity in anesthetised rabbits. Circ Res 1971; 28: 254–62.

21. Keatinge WR. Electrical and mechanical response of arteries to stimulation of sympathetic nerves. J Physiol London 1966; 185: 701–15.

22. Cox RH: Mechanics of canine iliac artery smooth muscle in vitro. Am J Physiol 1976; 230: 462–70.

23. O'Rourke MF: Arterial function in health and disease. Edinburgh: Churchill Livingstone, 1982: 116–35.

24. Peterson LH, Jensen RE, Parnell R. Mechanical properties of arteries in vivo. Circ Res 1960; 8: 622–39.

25. Bagshaw RJ, Peterson LH. Sympathetic control of the mechanical properties of the canine carotid sinus. Am J Physiol 1972, 222: 1462–8.

26. Dobrin PB. Vascular mechanics. In: Shepherd JT, Abboud FM, editors. The Cardiovascular system, Peripheral circulation and organ blood flow. Bethesda: American Physiological Society, Williams & Wilkins Company, 1983: 65–102.

27. Cox RH, Fronek A, Peterson LH. Effects of carotid hypotension on aortic hemodynamics in the unanesthetized dog. Am J Physiol 1975; 229: 1376–80.

28. Cox RH, Bagshaw RJ. Baroreceptor reflex control of arterial hemodynamics in the dog. Circ Res 1975: 37: 772–86.

29. Timmermans PMBWM, Van Zwieten PA. Alpha-adrenoreceptors antagonists. In: Van

Zwieten PA, editors. Handbook of hypertension, Vol. 3, Pharmacology of antihypertensive drugs. Amsterdam: Elsevier Science, 1984: 239–48.

30. Fitzgerald JD. Beta-adrenoreceptors antagonists. In: Van Zwieten PA, editor. Handbook of Hypertension, Vol. 3, Pharmacology of antihypertensive drugs. Amsterdam: Elsevier Science, 1984: 249–306.

31. Kiowski W, Hulthen UL, Ritz R, Bühler FR. Alpha[2] adrenoreceptor mediated vasoconstriction in human arterial vessels. Clin Pharmacol Ther 1983; 34: 565–9.

32. Jie K, Van Brummelen P, Vermey P, Timmermans PBMWM, Van Zwieten PA-Effects of exogenous adrenaline and noradrenaline on vascular post-synaptic alpha[1] and alpha[2] adrenoreceptors in man. J Hypertens 1984; 2(Suppl 3): 119–121.

33. Safar M, Peronneau J, Levenson J, Simon A. Pulsed Doppler: diameter velocity and flow of brachial artery in sustained essential hypertension. Circulation 1981, 63: 393–400.

34. Laurent S, Juillerat L, London GM, Nussberger J, Brunner H, Safar ME. Increased response of brachial artery diameter to norepinephrine in hypertensive patients. Am J Physiol 1988; 255: H36–H43.

35. Laurent S, Lacolley P, Brunnel P, Safar M. Effects of short-lasting mental stress on systemic and brachial hemodynamics in essential hypertension. Circulation 1988; 78(Suppl IV): IV175.

36. Safar ME, Daou JE, Safavian A, London GM. Comparison of forearm plethysmographic methods with brachial artery Doppler flowmetry in man. Clin Physiol 1988; 8: 163–70.

37. Laurent S, Brunel P, Lacolley P, Billaud E, Pannier B, Safar M: Flow-dependent vasodilation of the brachial artery in essential hypertension: preliminary report. J Hypertension 1988; 6(Suppl 4): S182–S4.

38. London GM, Pannier BP, Laurent S, Lacolley P, Safar ME. Brachial artery diameter changes associated with Cardiopulmonary baroreflex activation in humans. Am J Physiol 1990; 258 (Heart Circ. Physiol. 27): H773-H7.

39. Anderson EA, Mark AL. Flow-mediated and reflex changes in large peripheral artery tone in humans. Circulation 1989; 79: 93–100.

40. Safar ME, London GM, Asmar RG, Huges CJ, Laurent SA. An indirect approach for the study of the elastic modulus of the brachial artery in patients with essential hypertension. Cardiovasc Res 1986; 20: 563–7.

41. Hoeks APG, Brands PJ, Smeets FAM, Reneman RS. Assessment of the distensibility of superficial arteries. Ultrasound Med Biol 1990; 16: 121–8.

42. Hayoz D, Rutchsmann B, Perret F, et al. Conduit arteries compliance and distensibility are not necessarily reduced in hypertension. Hypertension 1992; 20: 1–6.

43. Madkour A, Levenson J, Bravo EL, Simon A, Fouad-Tarazi FM. Preload, adrenergic activity, and aortic compliance in normal and hypertensive patients. Am Heart J 1989; 118: 1243–47.

44. London GM, Levenson JA, Safar ME, Simon AC, Guerin AP, Payen D. Hemodynamic effects of head-down tilt in normal subjects and sustained hypertensive patients. Am J Physiol 1983; 245: H194–H202.

45. Roddie IC, Shepherd JT, Whelan RF. Reflex changes in vasoconstrictor tone in human skeletal muscle in response to stimulation of receptors in low-pressure area of the intrathoracic vascular bed. J Physiol (London) 1957; 139: 369–76.

46. Rubanyi GM, Romero JC, Van Houtte PM. Flow-induced release of endothelium-derived relaxing factor. Am J Physiol 1986; 250 (Heart Circ Physiol): H1145–H9.

47. Mark AL, Kerber RE. Augmentation of cardiopulmonary baroreflex control of forearm vascular resistance in borderline hypertension. Hypertension 1982; 4: 39–46.

48. Levenson J, Simon ACh, Bouthier JD, Benetos A, Safar ME. Post-synaptic alpha-blockade and brachial artery compliance in essential hypertension. J Hypertens 1984; 2: 37–41.

49. Falkner B: Reactivity to mental stress in hypertension and prehypertension. In: Julius S, Bassetts DR, eds. Handbook of hypertension, Vol. 9, Behavioral factors in hypertension. Amsterdam: Elsevier Science, 1987: 95–122.

50. Safar ME, Laurent S, Pannier B, Younsi FE, London GM. Arterial compliance and autonomic nervous system in hypertension. Curr Opinion Cardiol 1989; 4(Suppl 4): S23–S8.
51. Lacolley P, Boutouyrie P, Gired X, Beck L, Safar M, Laurent S. Sympathetic activation decreases arterial compliance through a direct effect on the arterial wall. (submitted for publication).

12. Large arteries and sodium in hypertension
Pathophysiological and therapeutic aspects

ATHANASE BENETOS and MICHEL E. SAFAR

Introduction

The concept that a high salt intake is related to increased prevalence of hypertension is an old one. There is enough epidemiological, clinical, historical and experimental evidence to support this concept [1–3]. Most authorities currently believe that excessive salt intake is the first environmental risk factor for hypertension [4]. It appears that approximately one out of four normotensive subjects and one-half of all hypertensive patients are sensitive to salt, with their blood pressure increasing following excessive salt intake [5–7].

This susceptibility to salt may be genetically determined in humans with a hereditary predisposition. The mechanism(s) by which salt intake may increase blood pressure is still not completely understood.

Indeed, sodium intake affects blood pressure causing hypertension either by an increase in blood flow (short-term effect) or an increase in vascular resistance (long-term effect), indicating a change in arteriolar tone in the latter case. The possibility that sodium intake may influence the totality of the cardiovascular system in hypertension, independently of the blood pressure changes has not been widely considered. However, recent animal studies suggest that decreased sodium intake may improve cardiac hypertrophy independently of blood pressure changes [8], and that elevated sodium intake is associated with structural alterations of the large arteries, particularly in the brain [9].

Arterial compliance and distensibility are reduced in patients with essential hypertension, indicating an alteration in the damping function of large arteries, principally at the site of the aorta. On the basis of experimental studies indicating a negative relationship between pressure and compliance, it was believed for a long time that the reduced visco-elastic properties of the arterial system in hypertensive patients was the simple mechanical consequence of the elevated distending blood pressure. However, recent studies in such subjects indicate that the magnitude of the reduction in compliance is not constantly correlated with the level of blood pressure, thus suggesting

M. E. Safar and M. F. O'Rourke (eds.), The arterial system in hypertension. pp. 195–207.
© 1993 *Kluwer Academic Publishers. Printed in the Netherlands.*

intrinsic alterations of the hypertensive arterial wall [10]. From this observation arises the possibility that sodium might act on arterial stiffness independently of the blood pressure level. There are several arguments in favor of this possibility. First, sodium modifies arterial smooth muscle tone through different mechanisms involving sodium-potassium pumps [11], calcium exchange [12], modification of the adrenergic nervous system [13, 14] and of natriuretic factors [15]. Second, changes in vasomotor tone affect the viscoelastic properties of the arterial wall both in experimental and in clinical studies [10, 16].

In the present report, clinical, epidemiological and pharmacological evidence for the effect of sodium on the mechanical properties of large arteries are analyzed, with particular emphasis on the action of diuretic agents.

Cross-sectional studies

Aging is associated with increased arterial stiffness, increased arterial pressure, and a higher prevalence of hypertension. All are usually regarded as normal aging phenomena, and it is considered appropriate to adjust the normal range of arterial pressure and arterial stiffness for age [17]. However, it is well known that in undeveloped societies with low dietary salt intake, arterial pressure rises to a lesser degree with increasing age, and the prevalence of hypertension is markedly less than in Western societies with regular salt intake [18]. Therefore, in order to establish an adequate relationship between arterial stiffness and salt intake, it is important to demonstrate that the relationship between arterial stiffness (measured non-invasively from pulse wave velocity) and salt intake is independent of, or additional to, the relationship between stiffness and mean arterial pressure for a given age range. Such relationships have been investigated in epidemiologic studies performed both in China and Australia by Avolio et al. [19, 20].

Arterial pulse wave velocity was measured together with arterial pressure in two groups of normal subjects living either in a rural or an urban community in China [19]. Serum cholesterol levels were similar and low in each group, whereas both the prevalence of hypertension and salt intake were significantly higher in the urban community. In the rural group, pulse wave velocity was consistently lower in the aorta, arm, and leg, and increased to a lesser degree with age compared with the urban group. This finding was observed even when subjects with the same arterial pressure and of the same age were compared. Thus, results in two ethnically similar populations with low serum cholesterol levels and low prevalence of hypertension and salt intake, suggested that salt intake had an independent effect on arteriolar tone and arterial wall properties, with the former indirectly and the latter directly contributing to increase arterial stiffness with age.

In Australia [20], pulse wave velocity was measured in 57 normotensive subjects who voluntarily followed a low-salt diet (mean intake, 44 mmol sodium per day for a period ranging from eight months to five years). Subjects who followed a regular diet were matched for age and mean arterial pressure with the low-salt group, and were used as a control group. For both samples, subjects were divided into three age subgroups. In subgroup 1 (age 2 to 19 years), pulse wave velocity was similar in the control and low-salt groups. In subgroups 2 (20 to 44 years) and 3 (45 to 66 years), pulse wave velocity measured in the aorta, arms, and legs was consistently lower in the low-salt than in the control group. The findings suggested that normotensive adult subjects who followed a low-salt diet have reduced arterial stiffness, and that this effect was independent of blood pressure.

In conclusion, a small number of cross-sectional epidemiologic studies suggests that salt intake may influence arterial stiffness in a manner that is independent of blood pressure, and that this influence is possibly more pronounced in older than in younger subjects.

Sodium induced changes in arterial diameter and stiffness: longitudinal studies

In the recent years, some longitudinal studies were focused on the sodium-induced changes in arterial diameter and stiffness and were performed in different populations (subjects with mild to moderate essential hypertension of the middle age; systolic hypertension in the elderly).

Recently we investigated the hemodynamic effect of a moderately low salt diet in a 2-month, randomized, double-blind, cross-over study, in 20 hypertensive ambulatory patients [21]. All subjects followed a 9-week low salt diet. During this period they received capsules containing either lactose or NaCl [70 mEq/day) in 4-week treatment periods, separated by one-week wash-out period. Hemodynamic and biological parameters were evaluated at the day of randomization and at the end of the forth and ninth weeks. Low sodium diet (LSD) was defined as a NaCl restriction period with lactose capsules, and normal sodium diet (NSD) as a NaCl restriction period with capsular salt supplementation. Blood pressure was significantly lower during the LSD as compared to the NSD group but the blood pressure changes were small: 6.5 ± 1.5 mmHg for systolic blood pressure ($p < 0.001$) and 3.7 ± 1.1 for diastolic blood pressure ($p < 0.001$) (Table 1). This decrease in blood pressure was associated with a decrease in peripheral resistance in the carotid and forearm circulations. Interestingly, the brachial artery diameter was larger during the LSD ($p < 0.01$), whereas the carotid artery diameter was unchanged (Table 1). The brachial artery diameter changes were not related to the blood pressure changes but were positively related to the age of the patients (Figure 1). These findings suggested that moderate low salt restriction was indeed capable of decreasing blood pressure and lowering peripheral resistance in the carotid and forearm circulations but caused in parallel a brachial, but not carotid, dilatation. These effects were

Table 1. Hemodynamic parameters following periods of low (LSD) and normal (NSD) salt diets in hypertensive subjects [21]

	LSD	NSD	P
SBP (mmHg)	142 ± 2.6	149 ± 2.3	<0.001
DBP	89.5 ± 1.5	93.2 ± 1.3	<0.001
HR (b/mn)	75.4 ± 1.8	75.3 ± 1.7	NS
Brachial artery-diameter (cm)	0.527 ± 0.020	0.460 ± 0.019	<0.001
Carotid artery diameter (cm)	0.609 ± 0.012	0.592 ± 0.11	NS
Forearm circ. periph. resistance (mmHg. sec/ml)	107 ± 15	142 ± 19	<0.01
Carotid circ. periph. resistance (mmHg. sec/ml)	17.7 ± 1.3	20.0 ± 1.3	<0.05

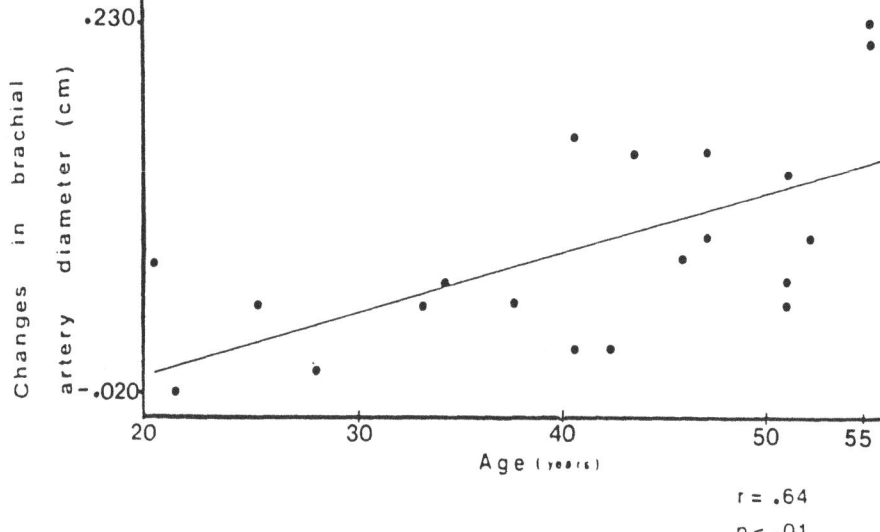

$r = .64$

$p < .01$

Figure 1. Correlation of changes in brachial artery diameter with age, in low and normal salt diet [21].

more pronounced in older than in younger patients. Moreover, this study showed that there are differences in salt dependence among different peripheral arteries, independently of blood pressure changes.

Since Myers and Morgan [22] have shown that salt intake was associated with larger increases in blood pressure in older than in younger subjects and that these changes were more pronounced with regard to systolic than diastolic blood pressure, it seems likely that the higher sensitivity of systolic pressure to sodium in old people might be mediated by a sodium-induced increase in the rigidity of the arterial wall. Further support for this hypothesis was obtained from the study of intravenous administration of isotonic saline to elderly subjects with systolic hypertension and arteriosclerosis obliterans of the lower limbs [23]. In such patients, isotonic saline caused a significant increase in systolic pressure, whereas diastolic and mean arterial pressure did not change significantly. No comparable results on blood pressure were observed in age-and sex-matched normotensive controls. Before saline infusion, forearm arterial compliance was found to be reduced, indicating that increased stiffness of the arterial wall participated to the mechanism of untreated systolic hypertension in these patients. Following saline infusion, a further decrease in forearm arterial compliance was observed in parallel with the increase in systolic blood pressure. Such findings indicate that the reduction in arterial compliance following isotonic saline was due to sodium-induced mechanisms acting on the arterial wall independently of the changes in blood pressure.

Salt sensitivity and arterial alterations

Some recent findings suggest that in genetically predisposed animals and subjects, arterial alterations exist even before salt loading.

Animal studies show that the blood pressure of genetically salt sensitive models increases after acute or chronic excessive ingestion of sodium chloride [24, 25]. Dahl developed two strains of rats with different responses to salt loading [24]: a salt-sensitive strain (DS) which becomes hypertensive when fed a high NaCl diet, and a salt resistant (DR) strain which does not. Chronic elevation of blood pressure in Dahl sensitive rats, on a high salt diet, is related to an increase in vascular resistance, whereas blood volume, after a transient increase, returns to normal values [25]. Different mechanisms have been proposed to explain this arteriolar vasoconstriction. It has been suggested that the effects of chronic NaCl loading on sympathetic activity are different in DS and DR rats [26, 27]. Other mechanisms, such as changes in baroreceptor activity [28], renal function [29] or responsiveness to various vasoconstrictive or vasodlilating [31, 32] have been proposed. Recent studies even showed that NaCl loading can suppress, in some experimental models, the bradykinin-kallikrein plasma or tissue activity [29, 30]. Independently of the mechanisms involved in salt sensibility, it should be emphasized that, in this experimental model, rats develop substantial arterial and arteriolar lesions [33–35].

In a recent study [36], we evaluated the mechanical properties of the carotid arteries in Dahl sensitive rats with or without salt loading using a method able to measure the arterial compliance in vivo, in situ with respect to the anatomical vascularization and innervation of the carotid artery [37, 38]. We observed that the pressure-volume curves in Dahl sensitive rats compared to Dahl resistant rats was shifted to the right, showing an increased

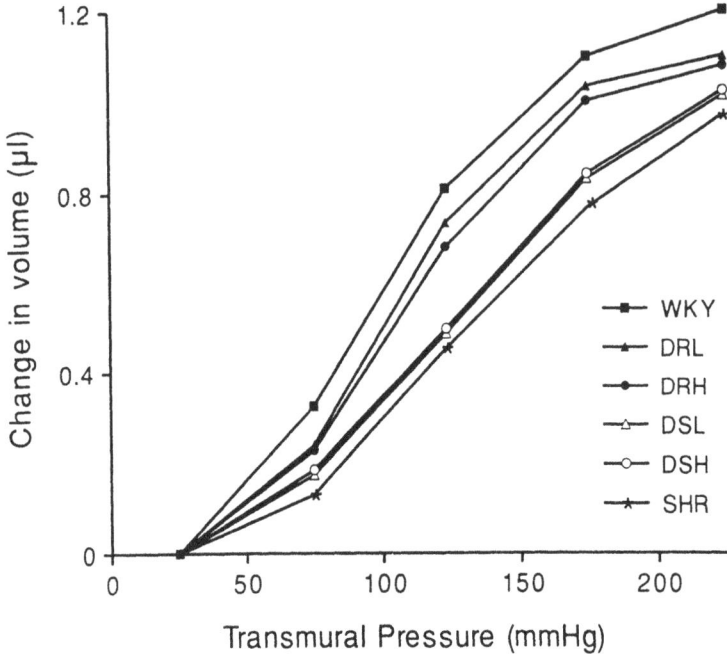

Figure 2. Pressure to volume relationship in Dahl sensitive rats fed a low (DSL) or a High (DSH) salt diet Dahl resistant (DRL and DRH) and in WKY and SHRs [36].

arterial stiffness in the salt sensitive strain (Figure 2). The values of compliance were very close to those observed in previous studies in spontaneously hypertensive rats (SHR) and significantly lower than the values recorded in normotensive Wistar-Kyoto rats [36].

The shift of the carotid pressure-volume relationship in Dahl sensitive (DS) rats exhibited two dominant characteristics. Firstly, the alteration was observed in all DS rats, either on low or high NaCl diet. Secondly, salt loading induced a more pronounced decrease in arterial compliance which was mainly due to the increase in blood pressure. This could be explained by the fact that since the compliance (V/P) curve is curvilinear, increased in arterial pressure can, by itself, reduce the compliance (Figure 2) corresponding to the mean blood pressure values (operating compliance). The results of this study suggest that in this particular model of salt sensitivity, carotid artery wall alteration exist even before the development of hypertension produced by increased sodium intake and due to arteriolar constriction.

Similar results have been recently reported in a clinical study by Draaijer et al. [39]. The authors evaluated the arterial compliance of salt sensitive and salt resistant borderline hypertensive patients under normal salt diet. Both populations had the same levels of blood pressure. Their results clearly showed that salt sensitive patients exhibited an increased arterial stiffness as compared to the SR patients even without salt loading.

Diuretic-induced changes in arterial stiffness

Studies of the effects of diuretics on arterial stiffness in hypertension are based on both experimental and clinical recent data.

Experimental data

Two different diuretic compounds were investigated by our group: the Indapamide and the Cicletanine.

Recently, we evaluated the arterial effects of chronic treatment with Indapamide in Dahl sensitive (DS) or resistant (DR) fed a high (H) or a low (L) NaCl diet rats. Indapamide completely prevented the development of salt dependent hypertension in Dahl rats [37]. Previous studies showed that treatment of Dahl rats with other diuretic agents was able to prevent the development of salt sensitive hypertension [35, 40]. However these studies also indicated that the different diuretic agents had various effects on arterial smooth muscle. Uehara et al. [40] showed that Cicletanine was able to release vasorelaxant prostaglandins in Dahl sensitive rats, whereas treatment with thiazides had no effect on these vasodilating substances. On the other hand, Indapamide is known to have vascular effects which may be dissociated from its natriuretic effect [41, 42].

The principal finding of this study was that Indapamide improved the mechanical properties of the carotid artery and that an increase in the operating compliance was observed even in the groups in which no significant change in blood pressure was observed (Figure 3). Particularly for the Dahl sensitive rats fed a high NaCl diet, the increase in operating compliance (corresponding to the mean blood pressure levels) was due to both a reduction in blood pressure and a shift of the pressure-volume curve to the left (Figure 3). Using the same experimental procedure, Levy et al. [43] showed that local intra carotid applications of Indapamide improved arterial mechanical properties in DOCA-salt hypertension independently of transmural pressure changes. In addition to these findings, in the Dahl rats, chronic treatment with Indapamide was able to improve the elastic properties of the carotid artery wall even in animals without salt loading. This result supports the hypothesis that Indapamide has other properties than natriuretic effects [38, 44]. Indeed Schini et al. [41] reported that Indapamide was able to increase the release of vasodilators in isolated arterial segments and to improve the endothelial functions. In addition, previous experiments [43] have shown that Indapamide might modify the local vascular production of the prostaglandin PGI_2. In the recent study (unpublished data), we observed that Indapamide enhanced the activity of endogenous bradykinin in Dahl sensitive

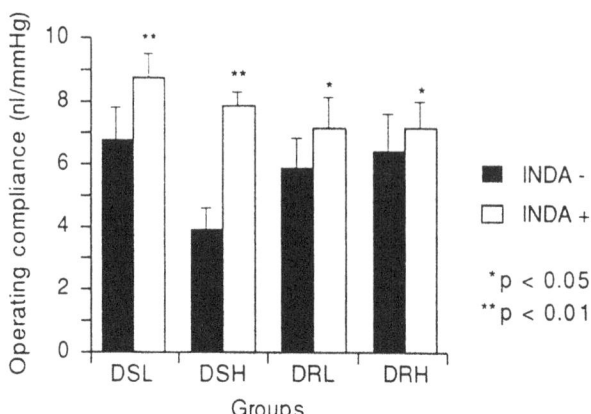

Figure 3. Effects of chronic treatment with Indapamide on the operating compliance in Dahl rats (operating compliance: changes in arterial volume for pressure levels close to the mean blood pressure of the animal [37].

rats. Therefore, we can tentatively suggest that the effects of Indapamide after acute or chronic treatment are related to a drug-induced activation of vasorelaxant factors at the site of the large arteries.

In another study [45], the effects of cicletanine (3 mg/Kg) on the systemic hemodynamics and the mechanical properties of the arterial wall were tested in 12-week-old normotensive Wistar Kyoto (WKY) rats and spontaneously hypertensive rats (SHR). The mechanical properties of the arterial wall were assessed using three independent methods: the characteristic impedance of the ascending aorta, systemic arterial compliance, and compliance of the carotid artery. Characteristic impedance and systemic compliance were calculated from phasic records of pressure and flow in the ascending aorta; carotid compliance was measured in situ with or without smooth muscle cell activity (obtained using potassium cyanure). After chronic therapy by daily gavage for 15 days, there were no significant changes in either WKY and SRH in terms of arterial blood pressure, cardiac output, and heart rate. In contrast, characteristic impedance, systemic compliance, and passive distensibility of the isolated carotid arteries were significantly improved in treated groups. From the effect of potassium cyanure, it appeared that the increase in carotid compliance reflected modifications in the smooth muscle tone of the arterial wall after cicletanine chronic therapy. Although the exact mechanisms of the observed changes in arterial mechanics remained unclear, the study showed that, in experimental hypertension, cicletanine affected distensibility and compliance of large arteries independently of significant changes in blood pressure.

Table 2. Arterial changes following hydrochlorothiazide versus félodipine in subjects with essential hypertension [46]

	Baseline	Felodipine	HCTZ	Felodipine vs HCTZ
Systolic blood pressure (mmHg)	162 ± 12	140 ± 17	150 ± 13	<0.02
Diastolic blood pressure (mmHg)	96 ± 9	85 ± 9	89 ± 9	<0.05
C.F.–P.W.V. (m/s)	10.9 ± 2.0	9.2 ± 1.8	10.1 ± 2	<0.005
F.T.–P.W.V. (m/s)	12.8 ± 1.7	11.1 ± 1.9	12.2 ± 1.7	<0.005
C.R.–P.W.V. (m/s)	11.7 ± 1.9	10.0 ± 2	11.8 ± 1.8	<0.005
Brachial arterial diameter (cm)	0.437 ± 0.06	$0.449 = 0.06$	0.431 ± 0.05	<0.05
Brachial vascular resistance (dyn.sec.cm^{-4})	104 ± 40	72 ± 30	92 ± 46	<0.05
Brachial artery compliance (dyn.cm$^{-4}.10^{-7}$)	1.13 ± 0.48	1.71 ± 0.83	1.19 ± 0.57	<0.005

± 1 standard deviation; PWV = pulse wave velocity; CF = carotido-femoral; FT = femoro-tibial; CR = carotido radial.

Clinical data

This issue has been recently reviewed on the basis of data of our group on hydrochlorothiazide [46] and recent studies on indapamide [47].

The antihypertensive and the arterial effects of the diuretic compound Hydrochlorothiazide (HCTZ) was compared to those of the calcium-entry blocker, Felodipine, in patients with essential hypertension [46]. After one month placebo-period, the patients were included in a double blind, cross over and randomized study. All received either Hydrochlorothiazide (25 to 50 mg) or Felodipine (5 to 10 mg) once a day for 6 weeks. Hemodynamic investigations at the end of placebo and each treatment period included: blood pressure, regional pulse wave velocities (P.W.V.) using a doppler technique for the carotid-femoral (C.F.), femoro-tibial (F.T.) and carotid-radial (C.R.) areas. Arterial diameter, blood flow, vascular resistance and compliance were measured at the site of the brachial artery using a bidimensional Doppler system [10] The study showed that, whereas Felodipine decreased more substantially blood pressure than HCTZ and improved arterial distensibility in the aortic and limbs circulations, the diuretic compound had absolutely no arterial effect despite significant but modest blood pressure reduction (Table 2).

In another study using indapamide [47], systemic arterial compliance, assessed by the ratio between stroke volume and pulse pressure, was determined in ten patients with essential hypertension, treated with placebo or indapamide (2.5 mg/day), in a cross-over, single blind study. After three months of therapy, mean arterial pressure and total peripheral resistance were significantly reduced, whereas cardiac index and arterial compliance increased. The results supported the conclusion that chronic treatment with

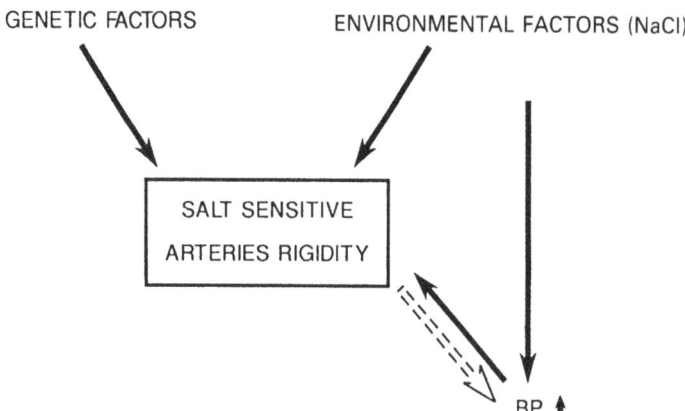

Figure 4. The arterial stiffness of NaCl sensitive subjects is related to the combination of genetic predisposition and NaCl loading. It is possible that reduction in compliance observed even before the salt loading participate to the BP increase in these subjects.

indapamide enhanced arterial compliance. Whether this was due to blood pressure reduction or to a drug-induced arterial effect remained to be investigated.

The arterial effect of indapamide on systemic compliance was not observed on other arteries, as the brachial artery. In this particular case, indapamide did not change brachial artery diameter despite a significant blood pressure reduction [48]. Compliance and distensibility were unchanged [48] or poorly modified [49]. Nevertheless, the lack of change in arterial diameter in the presence of the fall in blood pressure proved a shift of the pressure-diameter curve toward lower values of blood pressure and therefore indicated diuretic-induced changes of the arterial wall [47]. A similar finding was observed with the anti aldosterone compound, canrenone [50].

Therefore, it seems that sodium acts undoubtedly on the arterial wall partially independently of blood pressure changes. However the arterial modifications produced by diuretic agents are relatively small in hypertensive humans and this point remains difficult to explain. Potassium changes are an unlikely explanation since indapamide and canrenone, which have opposite effects on serum potassium, induce the same arterial effects [48]. A more satisfying explanation is that diurectics and especially thiazides induce counterregulatory mechanisms involving an activation of the renin-angiotensin system and of the autonomic nervous system, which both favour arterial constriction [51]. It is so suggested that all these factors contribute to modulate the relaxing process induced by salt and water depletion.

Conclusion

Sodium chloride plays an important role in the regulation not only of the arteriolar tone but also of the large arteries elastic properties. Salt sensitive subjects may present genetically increased arterial stiffness even without salt loading (Figure 4). These arterial alterations are aggravated by salt NaCl loading and may participate in the development of salt dependant hypertension. Diuretics lack of improvement of arterial compliance, despite sodium depletion and blood pressure reduction, may be related to an overactivation of renin angiotensin system.

Acknowledgement

We thank Mrs Annette Seban for her excellent assistance.

References

1. Morgan T, Gilles A, Morgan G, Adam W, Wilson M, Carney S. Hypertension treated by salt restriction. Lancet, 1978, i: 227–30.
2. McGregor GA, Markandu N, Best FE, et al. Double-blind randomized cross-over trial of a moderate sodium restriction in essential hypertension. Lancet 1982, i: 351–5.
3. Hollenberg NK, Williams GH. Sodium-sensitive hypertension. Implication of pathogenesis for therapy. Am J Hyperten 1989; 2: 809–15.
4. Horan MJ, Lenfant C. Epidemiology of blood pressure and predictors of hypertension. Hypertension 1990 15(Suppl 1): 10-1-24.
5. Dahl LK. Metabolic aspects of hypertension. Ann Rev Med 1963; 14: 69–98.
6. Kawasaki T, Delea CS, Batter FC, Smith H. The effect of high-sodium and low-sodium intakes on blood pressure and other related variables in human subjects with idiopathic hypertension. Am J Med 1978; 68: 193–8.
7. Fujita T, Henrt WL, Batter FC, Lake CR, Delea CS. Factors influencing blood pressure in salt-sensitive patients with hypertension. Am J Med 1980; 69: 334–44.
8. Lindpaintner K, Sen S. Role of sodium in hypertensive cardiac hypertrophy. Circ Res 1985; 57: 1610–7.
9. Tobian L. Salt and hypertension lessons from animal models that relate to human hypertension. Hypertension 1991; 117(Suppl. 1): 1152–8.
10. Safar ME, Bouthier JA, Levenson JA, Simon AC. Peripheral large arteries and the response to antihypertensive treatment. Hypertension 1983; 5(Suppl 3): 63–8.
11. Haddy FJ. The role of a humoral Na^+, K^+-ATPase inhibitor in regulating precapillary vessel tone. J Cardiovasc Pharmacol 1984; 6: S439–S56.
12. Brading AF, Lategan TW. Editorial review: Na-Ca exchange in vascular smooth muscle. J Hypertens 1985; 13: 109–16.
13. Clausen T. Adrenergic control of Na^+ K^+ homeostasis. Acta Med Scand 1983; 672 (Suppl): 111–5.
14. Benetos A, Breshahan M, Gavras I, Gavras H. Central catecholamines and alpha-adrenoreceptors in acute hypertension induced by intracerebroventricular hypertonic saline. J Hypertens 1987; 5: 767–71.
15. McGregor GA, de Wardener HE. A circulation sodium transport inhibitor and essential hypertension. J Cardiovasc Pharmacol 1984; 6: S55–S60.

16. O'Rourke MF. Arterial function in health and disease. Edinburgh: Churchill Livinstone 1982: 24–357.

17. Roberts J ed. Blood pressure levels of persons 6–74 years. United states 1971–74. Department of Health. Education and Welfare publication No. HRA 78. Washington DC: United States Government Printing Office 1977.

18. Oliver WJ. Sodium homeostasis and low blood pressure populations. In: Kesteloot H, Joosens JV, editors. Epidemiology of arterial pressure. The Hague: Martinus Nijhoff, 1980: 229–41.

19. Avolio AP, Deng FQ, Li WQ, et al. Effects of aging on arterial distensibility in populations with high and low prevalence of hypertension: comparison between urban and rural communities in China. Circulation 1985; 71: 202–10.

20. Avolio AP, Clyde CM, Beard TC, Cooke HM, Kenneth KL, O'Rourke MF. Improved arterial distensibility in normotensive subjects on a low salt diet. Arteriosclerosis 1986; 16: 166–9.

21. Benetos A, Yang-Yan X, Cuche JL, Hannaert P, Safar M. Arterial effects of salt restriction in hypertensive patients. A 2-month randomized double-blind, cross-over study. J Hypertens 1992; 10: 355–60.

22. Myers JB, Morgan TO.The effect of sodium intake on the blood pressure related to age and sex. Clin Exp Hypertens 1983; 5: 99–118.

23. Levenson JA, Simon AC, Maarek BE, Gitelman GJ, Fiessinger JN, Safar ME. Regional compliance of brachial artery and saline infusion in patients with arteriosclerosis obliterans. Arteriosclerosis 1985; 5: 80–7.

24. Dahl LK, Heine M, Tassinari L. Role of genetic factors in susceptibility to experimental hypertension due to chronic excess salt ingestion. Nature 1962; 194: 480–2.

25. Ganguli M, Tobian L, Iwai J. Cardiac output and peripheral resistance in strains of rats sensitive and resistant to NaCl hypertension. Hypertension 1979; 1: 3–7.

26. Racz K, Kuchel O, Buu NT. Abnormal adrenal catecholamine synthesis in salt-sensitive dahl rats. Hypertension 1987; 9: 76–80.

27. Chen YF, Meng Q, Wyss JM, Jin H, Rogers CF, Oparil S. NaCl does not affect hypothalamic noradrenergic input in deoxycorticosterone acetate/NaCl and Dahl salt-sensitive rats. Hypertension 1987; 9: 76–80.

28. Ferrarie AU, Mark AL. Sensitization of aortic baroreceptors by high salt diet in dahl salt-resistant rats. Hypertension 1987; 10: 55–60.

29. Rapp JP. Dahl salt-susceptible and salt-resistant rats. Hypertension 1982; 4: 1753–63.

30. Kong JQ, Taylor DA, Fleming WW, Kotchen TA. Specific supersensitivity of the mesenteric vascular bed of Dahl salt-sensitive rats. Hypertension 1991; 17: 1349–56.

31. Lischer TF, Raij, Van Houtte PM. Endothelium-dependent vascular responses in normotensive and hypertensive Dahl rats. Hypertension 1987; 9: 1 57–63.

32. Benetos A, Bouaziz H, Safar M. Endogenous bradykinin activity in Dahl rats. J CV Pharmacol 1993; 21: 101–104.

33. Boegehold M, Kotchent T. Effect of dietary salt on the skeletal muscle microvasclarture in Dahl rats. Hypertension 1990; 15: 420–6.

34. Lee RMKW, Triggle CR. Morphometric study of mesentereic arteries from genetically hypertensive Dahl strain rats. Blood Vessels 1986; 23: 199–224.

35. Tobian L, Lange J, Iwai J, Hiller K, Johnson MA, Grossen P. Prevention with thiazide of NaCl-induced hypertension in Dahl "S" rats. Hypertension 1979; 1: 316–23.

36. Bouaziz H, Benetos A, Levy BI, Safar ME. Arterial mechanical properties of Dahl sensitive rats. In: Sassard J, editor. Genetic Hypertension. Colloque INSERM 1992; 218: 273–5.

37. Bouaziz H, Benetos A, Albaladejo P, Guez, Safar ME. Arterial mechanical properties of Dahl sensitive rats: effects of indapamide. (Submitted for publication.)

38. Benetos A, Bouaziz H, Albaladejo P, Levy BI, Safar ME. Physiological and pharmacological changes in the carotid artery pressure-volume in situ in rats. J Hypertens 1992; 10(Suppl 6): S127–S31.

39. Draaijer P, Kool M, Van Bortel L, De Leeuw P, Leunissen KML. Salt sensitive borderline

hypertensive patients (SRBHT vs SSBHT). J Hypertens 1992; Vol. 10(Suppl 4): 74 (Abstract).

40. Uehara Y, Numabe A, Hirawa N, et al. Antihypertensive effects of cicletanine and renal protection in Dahl salt-sensitive rats. J Hypertens 1991; 9: 1719–28.

41. Schini VB, Dewey J, Van Houtte PM. Effects of indapamide on endothelium-dependent relaxations in isolated canine femoral arteries; Am J Cardiol 1990; 65: 6H–10H.

42. Uehara Y, Shirahase H, Nagata T, et al. Radical scavenging effects of indapamide on prostacyclin generation in vascular smooth muscle cells in rats. Hypertension 1990; 15: 216–24.

43. Levy BI, Poitevin P, Safar M. Effects of Indapamide on the mechanical properties of normotensive and hypertensive rats without arterial pressure changes. J Card Pharmacol 1989; 14: 253–9.

44. Kraetz J, Criscione L, Hedwal PR. Dissociation of vascular and natriuretic effects of diuretic agents. Naumyn Schmiedeberg's Arch Pharmacol 1978; 302 (Suppl) R42.

45. Levy BI, Curmi P, Poitevin P, Safar ME. Modifications of the arterial mechanical properties of normotensive and hypertensive rats without arterial pressure changes. J Cardio Pharmacol 1989; 14: 253–9.

46. Asmar R, Benetos A, Chaouche K, Raveau-Landon C, Safar M. Arterial changes following diuretic therapy versus calcium blockade hypertension. 14e Scientific Meeting of the International Society of Hypertension.(Abstract), Madrid 1992.

47. Carretta R, Fabris B, Bardelli M, et al. Arterial compliance and baroreceptor sensitivity after chronic treatment with indapamide. J Human Hypertension 1988; 2: 171–5.

48. Laurent S, Lacolley PM, Cuche JL, Safar ME. Influence of diuretics on brachial artery diameter and distensibility in hypertensive patients. Fundam Clin Pharmacol 1990; 4: 685–93.

49. Smulyan H, Vardan S, Griffiths A, Gribbin B. Forearm arterial distensibility in systolic hypertension. J Am Coll Cardiol 1984; 3: 387–93.

50. Laurent S, Hannaert PA, Girerd XJ, Safar ME, Garay R. Chronic treatment with canrenone potentiates the acute pressor effects of ouabain in essential hypertensive patients. J Hypertens 1987; 5(Suppl 5): S1 73–S5.

51. Safar ME, Levy BI, Laurent S, London GM. Hypertension and the arterial system: clinical and therapeutic aspects. J Hypertens 1990; 8(Suppl 7): S113–S9.

13. Large arteries and calcium in hypertension
Pathophysiological and therapeutic aspects

GERARD M. LONDON and BERNARD I. LÉVY

Introduction

Epidemiological studies have emphasized the close relationship between the level of blood pressure and the incidence of cardiovascular diseases [1]. Clinical hypertension is usually classified on the basis of diastolic blood pressure and the high blood pressure is attributed to a reduction in the lumen area of small arteries resulting in an increase in hemodynamic resistances. This definition does not account for the fact that the large systemic arteries play an important role in determining the shape and the amplitude of the blood pressure wave, influencing the level of systolic, diastolic and pulse pressure [2] Some studies have directed attention to systolic pressure as a better guide than diastolic pressure to cardiovascular mortality [3, 4]. In the same way, increased pulse pressure has been reported as an independent cardiovascular risk factor in hypertension [5–7]. Therefore, arterial compliance and other factors influencing the systolic and the pulse pressure could be important cardiovascular risk factors. The implication of large arteries in the morbid events of patient treated for hypertension has also resulted in an extensive investigation of the effects of antihypertensive drugs on arterial compliance [8–12].

With aging the arterial wall thickens, the artery dilates and become less compliant (13–15] The principal changes occur in the media and intima and concern the elastic fibers and laminae which are principally responsible for the vessel distensibility. The degeneration of elastic tissue is associated with an increase in collagen content in the media and deposition of calcium [16] Deposition of calcium salts in the walls of human arteries is a normal process which starts in childhood and progress with age. Blumenthal et al. [17] were among the first to present evidence that calcium concentration in the human aorta increased with age even before the development of fibrous or atherosclerotic plaques. Therefore, calcinosis appears to be an inevitable consequence of aging even in the absence of atherosclerotic plaques and occlusive lesions [18, 19] Arterial calcinosis 'per se' was considered as a phenomenon of secondary importance, since it does not compromise the down-stream

M. E. Safar and M. F. O'Rourke (eds.), The arterial system in hypertension. pp. 209–219.
© 1993 *Kluwer Academic Publishers. Printed in the Netherlands.*

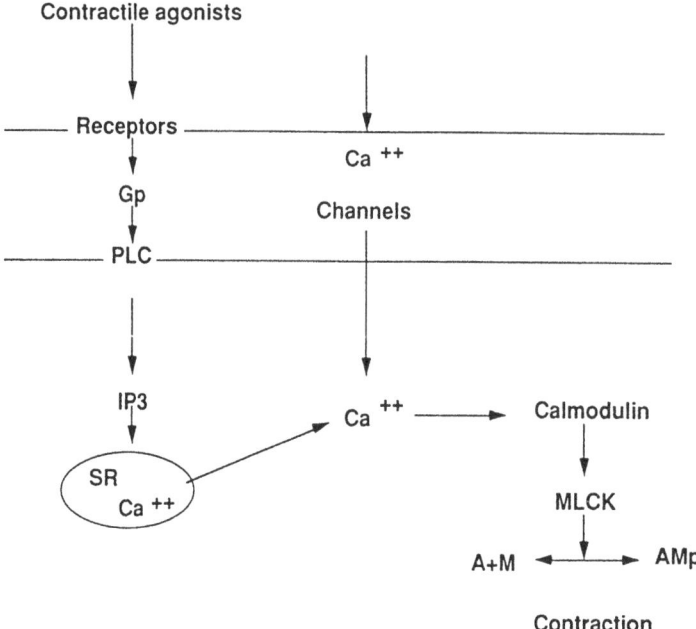

Figure 1. Schematic mechanisms for contraction in vascular smooth muscle. Gp = phospholipase C activating G protein; PLC = phospholipase C; IP3 = inosistol tri-phosphate; SR = sarcoplasmic reticulum; MLCK = myosin light chain kinase; A = actine; M = myosin; AMp = attached phosphorylated myosin.

perfusion. Nevertheless, cross sectional studies in normal population have shown that calcinosis decreases the distensibility of the aorta even after adjustment for age and blood pressure [20] Interestingly, several authors reported that calcium antagonists could prevent the development of experimental arterial calcinosis and could retard the calcium accumulation in aging, hypertensive, and alloxan-diabetic rats [18, 19].

Calcium and smooth muscle cells

Calcium ion (Ca^{++}) has an essential role in the contraction of vascular smooth muscle (Figure 1). Cellular Ca^{++} is increased by an activation of influx and the release of calcium from store sites in the smooth muscle cell. Most contractile stimuli induce arterial smooth muscle contraction by increasing myoplasmic calcium concentration [21] Ca^{++} binds to calmodulin and the Ca^{++}-calmodulin complex removes the auto-inhibition of myosin light chain kinase [22]. The activated myosin light chain kinase phosphorylates the 20-kd light chain of myosin and activates the myosin's ATPase [23] Finally, the phosphorylated myosin binds to actin filaments producing force and shortening of the smooth muscle cell [24] However, the theory of myosin phosphorylation probably cannot entirely explain vascular smooth muscle contraction: there is evidence that the regulatory mechanism for tension does not depend solely on the phosphorylation of myosin [25]; furthermore, neurotransmitters transiently increase cellular Ca^{++} but maintain the contraction [26]. Based on the results obtained from measurements of tension and cellular Ca^{++}, it has been suggested that the agonist activates Ca^{++} influxes in both voltage-dependent and voltage-independent manners in vascular smooth muscle cells. This hypothesis is mainly supported by the following:

- nor-epinephrine or acetylcholine can produce tonic contraction without altering membrane depolarization; and,
- organic Ca^{++}-antagonists, such as nifedipine, nimodipine, nisoldipine, completely block the tonic increase of $[Ca^{++}]i$ and tension induced by high potassium concentration, but only partially inhibit the tonic responses induced by an agonist [27].

To test the mechanisms of pharmaco-mechanical coupling in the vascular smooth muscle, two methods have been used. First, the relation between the level of myosin light chain phosphorylation, tension and the shortening velocity of smooth muscle strips were studied, in vitro. Secondly, using membrane permeabilized smooth muscle (skinned smooth muscle) strips, the relation between tension and level of myosin light chain phosphorylation was more directly compared in clamped cellular Ca^{++} concentration. Since Ca^{++} concentration is supposed to be constant under a steady state condition in skinned muscle cells, the data obtained could give more direct evidence about the Ca^{++} dependent relation between tension and MLC phosphorilation. Reviewing results obtained from both types of experiments, Itoh [27] concluded that the phosphorylation of myosin light chain may be the mechanism for the Ca^{++} induced contraction in smooth muscle. However, additional high Ca^{++} sensitive mechanisms are no doubt involved in the contraction of vascular smooth muscle.

By blocking the transport of calcium across cell membrane, calcium entry blockers (CEB) reduce the tone of vascular smooth muscle and produce relaxation of vascular smooth muscle. Calcium entry blockers are now widely used in the treatment of patients with cardiovascular diseases, e.g., ischemic heart disease, heart failure, arterial hypertension, Raynaud's disease. Their therapeutic action is based upon a range of hemodynamic actions, including effects on blood vessels, the heart and the kidney as well as different neural and endocrine mechanisms involved in cardiovascular control. The reduction of left ventricular afterload is classically attributed to peripheral arteriolar dilation [28]. However, the effects of calcium blockers on large arteries could markedly influence the left ventricular afterload.

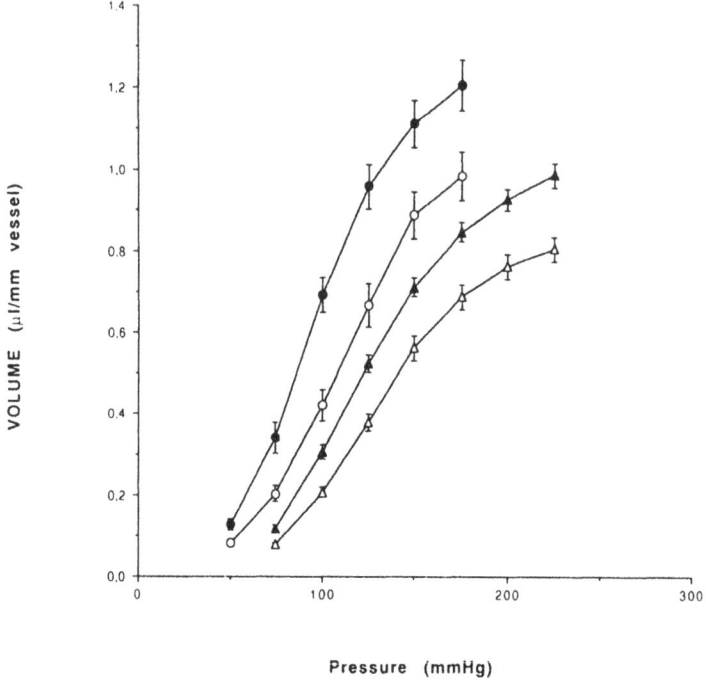

Figure 2. Pressure-volume (mean values ± sem) relationships in carotid arteries under control conditions (open symbols) and after total abolition of smooth muscle tone (closed symbols). Normotensive WKY rats: open and closed circles, Spontaneously hypertensive rats (SHR) open and closed triangles. The slope of the pressure-volume curves represent the compliance of the carotid artery. In SHRs, under control conditions and after abolition of smooth muscle tone, the carotid compliance is significantly smaller than in WKY rats.

Large arteries in hypertension and the role of calcium

An experimental model was developed in our laboratory, allowing a precise measure of pressure-volume relation in the 'in situ' isolated rat carotid artery [29, 30]. Investigations were carried out in living reno-vascular hypertensive rats and spontaneously hypertensive rats (SHR) with Wistar Kyoto (WKY) normotensive rats used as controls. For varying pressures from 50 to 200 mmHg, the carotid artery compliance values were significantly lower in SHR than in WKY rats, indicating that there had been intrinsic, pressure independent, modifications of the arterial wall in hypertensive rats. These changes may be due to structural changes or modifications in arterial smooth muscle tone. Abolition of vascular smooth muscle by potassium cyanide poisoning resulted in a significant increase in compliance in both WKY and SHR. The compliance of the totally relaxed carotid arteries was still smaller in SHRs than in WKY rats (Figure 2) suggesting that structural changes, and not only vasomotor tone, were important in reducing the compliance observed in hypertensive animals [29–31] Several studies in man showed that the damping function of the arteries is altered in essential as well as in secondary hypertension [32–34] and that age-related changes of arterial wall are accelerated. These studies agree to suggest that arterial compliance is reduced in hypertension not only because of high blood pressure but also in relation with intrinsic alterations of the viscoelastic properties of the arterial walls.

The role played by calcium in the alteration of the function of human large arteries was demonstrated in hypertensive and normotensive patients with end-stage renal disease [20, 35]. It has been shown that the use of high-calcium dialysate produces acute hypercalcemia and a decrease in arterial compliance occurring despite a decrease in arterial pressure. This decrease in compliance was not observed in patients with low calcium concentration dialysate and in patients receiving CEB [35]. These results provided evidence that increase extracellular calcium decreases arterial distensibility by increasing the vasomotor tone. Calcium also alters the structure of arteries, with increase of incidence of calcinosis in patients with end-stage renal disease.

Response of the large arteries to calcium entry blockers

Experimental data

There are few reports in which the large arteries response to CEB was evaluated. The usual response which is evaluated is the aortic pressure-diameter relationship during acute administration of drugs. Yano et al. [36] studied the effects of acute administration of diltiazem on aortic pressure-diameter relationship in anesthetized dogs. They reported that the aortic diameter and pressure were reduced by diltiazem, and that the aortic pressure-diameter curves was shifted towards higher diameters for any given pressure. The significant increase in aortic wall distensibility was attributed to a decrease in aortic smooth muscle tone. Using an 'in situ' model of isolated carotid arteries in normotensive and spontaneously hypertensive rats, we observed that calcium blockade by clentiazem induced in both strains a significant shift of the pressure-volume curve so that volume was significantly higher after calcium blockade than under control conditions. In normotensive rats, the carotid mechanical properties were similar after calcium blockade and after abolition of the smooth muscle tone by potassium cyanide poisoning. In spontaneously hypertensive rats, the carotid compliance measured after incubation with clentiazem was significantly lower than that measured after KCN poisoning (Figure 3). These results suggests that, in hypertensive rats, constrictive factors non sensitive to calcium blockers could participate to the high vasomotor tone [37].

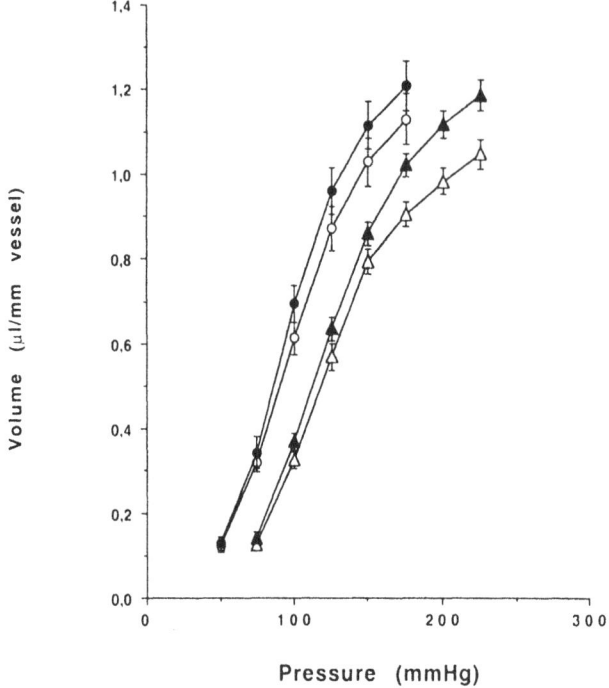

Figure 3. Pressure-volume (mean values ± sem) relationships in carotid arteries after local incubation with calcium entry blocker (open symbols) and after total abolition of smooth muscle tone (closed symbols). Normotensive WKY rats: open and closed circles, Spontaneously hypertensive rats (SHR) open and closed triangles. The slope of the pressure-volume curves represent the compliance of the carotid artery. In WKY rats, calcium entry blocker completely relaxed the carotid. but in SHRs, a significant reserve of relaxation remained after CEB.

Effects of CEB on arterial diameter in hypertensive patients

The fall in arterial pressure produced by antihypertensive drugs may be associated with active changes in the geometry of large arteries; this was demonstrated in healthy volunteers as well as in hypertensive patients [38–40]. In a double blind placebo controlled study in healthy volunteers maintained on an ad libitum sodium intake, acute administration of increasing doses of nicardipine increased the diameters of the carotid and brachial arteries in a dose dependent manner. Systemic blood pressure did not significantly change, suggesting that CEB acted on the arterial wall independently of pressure-induced mechanical factors. When healthy volunteers received verapamil, arterial diameter did not increase but blood pressure significantly decreased suggesting also a direct action on the arterial wall [40]. Similar observations were performed on brachial artery in essential hypertension with diltiazem [38]. For an equipotent antihypertensive effect, dihydralazine reduced the diameter of brachial artery whereas diltiazem caused an increase in brachial arterial diameter. In patients with sustained essential hypertension, acute oral administration of dihydropyridine derivatives such as nifedipine, nicardipine, and nitrendipine caused a significant increase in arterial diameter in the brachial artery [41–43]. With nicardipine given orally, the brachial artery diameter increase persisted for several weeks [43]. As such findings were obtained in the presence of a significant reduction of blood pressure, it appeared that the passive mechanical effect of blood pressure (decrease in diameter) was offset by the direct arterial dilatation effect of CEB. In a 24 week, double blind placebo controlled study of nitrendipine in patients with end-stage renal disease and arterial calcinosis, treatment with CEB did not induce any changes in aortic diameter despite a significant decrease in arterial pressure [20].

Several studies showed that dihydropyridine derivatives significantly increase forearm and brachial blood flow in both normotensive and hypertensive subjects with a larger effect in hypertensive than in normotensive [44, 45]. Since CEBs cause an increase in blood flow, the simultaneous increase in the diameter of large arteries could be related to mechanisms of 'high flow dilation' due to the increase in endothelial shear stress. At the site of brachial artery, this possibility seems likely with dihydropyridines [41, 42] but less plausible with diltiazem which does not increase flow velocity and therefore shear stress [38]. The possible role of high blood flow dilation on the mechanism of the diameter alterations following calcium blockade remains difficult to assess in patients.

Calcium and endothelium functions

Since Furchgott and Zawadzki [46] in 1980, it has been widely established that endothelial cells can secrete both relaxing and contracting factors that influence the responsiveness of the underlying vascular smooth muscle [47]. It has been suggested that calcium antagonists can interfere with the endothelium-dependent vasomotor tone [48]. The Ca^{++} ionophore A23187 evokes endothelium dependent relaxations in different isolated arteries and veins [49] and stimulates the release of endothelium derived relaxing factor from the perfused arteries [50, 51]. In the same way, removal of the extracellular Ca^{++} reduces endothelium-dependent relaxation [52, 53] in response to muscarinic activation in the aorta of the rat and rabbit. Incubation of isolated blood vessels in Ca^{++} free solution does not affect the increase in cyclic GMP levels caused by sodium nitroprussiate, but prevents that caused by basal or acetylcholine induced release of endothelium derived relaxing factor [54]. Theses findings suggest that an increase in cytosolic Ca^{++} is an essential step in the synthesis and/or release of endothelium-derived relaxing factor [55].

Endothelial cells can contain voltage-operated Ca^{++} channels that allow enough Ca^{++} to enter the cell to cause the release of endothelium-derived relaxing factor. This conclusion is reached from the observation that, in the canine femoral artery, Ca^{++}-channel agonists such as BAY K 8644 cause the release of endothelium-derived relaxing factor. This effect can be prevented by Ca^{++} antagonists such as nitrendipine [56].

Even if there are voltage-operated Ca^{++} channels on endothelial cells, these seem not to be involved in the release of endothelium-derived relaxing factor evoked by acetylcholine and other endothelium-dependent dilators [56–59]. The inhibitory effects of Ca^{++} and that of endothelium-derived relaxing factor seem to be additive. This is suggested by studies in canine coronary arteries that show that the dihydropryridine derivative nisoldipine is more effective in the presence than in the absence of endothelium in preventing contractions caused by alpha-1 adrenergic agonists [60]. The synergism between Ca^{++} antagonists and endothelium-derived relaxing factor may be explained by a simultaneous action on voltage-and receptor-operated Ca^{++} channels, respectively [61, 62].

Using our experimental model of 'in situ' isolated carotid artery in WKY and SHR rats, we have recently observed [37] that removal of the endothelium induced a significant shift of the pressure-volume curve toward the volume axis in both strains and an increase in carotid compliance. Local incubation with clentiazem or total abolition of smooth muscle tone did not induce further modifications of the pressure-volume relation either in WKY or in SHR.

Furthermore, in SHR and in WKY carotid arteries, the pressure-volume relationship and the compliance measured after incubation with clentiazem were identical in the presence and in the absence of endothelium. Finally, part of the compliance enhancement induced by calcium antagonist could be related to an antagonizing mechanism of the production of endothelial constricting factor(s) [37].

In conclusion, this chapter reviews the interaction between calcium and calcium antagonists in the physiology and the physiopathology of the large peripheral arteries. These latter are an important site of action for calcium entry blockers, causing an increase in arterial compliance and/or in diameter together with blood pressure reduction in patients treated for sustained essential or secondary hypertension. Interaction between calcium, calcium entry blockers in one hand and paracrine and autocrine functions of the endothelial cells on the other hand is of major interest and needs further investigations.

References

1. Tverdal A. Systolic and diastolic blood pressure as predictor of coronary heart disease in middle aged Norwegian men. Br Med J 1987; 294: 671–3.
2. O'Rourke MF. Vascular impedance: the relationship between pressure and flow. In: Arterial Function in Health and Disease. Edinburgh: Churchill Livingstone 1982;: 94–132.
3. Curb JD, Borhani NO, Entwisle G, et al. Isolated systolic hypertension in 14 communities. Am J Epidemiol 1985; 121: 362–70.

4. Kannel WB, Gordon T, Schwartz MJ. Systolic versus diastolic blood pressure and risk of coronary heart disease: The Framingham study. Am J Cardiol 1971; 27: 335–46.
5. Darne B, Girerd X, Safar ME, Cambien F, Guize L. Pulsatile versus steady component of blood pressure: a cross sectional an a prospective analysis on cardiovascular mortality. Hypertension 1898; 13: 392–400.
6. Dyer AR, Stamler J, Shekelle RB, et al. Pulse pressure. III. Prognostic significance in four Chicago epidemiologic studies. J Chron Dis 1985; 35: 283–94.
7. Rutan GH, Kuller LH, Neaton JD. Mortality associated with diastolic hypertension among men screened for the Multiple Risk Factor Intervention Trial. Circulation 1988; 77: 504–14.
8. Asmar RG, Pannier B, Santoni JP, et al. Reversion of cardiac hypertrophy and reduced arterial compliance after converting enzyme inhibition in essential hypertension. Circulation 1988; 78: 941–50.
9. London GM, Marchais SJ, Guerin AP, et al. Salt and water retention and calcium blockade in uremia. Circulation 1990; 82: 105–113.
10. Simon AC, Levenson JA, Levy BI, Bouthier JE, Peronneau PP, Safar ME., Effect of nitroglycerin on peripheral large arteries in hypertension. Br J Clin Pharmacol 1982; 14: 241–6.
11. Smulyan H, Moorkerherjee S, Warner RA. The effect of nitroglycerin on forearm arterial distensibility. Circulation 1986; 73: 1264–9.
12. Van Merode T, Van Bortel L, Smeets FA, et al. The effect of verapamil on carotid artery distensibility and cross sectional compliance in hypertensive patients. J Cardiovasc Pharmacol 1990; 15: 109–13.
13. Avolio AP, Chen SG, Wang RP, Zhang CL, Li MF, O'Rourke MF. Effects of aging on changing arterial compliance and left ventricular load in a northern Chinese Urban community. Circulation 1983; 68: 50–8.
14. Mitchell JRA, Schwartz CJ. Arterial disease. Oxford: Bramwell 1965: 87–102.
15. Virmani R, Avolio AP, Mergner WJ, et al. Effects of aging on aortic morphology in populations with high and low prevalence of hypertension and atherosclerosis. Am J Pathol 1991; 139: 1119–29.
16. O'Rourke MF, Avolio AP, Lauren PD, Young J. Age related changes of elastic lamellae in the human thoracic aorta. J Am Coll Cardiol 1987; 9: 53A.
17. Blumenthal HT, Lansing AI, Wheeler PA. Calcification of the human aorta and its relation to intimal atherosclerosis, aging and disease. Am J Pathol 1944; 20: 665–87.
18. Fleckenstein A. Frey M, Fleckenstein-Grn G. Protection by calcium antagonists against experimental arterial calcinosis. In: Pyrl K, Rapaport E, Knig K, Schettler G, Diehm C, editors. Secondary prevention of coronary heart disease. Stuttgart: Georg Thieme Verlag 1983: 109–22.
19. Fleckenstein A. Calcium antagonism: History and prospect for a multifaceted pharmacodynamic principle. In: Opie LH, editor. Calcium antagonists and cardiovascular disease. New York: Raven Press 0000: 9–28.
20. London GM, Marchais SJ, Safar ME, et al. Aortic and large artery compliance in end-stage renal failure. Kidney Int 1990; 37: 137–42.
21. Rembold CM. Regulation of contraction and relaxation in arterial smooth muscle. Hypertension 1992; 20: 129–37.
22. Means AR, Van Berkum MFA, Bagchi I, Lu KP, Rasmussen CD. Regulatory functions of calmodulin. Pharmacol Ther 1991; 50: 255–70.
23. Ikebe M, Koretz J, Hartshorne DJ. Effects of phosphorylation of light chain residues threonine 18 and serine 19 on the properties and conformation of smooth muscle myosin. J Biol Chem 1988; 263: 6432–7.
24. Hai CM, Murphy RA. Ca^{++}, crossbridge phosphorylation, and contraction. Ann Rev Physiol 1989; 51: 285–98.
25. Kamm KE, Stull JT. The function of myosin and myosin light chain kinase phosphorylation in smooth muscle. Ann Rev Pharmacol Toxicol. 1985; 25: 593–620.

26. Morgan JP, Morgan KG. Stimulus-specific patterns of intracellular calcium levels in smooth muscle of ferret portal vein. J Physiol (Lond) 1984; 351: 155–67.

27. Itoh T. Pharmacological coupling in vascular smooth muscle cells. An overview. Japan J Pharmacol 1991; 55: 1–9.

28. Gross R, Kirchhaim H, von Olshausen K. Effects of nifedipine on coronary and systemic hemodynamics in the conscious dogs. Arzneim Forsch 1979; 29: 1361–7.

29. Levy BI, Michel JB, Salzmann JL, et al. Effects of chronic inhibition of converting enzyme on the mechanical and structural properties of arteries in rat renovascular hypertension. Circulation Res 1988; 63: 227–39.

30. Levy BI, Benessiano J, Poitevin P, Safar ME. Endothelium dependent mechanical properties of the carotid artery in WKY and SHR: Role of angiotensin converting enzyme inhibition. Circulation Res 1990; 66: 321–8.

31. Levy BI, Curmi P, Poitevin P, Safar ME. Modifications of arterial mechanical properties of normotensive and hypertensive rats without arterial pressure changes. J Cardiovasc Pharmacol. 1989; 14: 253–9.

32. Arcaro G, Laurent S, Jondeau G, Hoeks AP, Safar ME. Stiffness of the common carotid artery in treated hypertensive patients. J Hypertens 1991; 9: 947–54.

33. Hugue CJ, Safar ME, Aleferakis MC, Asmar RG, London GM. The ratio between ankle and brachial systolic pressure in patients with sustained uncomplicated essential hypertension. Clin Sci 1988; 174: 179–2.

34. Nichols WW, O'Rourke MF. Vascular impedance. In: McDonald's Blood Flow in Arteries: Theoretic, experimental and clinical principles (3rd ed). London: Edward Arnold Publisher 1991: 283–329.

35. Marchais S, Guerin A, Safar ME, London GM. Arterial compliance in uremia. J Hypertens 1989; 7(Suppl 6): S84–S5.

36. Yano M, Kumada T, Matsuzaki M, et al. Effect of diltiazem on aortic pressure-diameter relationship in dogs. Am J Physiol 1989; 256: H1580–H7.

37. Levy BI, El Fertak L, Piedeloup C, Barouki F, Safar ME. Role of endothelium in the mechanical response of the carotid arterial wall to calcium blockade in SHR and WKY rat. J Hypertens (in press).

38. Safar ME, Simon AC, Levenson JA, Cazor JI. Hemodynamic effect of diltiazem in hypertension. Circ Res 1983; 52(Suppl 1): 169–73.

39. Thuillez C, Gueret M, Duhaze P, Lhoste F, Kiechel JR, Giudicelli JF. Nicardipine: pharmacokinetics and effects on carotid and brachial blood flow in normal volunteers. Brit J Clin Pharmacol 1984; 18: 837–47.

40. Thuillez C, Duhaze P, Fournier C, Lapierre V, Giudicelli JF. Arterial and venous effects of verapamil in normal volunteers. Fundam Clin Pharmacol 1987; 1: 35 44.

41. Bouthier JD, Safar ME, Benetos A, Simon AC, Levenson JA, Hugues CM. Haemodynamic effects of vasodilating drugs on the common carotid and brachial circulations of patients with essential hypertension. Br J Clin Pharmacol 1986; 21: 137–42.

42. Levenson JA, Simon AC, Safar ME, et al. Large arteries in hypertension: acute effects of a new calcium.entry blocker, nitrendipine. J Cardiovasc Pharmacol 1984; 6(Suppl 7): S1006–S10.

43. Levenson JA, Simon AC, Bouthier J, Maarek BC, Safar ME. The effect of acute and chronic nicardipine therapy on forearm arterial hemodynamics in essential hypertension. Br J Clin Pharmacol 1985; 20: 107–13.

44. Hulthen UL, Bolli P, Buhler FR. Vasodilatory effect of nicardipine and verapamil in the forearm of hypertensive as compared with normotensive man. Br J Clin Pharmacol 1985; 20(Suppl 1): 62S–6S.

45. Robinson BF, Collier JG, Dobbs RJ. Comparative dilator effect of verapamil and sodium nitroprussiate in forearm vascular bed and dorsal hand veins in man: functional differences between vascular smooth muscles in arterioles and veins. Cardiovasc Res 1979; 13: 16–21.

46. Furchgott R, Zawadzki JV. The obligatory role of endothelial cells in the relaxation of arterial smooth muscle by acetylcholine. Nature (Lon) 1980; 288: 373–6.

47. Vanhoutte PM. Endothelium and the control of vascular tissue. News Pharmacol Sci 1987; 2: 18–22.
48. Vanhoutte PM. Vascular endothelium and Ca^{++} antagonists. J Cardiovasc Pharmacol 12(Suppl 6): S21–S8.
49. Miller VM, Reigel MM, Hollier LH, Vanhoutte PM. Endothelium-dependent responses in autogenous femoral veins grafted into the arterial circulation of the dog. J Clin Invest 1987; 80: 1350–7.
50. Griffith TM, Edwards DH, Lewis MJ, Newby AC, Henderson AH. The nature of the endothelium-derived relaxing factor. Nature (Lond) 1984; 308: 645–7.
51. Rubanyi GM, Schwartz A, Vanhoutte PM. The effect of diltiazem and verapamil on endothelium-dependent responses in canine blood vessels. Pharmacologist 1985; 27: 290.
52. Singer HA, Peach MJ. Calcium and endothelial mediated vascular smooth muscle relaxation in rabbit aorta. Hypertension 1982; 14(Suppl): 19–25.
53. Winquist RJ, Bunting PB, Schofield TJ. Blockade of endothelium dependent relaxation by the amiloride analog dichlorobenzamil: possible role of Na^+/Ca^{++} exchange in the release of.endothelium derived relaxing factor. J Pharmacol Exp Ther 1985; 235: 644–50.
54. Rapoport RM, Murad F. Agonist-induced endothelium dependent relaxation in rat thoracic aorta may be mediated through cGMP. Circ Res 1983; 52: 352–7.
55. Rubanyi GM, Vanhoutte PM. Calcium and activation of the release of endothelium derived relaxing factor. Proc NY Acad Sci 1988; 1552: 226–33.
56. Rubanyi GM, Schwartz A, Vanhoutte PM. The calcium agonist BAY K 8644 stimulates the release of endothelium-derived relaxing factor from canine femoral arteries. Eur J Pharmacol 1985; 117: 143–4.
57. Rubanyi GM, Vanhoutte PM. Calcium and activation of the release of endothelium derived relaxing factor. Proc NY Acad Sci 1988; 552: 226–33.
58. Schoeffler P, Miller RC. Role of sodium-calcium exchange and effect of calcium entry blockers on endothelial mediated responses in rat isolated aorta. Mol Pharmacol 1986; 30: 53–7.
59. Nagase H, Karaki H, Urakawa N. The inhibitory effects of calmodulin antagonists on the endothelium-dependent relaxation in rabbit aorta. Jpn J Smooth Muscle 1986; 22: 97–102.
60. Duprez DA, Flavahan NA, Vanhoutte PM. Effects of nisoldipine on contractions of isolated canine coronary arteries. In: International Symposium on Calcium Antagonists: Pharmacology and Clinical Research, February 1987, New York (Abstract).
61. Oshiro MEM, Paiva ACM, Paiva TB. Endothelium dependent inhibition of the use of extracellular calcium for the arterial response to vasoconstrictor agents. Gen Pharmacol 1985; 16: 567–72
62. Godfrain T. EDRF and cyclic GMP control gating of receptor operated calcium channels in vascular smooth muscle. Eur J Pharmacol 1986; 126: 341–3.

14. Wave reflections
Clinical and therapeutic aspects

GÉRARD M. LONDON and TOSHIO YAGINUMA

Introduction

Ejection of blood during contraction of the left ventricle generates a pressure wave which is propagated along the arterial tree and which is perceived in the peripheral arteries as the arterial pulse. As the pressure wave moves away from the heart, part of the energy is reflected back at various sites of the arterial tree. The forward and backward pressure waves merge to produce a characteristic arterial pressure wave [1–3] (Figure 1). The existence of wave reflections is demonstrated by at least two fundamental phenomena:
- the radically different shapes of flow and pressure waves in the ascending aorta, since in the absence of reflected waves the flow and pressure waves would be almost identical [1–3]; and
- the different pressure amplitudes and waveforms in the aorta and peripheral arteries, with an increased pulse amplitude along the arterial tree with systolic pressure usually higher and diastolic pressure lower in the peripheral arteries [1–3]. This peripheral amplification of pulse and systolic pressures contrasts with an almost constant mean blood pressure whose pressure drop between ascending aorta and radial artery does not exceed 3 mmHg [4, 5].

Basic physiological concepts

The pressure waveform in the ascending aorta and central arteries is determined by the pattern of left ventricular ejection and aortic input impedance [1–3]. The ascending aortic flow wave is variable in amplitude and duration, but its contour is almost similar in different animal species and under different physiological conditions [3]. In contrast, the pressure wave is variable under different conditions illustrating the importance of the aortic input impedance as a determinant of the arterial pulse shape [3]. Aortic input impedance which describes the relationship between the steady and pulsatile components of ventricular ejection and resulting pressure wave, is a complex, frequency

M. E. Safar and M. F. O'Rourke (eds.), The arterial system in hypertension. pp. 221–237.
© 1993 *Kluwer Academic Publishers. Printed in the Netherlands.*

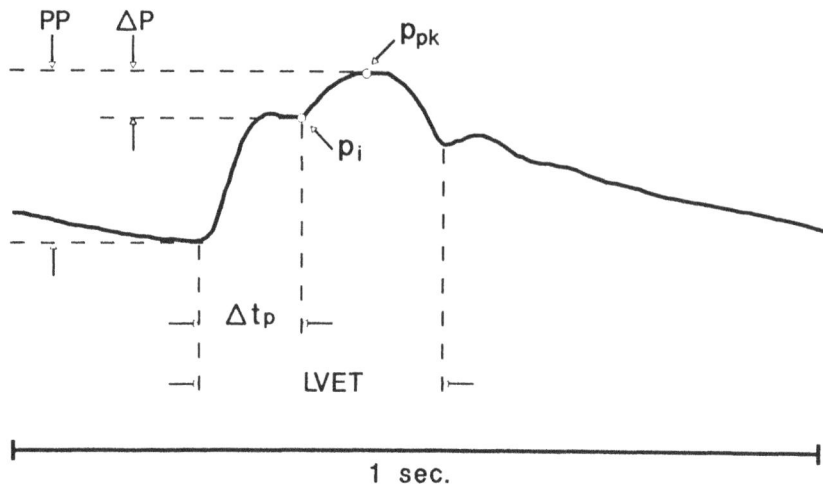

Figure 1. Carotid pressure waveform contour recorded by applanation tonometry. PP-pulse pressure; dP = Ppk-Pi (amplitude of late systolic peak); Pi = early systolic peak; dtp = time travel of reflected wave; dP/PP = augmentation index; LVET = left ventricular ejection time.

dependent quantity determined by the aortic diameter and distensibility, arteriolar tone, and intensity and timing of arterial wave reflections [1–3]. Thus, as a determinant of aortic impedance/arterial wave reflections play an important role in physiology and pathophysiology [1–3].

In the systemic arterial tree, wave reflections are generated wherever there is a discontinuity of arterial caliber(s), distensibility, or any mismatch in the vascular impedances [1–3]. Possible reflecting sites include branching points, sites of diameter and distensibility changes, and the high resistance arterioles which are a major site of wave reflections [1–3]. As the pressure waves travel at a finite velocity, the character and amplitude of arterial wave reflections are somewhat dependent on the location within the arterial tree at which the pressure wave is recorded [1–9]. An important point of observation is the ascending aorta [10–12]. Viewed from the aortic arch, there appears to be a prominent reflecting site in the descending aorta in the region of aortic bifurcation [10–11] in addition to reflection returning from the periphery in the lower body [1–3].

Both the magnitude and timing of the reflected wave(s) are important in assessing their significance and physiological role. Due to spatial dispersion of the reflecting sites and to viscosity of fluids, part of the energy of the forward traveling (incident) pressure wave would be dissipated and pressure wave would decrease continuously along the aorta and arterial tree [1–3]. On the other hand, as pressure travels down, the reflected waves are closer in phase with the incident waves which is therefore reinforced [1–3, 8]. The effect of reflected waves outweighs the viscous damping [1, 2]. Therefore, the wave reflections physiologically limit the (mean) pressure drop along the large conduit arteries having, thus, a beneficial effect on tissue perfusion. The reinforcement of the peripheral pressure by the wave reflections limits the pressure which must be developed by the left ventricle, and thus decreases the fluctuation of pulsatile aortic pressure and left ventricular pressures [3]. As already mentioned, the magnitude of arterial pressure wave reflection, i.e. the reflection coefficient, depends on the relationships of the diameters and distensibility of the successive arterial segments and on arteriolar tone and corresponding peripheral resistances [1–3]. Changes in peripheral resistances have been shown to result in corresponding changes in the wave reflections. An increase in peripheral resistances increases the magnitude of wave reflections, whereas a decrease in resistances induces a decrease in wave reflections [1–3].

An important aspect of arterial wave reflections is the timing of incident and reflected waves. This is particularly true for wave reflections as seen from the aorta and central arteries with regard to the duration of left ventricular ejection. Since a reflected pressure wave adds to the forward wave, a wave returning during systolic ejection would increase the end systolic pressure and ventricular afterload and would be disadvantageous for ventricular ejection (since the reflected flow wave which is theoretically generated by the backward pressure would subtract from the forward flow wave) [2, 3, 6, 12, 13]. Opposing the disadvantageous influence of a pressure wave returning early during systole, a wave returning after the peak forward pressure (Figure 1, lower panel) or during the early diastole would increase the diastolic pressure time index creating favorable conditions for the coronary perfusion and improving the ventricular/vascular coupling [2, 3, 12]. The timing of wave reflections in the ascending aorta is under the influence of three principal factors: (1) the propagation velocity of the pulse wave; (2) the distance of the reflecting site(s); and (3) the duration of the left ventricular ejection [1–3, 13, 14].

In recent years many excellent books and reviews have been devoted to fundamental physical and mathematical aspects of arterial pressure wave reflections and their influence on cardiovascular physiology [1–3, 5, 6, 11–16]. The present brief review will be limited to more clinical aspects of wave reflections, as those accessible to internist and cardiologists in their everyday practice.

The measurement of pressure wave reflections

The most precise information on wave reflections can be obtained from studies of vascular impedance [1–3]. The calculation of aortic input impedance requires measuring simultaneously pulsatile pressure and flow waves and deriving their respective sinusoidal components by Fourier analysis. The necessity to use an invasive catheterisation and complicated mathematical analysis has limited the clinical usefulness of these measurements.

Aortic impedance and the ejection pattern of the left ventricle determine the pulse pressure waveform in the ascending aorta and central arteries, and it has been demonstrated that the pulse pressure contour analysis provides information about the characteristics of arterial system in accepting pulsatile flow from the heart [1–3, 10, 11, 16]. The aortic and central arteries pulse pressure waveform in man has been well characterized and generally shown to manifest an inflection point which divides the pressure wave into an early (Pi) and mid-to-late systolic peak (Ppk) (Figure 1). The measured pressure waveform consists of both a forward incident, and backward reflected wave [5, 6, 10, 11, 14, 16]. The mid-to-late systolic peak is taken to be the result of the reflected wave returning from the peripheral site(s) and causing an increase in pulse pressure and systolic pressure [10, 11, 16]. This increase is the height of Ppk above Pi (Ppk-Pi = dP in mmHg). The ratio of dP to the pulse pressure (PP) defines an augmentation index (dP/PP) [5–7, 11, 12, 16]. The time (dtp) from the foot of the pressure wave to the foot of late systolic peak has been interpreted to represent the time of travel of the pulse wave to peripheral reflecting site(s) and its return back [5, 6, 7, 11, 12, 16] (Figure 1). The dtp is theoretically determined by the distance (L) to reflecting site(s) and the pulse wave velocity (PWV). Using the measurement of aortic PWV, the 'effective' length of arterial segments to reflecting site(s) could be determined as: $L = PWV*dtp/2$ [1–3, 10, 16]. Murgo et al. [11, 16] demonstrated a good correlation between this formula and the quarter-wave length formula, which is the method for estimating the distance to the reflection site(s) in the frequency domain: $L = PWV/4 f_{min}$, (where f_{min} is the frequency of the first minimum of the modulus of systemic input impedance). From these equations it can be derived that $f_{min} = 1/(2 dtp)$ [5–7, 10, 16]. According to the shape of aortic pressure wave and dP/PP ratio, Murgo et al. [11, 16] have divided patients in three subgroups: Type A where the Ppk occurs in late systole after inflection Pi and dP/PP > to 12%; Type C where inflection point Pi occurs after the systolic peak and dP/PP < 0, i.e. negative (Figure 1, lower panel)); Type B having the same characteristics as type A but with values of dP/PP between 0% and 12%. Study of the relationship between the aortic pressure waveform and aortic input impedance has shown that a larger secondary rise of pulse pressure (increase in dP/PP) is associated with an enhanced oscillatory impedance spectrum due to magnitude of wave reflections [10, 11, 16].

Recent developments in high fidelity applanation tonometry allow noninvasive recording of the arterial pressure waveform and magnitude in both peripheral and central arteries [5, 6, 7, 12, 17]. The high fidelity applanation tonometry has provided the opportunity for more accurate and extensive clinical studies of the effects of arterial wave reflections on cardiovascular function. Principles and details concerning the applanation tonometry have been published in detail [5, 6, 17]. Arterial pressure waveform and amplitude is recorded noninvasively with a pencil-type probe incorporating a high fidelity Millar strain gauge transducer in the tip of the probe (SPT 301, Millar

Instruments, Houston, Texas). The Millar strain gauge transducer possesses a small pressure-sensitive ceramic sensor (0. 5*1. 0 mm) incorporating piezoresistive elements forming two arms of a Wheatstone bridge. The frequency response of the sensor is more than 2 kHz coplanar with a larger area (7 mm diameter) of flat surface, which is in contact with the skin overlying the site of arterial pulse measurement. The tonometer is internally calibrated (1 mV = 1 mmHg) using a conventional Millar preamplifier (TCB 500). The instrument is based on the principles of applanation tonometry as used in ocular tonometry for measuring intraocular pressure. In theory, applanation of a curved surface of a pressure-containing structure equalizes the circumferential stress of the structure wall and allows the sensor to measure true intraarterial pressure. The accuracy of the probe has been validated in humans by comparing direct intra-aortic pressure recordings with indirectly recorded carotid pressure waves [5–7, 17]. A direct and indirect validation of recorded brachial and radial artery pressure were also performed. Comparisons making use of spectral analysis showed an excellent correlation between the direct intraarterial and indirect recordings. Tonometry recordings show a pressure wave with harmonic content that does not significantly differ from that of intra-arterially recorded waves [5–7, 17].

Arterial pulse and wave reflections in man

The principal factors determining the amplitude and timing of pressure wave reflections and their effect on the contour of the pulse wave in ascending aorta are:
– distensibility of the vessels and resulting PWV;
– body shape and height;
– vasomotor tone of resistive vessels; and
– duration of ventricular systole [1–3, 13].
A decrease in arterial distensibility causes an increase in PWV [1–3, 18, 19]. Increased PWV results in a shorter travel time of pressure wave and permits an early return of reflected waves during systole (Figure 2). The reflected wave(s) merge with the systolic part of the incident pulse wave, contributing to an increase in pulse pressure and systolic peak pressure, and the disappearance of the diastolic wave [2, 3, 5, 6]. The role of PWV on the timing of wave reflections could be well documented in certain acute physiological conditions. For example, during the Valsalva maneuver the aortic transmural pressure and PWV decrease, inducing a delayed return of wave reflections [10, 11, 16]. This alteration changes the shape of aortic flow and pressure waves and displaces the late systolic peak through the incisura to form a single wave in diastole. These changes are reversed on release of the Valsalva strain. The reverse of the Valsalva maneuver, the Muller maneuver which increases the aortic transmural pressure and PWV induces an increase in peak systolic pressure [10, 11, 16].

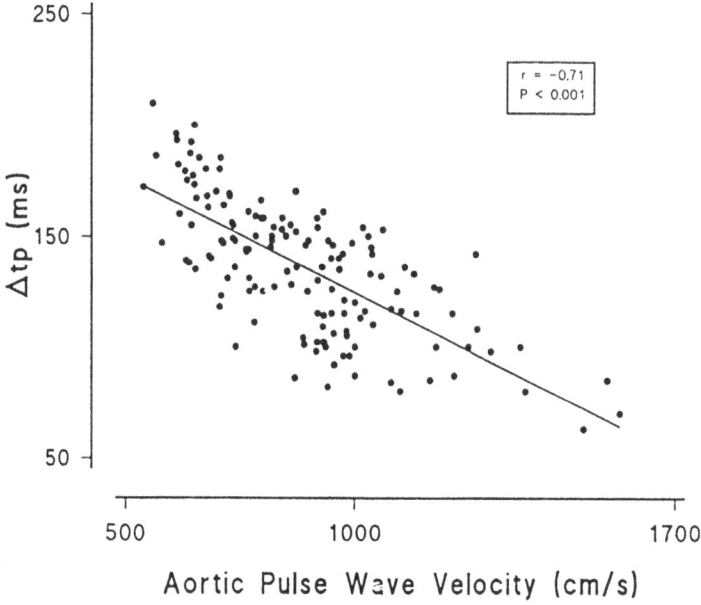

Figure 2. Scatterplot showing the correlation between aortic pulse wave velocity and dtp.

The increased effect of wave reflections and higher systolic pressure which develops with aging (Figures 3 and 4) and hypertension are attributed to the early return of reflected wave(s) due to stiffening of arteries, especially of the aorta [3, 5, 6, 7, 18, 19]. With the increased PWV the sites of reflections 'are closer' to the ascending aorta where the reflected waves tend to be more closely in phase with the incident waves. In these conditions systolic and pulse pressures are already amplified in the aorta itself instead of in the peripheral arteries, as is observed in younger subjects with slow PWV. As a consequence, during aging the pulse pressure amplification between central and peripheral arteries is less pronounced or absent (Figure 5) while the frequency of the first minimum of impedance ($f_{min} = 1/(2$ dtp) increases [1–3, 14]. Besides the alterations in the timing of pressure waves, the changes in arterial pulse during aging, as those described, are also due to alterations in the magnitude of the reflections [1–3]. The appreciation of the role of changes in the magnitude is more difficult [20]. On the one hand, the increase in peripheral vascular resistances and the changes of the diameter of the abdominal aorta during aging could increase the reflection coefficient [1–3, 20]. On the other hand, in the elderly there is an equalisation of the distensibility of the aorta and peripheral conduit arteries [1, 18–20]. This results in an improved matching of proximal to distal impedance which tends to diminish the amount of reflected energy and could partially offset the effects of the increased aortic stiffness [1–3, 20]. Hypertension is a situation of an accelerated aging process [2, 3, 5]. Due to peripheral 'vasoconstriction' and

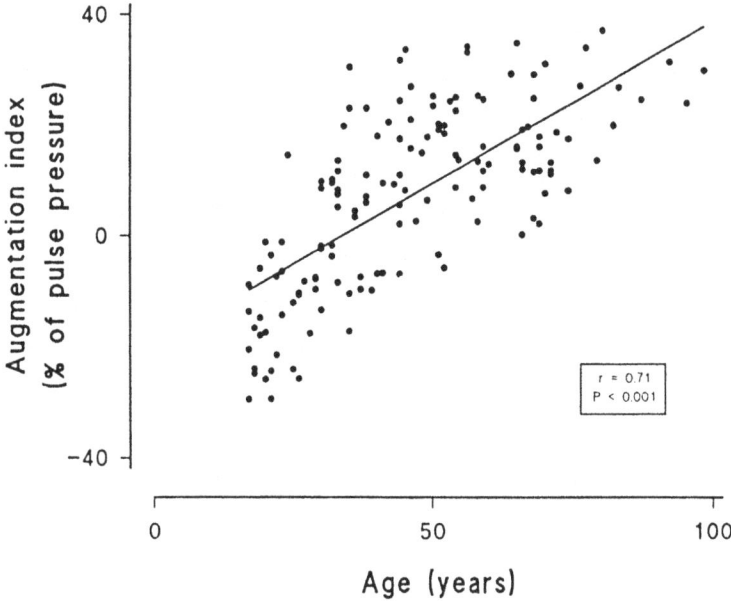

Figure 3. Scatterplot showing the correlation between the carotid augmentation index and age.

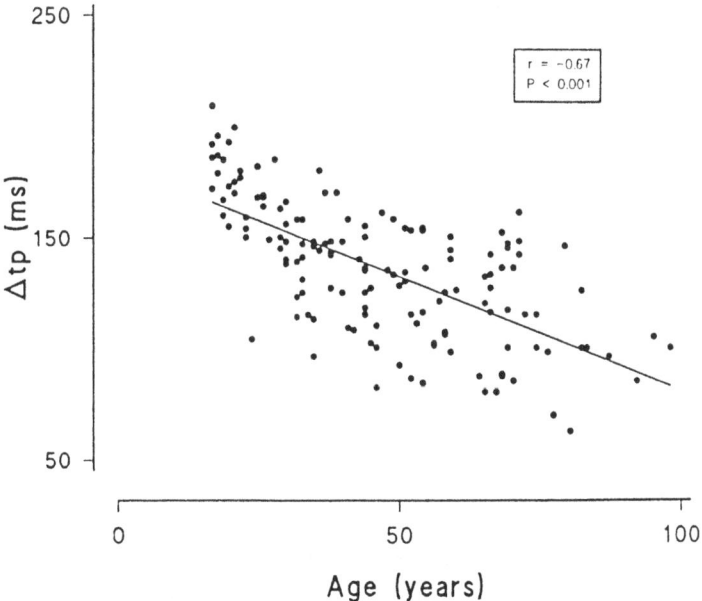

Figure 4. Scatterplot showing the correlation between age and dtp.

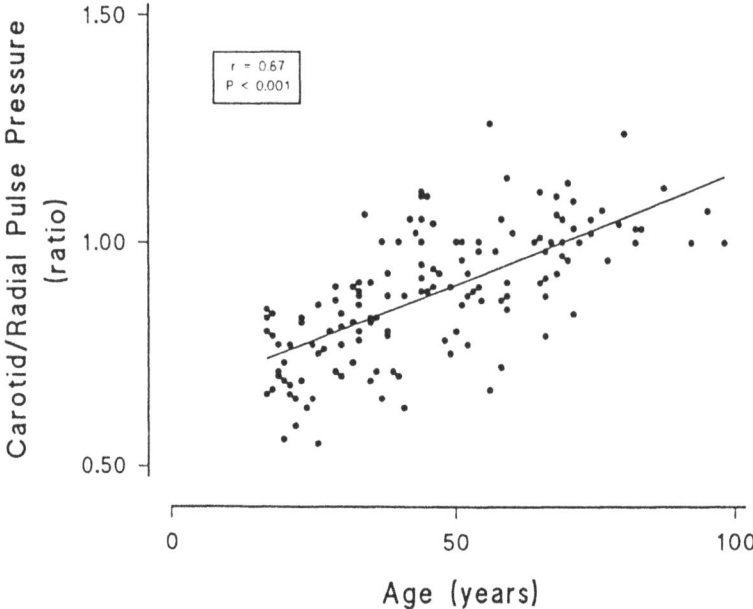

Figure 5. Scatterplot showing the correlation between age and carotid/brachial artery pulse pressure ratio.

increased vascular resistances the pressure amplification in hypertensive patients is related both to a decreased distensibility with altered timing and to an increase in the magnitude of reflections [2, 3, 5, 12].

Comparative physiology has shown that while ventricular ejection, arteriolar tone and arterial PWV are similar in the different mammal species, the shape, amplitude and frequency of the arterial pulse show important interspecies variability, indicating that body size and shape are determinants of vascular impedance, pulse contour and ventricular/vascular coupling [2, 3, 22, 23]. The influence of body size and body shape on wave reflections has several reasons. First, the reduced diameter of the major vessels in small subjects increases the effect of fluid viscosity and increases the resistance to flow [1]. This is evident from the constancy of mean and pulse pressure in subjects of different size and the contrasting direct relationship between the mean and pulsatile flow and body size [1, 22]. Second, in smaller subjects the path length to reflecting sites is shorter with two consequences: a lesser dispersion of reflecting sites and a more intense effect of reflections, and for any given PWV a shorter travel time of the reflected wave (dtp); thus, a higher first minimum of impedance [$f_{min} = 1/(2\ dtp)$] (Figures 6 and 7) [7, 22, 24]. This observation brings to mind the well-known fact that body length is a determinant of optimal heart rate (Figure 8) [22, 23, 25, 26]. This is directly related to the optimal matching of the left ventricular ejection to its hydraulic load, i.e. vascular impedance [2, 3]. The coupling would be optim-

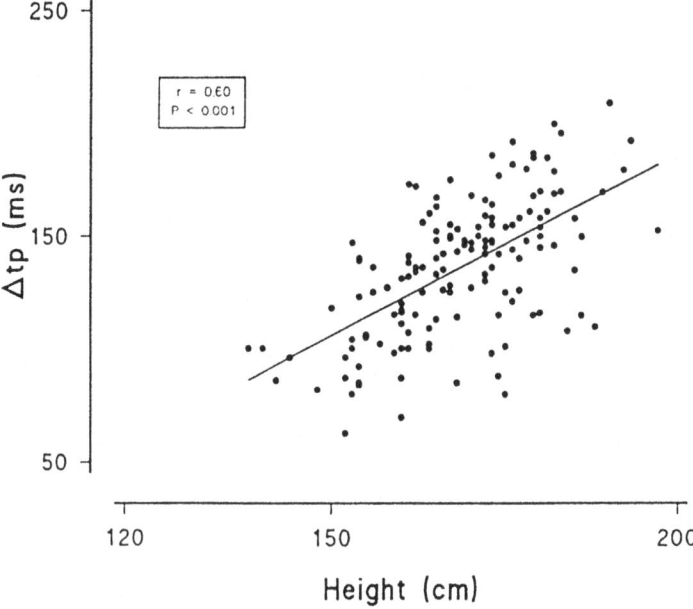

Figure 6. Scatterplot shows the correlation between body height and dtp.

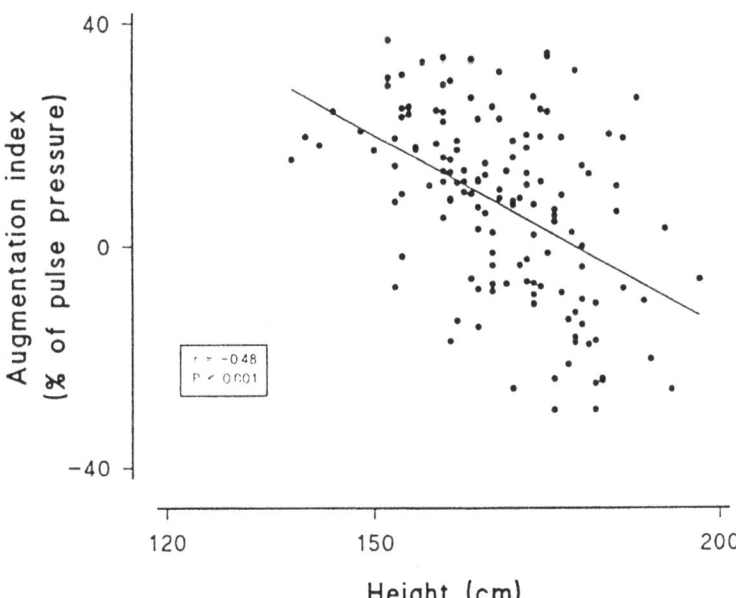

Figure 7. Scatterplot shows the correlation between body height and augmentation index.

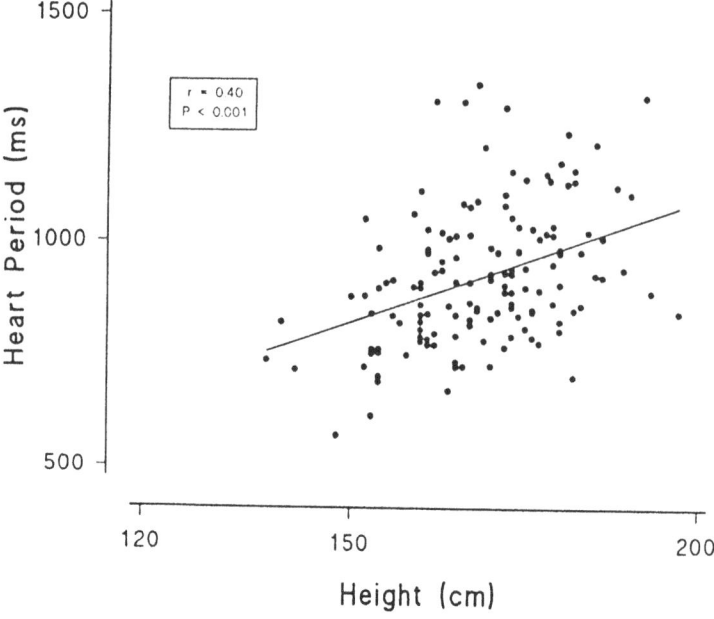

Figure 8. Scatterplot showing the correlation between body height and heart period.

ized when the lower harmonic of the flow wave (corresponding to heart rate-f, and containing the maximum flow) occur at the frequency of f_{min} (minimal value of impedance modulus i.e maximal flow for minimal pressure) [2, 3]. The ventricular/vascular coupling could be expressed in the frequency domain by the f_{min}/f ratio (or in the time domain by the ratio between heart period and dtp). For an optimal f_{min}/f ratio, f_{min} and f should change in parallel. Thus, as f_{min} is determined by body height, body height also determines f. With aging and in hypertension the favorable matching is degraded with 'detuning' [5] of the systemic circulation from the heart as expressed by the increase of f_{min}/f (Figure 9).

The direct relationship between heart rate, f_{min} and body height has another 'positive' consequence on the timing between ventricular ejection and reflected waves. The duration of left ventricular ejection is directly related to the duration of the heart period. Thus, in small subjects with an early return of reflected waves (i.e. short dtp and high f_{min}), the left ventricular ejection time is shorter in relation to shorter heart period. The shortening of the systole limits the possibility of the return of reflected waves during the ventricular systole, and reflections are more readily identified during diastole [3, 7, 13].

Besides the physiological process of aging, the most common conditions characterised by an increased wave reflection and an early return of reflected waves in humans is hypertension [5–7, 12]. Clinical hypertension is usually

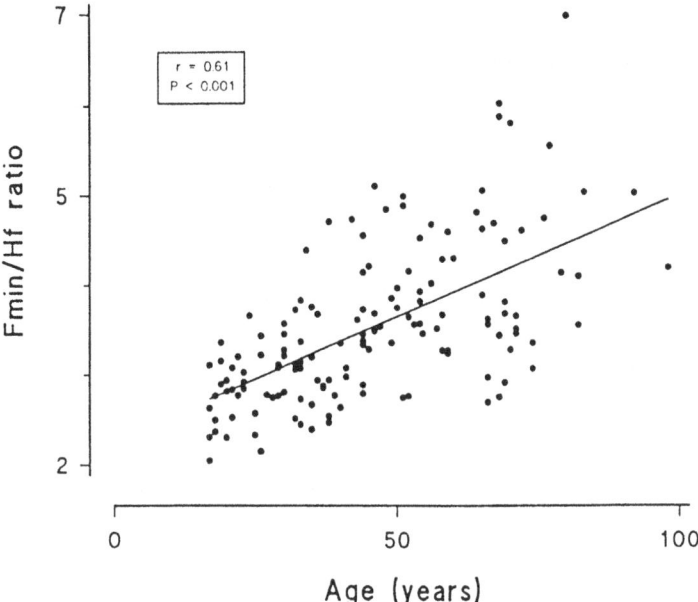

Figure 9. Scatterplot showing the correlation between the ratio of the first minimum of carotid impedance modulus [$f_{min} = 1/(2\ dtp)$] and heart frequency (Hf = 1/heart period).

classified on the basis of raised diastolic blood pressure. However, in recent years the extent of the systolic blood pressure has been reconsidered as being of prime importance in producing cardiovascular morbidity and mortality [27–29]. Analytical studies of arterial function treat blood pressure as a periodic phenomenon that can be divided into two components: a steady component (mean blood pressure) and a pulsatile component (pulse pressure) [1–3]. The mean blood pressure is determined exclusively by cardiac output and vascular resistances [1–3]. The pulse pressure represents the oscillation around this mean, and is determined by the interaction of the incident pressure wave generated by left ventricular ejection, and reflected waves [1–3].

Altered pulsatile arterial hemodynamics has serious ill effects on heart and arteries, and several experimental and clinical studies have shown that pulse pressure is an independent factor to cardiovascular lesions, morbidity and mortality [30–33].

A high prevalence of isolated systolic hypertension is observed in patients with end-stage renal disease (ESRD) [21, 34]. Furthermore, recent studies have shown that the relationship between the steady and pulsatile components of blood pressure is altered in ESRD where the pulse pressure is greater for any given mean pressure and age [7, 21]. Moreover, using applanation tonometry for the measurement of carotid pulse pressure amplitude, it has

Table 1. Carotid pulse wave analysis in ESRD patients and in control subjects

	Control subjects	ESRD patients
Radial artery PP (mmHg)$	60.7 ± 16.1	73.7 ± 22.0****
Carotid artery PP (mmHg)$	57.3 ± 19.6	73.2 ± 25.7****
Carotid PP/Radial PP (ratio)$	0.93 ± 0.14	0.99 ± 0.15**
P_i (mmHg)	47.4 ± 14.2	53.6 ± 15.8***
ΔP (mmHg)	7.5 ± 10.5	19.0 ± 15.2****
$\Delta P/PP$ (%)	9.8 ± 15.6	23.2 ± 15.0****
Δtp (ms)	131 ± 30	109 ± 24****
Heart period (ms)	909 ± 149	840 ± 145***
LVET (ms)	300 ± 26	310 ± 31*
Aortic PWV (cm/s)	930 ± 196	1035 ± 238***

Values are mean ± SD.
$Measurements with Millar micromanometer.
*P < 0.05; **P < 0.02; ***P < 0.01; ****P < 0.001.
Abbreviations: ESRD, end-stage renal disease; PP, pulse pressure; P_i, pressure at inflection point; a P (mmHg) = P_{PK}-P_i, amplitude of late systolic peak; $\Delta P/PP$ (%) = P_{PK}-P_i/PP, augmentation index; Δtp, travel time of reflected wave; LVET, left ventricular ejection time; PWV, pulse wave velocity.

been shown that for any given brachial artery pulse pressure, the carotid artery pulse pressure was increased in ESRD patients,. in comparison with nonuremic control subjects (Table 1) [7]. The increased aortic pulse pressure in ESRD was related to an increase in incident as well as reflected pressure waves, and to an early return of the reflected waves [7]. These alterations are due to a longer ejection of a higher stroke volume in a stiffer aorta which propagates the pressure wave at a higher velocity in an arterial tree of shorter 'effective' length [7]. The increased stroke volume is related to anemia, arteriovenous fistula used as an access to blood for dialysis [35]. The decreased aortic distensibility is related to accelerated arterial degeneration observed in these patients [21, 36], and the shorter arterial tree is associated to lesser body height due to growth retardation observed in azotemic children and in young adults [7]. Early wave reflection and resulting ventricular/vascular mismatch is an independent factor to left ventricular and septal hypertrophy [37] which is the most frequent cardiovascular abnormality in ESRD patients [35, 38, 39].

Therapeutic aspects

Many drugs used in the treatment of cardiovascular diseases exert their action by changing the intensity or timing of wave reflections brought about by alterations in vascular properties. In clinical studies of vasoactive drugs, the radial or brachial arterial pressure are assumed to reflect pressure changes in the overall arterial tree. This assumption can be accepted for the mean blood pressure which remains almost constant along the conduit arteries, but not for systolic and pulse pressures which are amplified toward the periphery by wave reflections. The effect of wave reflection on the augmentation of late systolic pressure is seen in the carotid pressure wave, the ascending aortic pressure wave, and the left ventricular pressure wave in mature humans [1–3, 5–7, 12, 40–42]. In contrast, the systolic fluctuation due to wave reflection occurs later in peripheral arteries than in central arteries, contributing little or nothing to the systolic peak and pulse pressure amplitude [1, 3, 5, 6, 12]. This is an important point since therapeutical efficiency of drugs is interpreted from pressure recordings in brachial artery, which do not necessarily reflect pressure changes in central arteries. Indeed, drugs which decrease or delay wave reflections would decrease aortic pressure (largely influenced by reflected waves) more than brachial or peripheral systolic and pulse pressure (less or not influenced by wave reflections). Recent studies have indeed shown that changes in systolic and pulse pressure in aorta and central arteries could be induced by various drug independently of changes in pressure in peripheral arteries [12, 39–43].

The hemodynamic effects of antihypertensive agents are usually analyzed in terms of a linear model of the circulation. Accordingly, antihypertensive agents are known to decrease mean blood pressure by alterations of cardiac output or vascular resistances. Studies of pulsatile arterial hemodynamics indicate that antihypertensive agents should not only affect mean blood pressure, but may also induce important changes in the pulsatile components of blood pressure dissociated from changes in mean pressure [40–44]. The antihypertensive drugs (and vasodilators in general) can change the intensity and/or the timing of wave reflection by several mechanisms.

The decrease in the intensity of wave reflection could be due to:
– decreased peripheral resistance and decreased reflection coefficient [1–3]; and
– an increase in the cross-sectional area ratio at arterial branching by dilation of smaller conduit arteries proximal to arterioles [5, 40, 43].

An alteration in the timing of wave reflection could be achieved by delaying the return of reflected waves and/or to a lesser degree by shortening the ventricular ejection [2, 3, 13, 44]. The delay in the return of reflected wave results from a decrease in arterial PWV whether related to decrease in blood pressure or to eventual alterations of the intrinsic viscoelastic properties of arterial walls.

With antihypertensive therapy in man, changes in arterial pressure wave contour and impedance are usually due to a combination of effects on intensity and timing of wave reflections. Antihypertensive agents with vasodilator properties (nitroprussite, ACE inhibitors, calcium channel blockers) reduce intensity of wave reflection by arteriolar vasodilation (decreased peripheral resistances) and by delay in the return of reflected waves (decreased PWV) [12, 40–44, 45]. As the reflected wave in mature adult humans constitutes

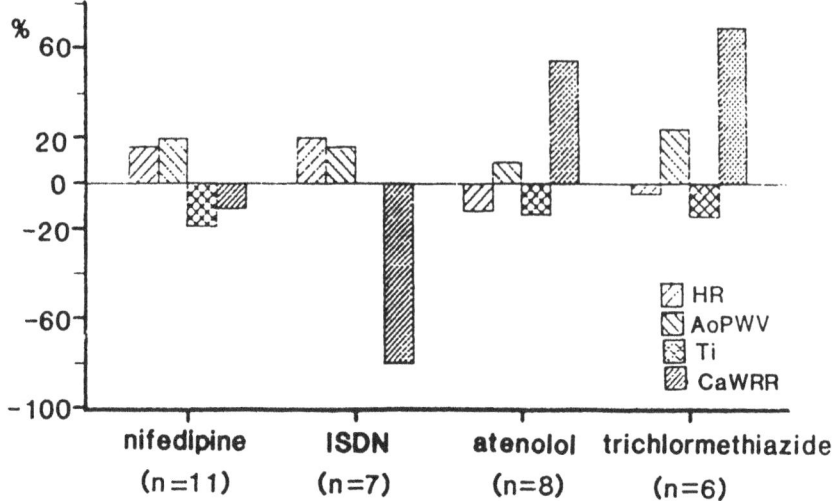

Figure 10. Effects of four antihypertensive drugs on carotid pulse waveform. Percent change in hemodynamic parameters taken from hypertensive patients after more than two weeks therapy were compared with age and mean blood pressure matched subjects. HR: heart rate; AoPWV: aortic pulse wave velocity; Ti = tp, CaWRR = P/PP as in Figure 1 [45].

the late systolic peak in central but not in peripheral arteries, the pressure recorded in brachial artery underestimate the pressure changes in the aorta and left ventricle [2, 3, 5, 6, 12, 40–43]. Atenolol, a beta blocking agent without vasodilator properties, increases peripheral resistances and the intensity of wave reflections (Figure 10) [12, 45, 46]. It decreases the aortic PWV and delays the return of the reflected wave [44]. This potentially beneficial effect is offset by the bradycardia and parallel increase in the duration of left ventricular ejection [44]. In contrast to atenolol, the vasodilating beta-blocking agent dilevalol consistently reduces the intensity of wave reflections with a greater fall in central aortic systolic pressure compared to atenolol [12].

In congestive heart failure, the peripheral resistances are increased and peripheral wave reflections augmented [14]. Beneficial effects of vasodilators in heart failure are explicable on the basis of reduction of the intensity and improved timing of wave reflection [14, 40–43]. In these patients the radial and brachial arterial pressure measurements may be a poor guide to the beneficial effect of these medications on left ventricular systolic pressure [40–43].

The effect of nitrates which are widely used in cardiovascular medicine appears to be strikingly different from the previously mentioned drugs. Indeed, the previously mentioned vasodilator and antihypertensive agents act by a combined effect on the intensity and timing of wave reflection, decreasing blood pressure and PWV, and reducing the peripheral resistances. Nitroglycerin decreases the ascending aortic and left ventricular pressure. This effect is not caused by arteriolar dilatation and fall in peripheral resistances, and it occurs without any change in aortic distensibility and/or PWV [40–42]. The major effect of nitrates is to decrease the intensity of reflected wave but without decreasing the terminal (arteriolar) reflection coefficient. Nitrates do that by increasing the caliber and distensibility of small conduit arteries proximal to the arterioles, increasing the cross-sectional area ratio at these arterial branching sites, thus decreasing the amplitude of reflected waves at this level [5, 40, 42]. As with other drugs which reduce the wave reflections, the effect of nitrates on systolic pressure is more pronounced in the ascending aorta and central arteries than peripheral arteries.

One of the best examples of the beneficial 'manipulation' of wave reflection in medical therapy is arterial counterpulsation. Arterial counterpulsation is a method of mechanical heart assistance in which a balloon, located in the descending aorta, is inflated and deflated in synchrony with the heart pulsation. The cycle is timed as to reduce the systolic pressure in the aorta, reducing the ventricular afterload and oxygen consumption. To the contrary, the balloon is inflated after the closure of aortic valves, generating a pressure wave in the descending aorta which returns centripetally in the diastolic interval, increasing the diastolic-pressure time index and boosting the coronary blood flow. Counterpulsation represents an exaggerated form of wave reflection but must be adequately timed so as to ensure an optimal ventricular/vascular coupling [3, 5]. Aging in man has the same effect as inappropriately timed counterpulsation, with increase in pressure during systole, and relative decrease during diastole [2, 3]. A logical therapeutic strategy in older humans is to offset this unfavorable effect of early wave reflection by reducing or delaying the reflected waves [5, 9, 40–44].

References

1. Milnor WR. Hemodynamics, 2nd ed. Baltimore: Williams & Wilkins 1989: 204–59.
2. Nichols WW, O'Rourke MF. In: McDonald's Blood Flow in Arteries: theoretic, experimental and clinical principles. 3rd ed. London; Edward Arnold 1991: 251–69; 281: 329.
3. O'Rourke MF. Arterial Function in Health and Disease. Edinburgh; Churchill Livingstone 1982: 77–182.
4. Kroeker EJ, Wood EH. Comparison of simultaneously recorded central and peripheral arterial pressure pulses during rest, exercise and tilted position in man. Circ Res 1955; 3: 623–32.
5. O'Rourke MF, Kelly R, Avolio A. The arterial pulse in cardiovascular disease. In: The arterial pulse. Philadelphia; Lea & Febiger 1992: 21–197.
6. Kelly R, Hayward C, Avolio A, O'Rourke M. Noninvasive determination of Age-Related Changes in the Human Arterial Pulse. Circulation 1989; 80: 1652–9.
7. London GM, Guerin AP, Pannier B, Marchais SJ, Benetos A, Safar ME. Increased systolic pressure in chronic uremia: Role of arterial wave reflections. Hypertension 1992; 20: 10–9.

8. Burattini R, Knowlen GG, Campbell KB. Two arterial effective reflecting sites may appear as one to the heart. Circ Res 1991; 68: 85–99.

9. O'Rourke MF, Yaginuma T. Wave Reflections and the Arterial Pulse. Arch Intern Med 1984; 144: 366–71.

10. Latham RD, Westerhof N, Sipkema P, Rubal BJ, Reuderink P, Murgo JP. Regional wave travel and reflection along the human aorta: a study with six simultaneous micromanometric pressures. Circulation 1985; 72: 1257–69.

11. Murgo JP, Westerhof N, Giolma JP, Altobelli SA. Aortic Input Impedance in Normal Man: Relationship to Pressure Wave Forms. Circulation 1980; 62: 105–16.

12. Kelly R, Daley J, Avolio A, O'Rourke M. Arterial Dilation and Reduced Wave Reflection: Benefit of Dilevalol in Hypertension. Hypertension 1989; 14: 14–21.

13. Fitchett H. LV-arterial coupling: interactive model to predict effect of wave reflections on LV energetics. Am J Physiol (Heart Circ. Physiol. 30); 1991; 261: H1026–H33.

14. Laskey WK, Kussmaul WG. Arterial wave reflection in heart failure. Circulation 1987; 75: 711–22.

15. Nichols WW, O'Rourke MF, Avolio AP, Yaginuma T, Pepine CJ, Onti R. Ventricular/vascular interaction in patients with mild systemic hypertension and normal peripheral resistance. Circulation 1986; 74: 455–62.

16. Murgo JP, Westerhof N, Giolma JP, Altobelli SA. Manipulation of ascending aortic pressure and flow wave reflections with the Valsalva maneuver: relationship to input impedance. Circulation 1981; 63: 122–32.

17. Kelly R, Hayward C, Ganis J, Daley J, Avolio A, O'Rourke M. Noninvasive Registration of the Arterial Pressure Pulse Wave form Using High-Fidelity Applanation Tonometry. J Vasc Med Biol 1989; 1: 142–9.

18. Avolio AO, Chen SG, Wang RP, Zhang Cl, Li MF, O'Rourke MF. Effects of Aging on Changing Arterial Compliance and Left Ventricular Load in a Northern Chinese Urban Community. Circulation 1983; 68: 50–8.

19. Avolio AP, Deng FQ, Li WQ, Luo YF, Huang ZD, Xing LF, O'Rourke MF. Effects of aging on arterial distensibility in populations with high and low prevalence of hypertension: comparison between urban and rural communities in China. Circulation 1985; 71: 202–10.

20. Greenwald SE, Carter AC, Berry CL. Effect of Age on the In Vitro Reflection Coefficient of the Aorto-iliac Bifurcation in Humans. Circulation 1990; 82: 114–23.

21. London GM, Marchais SJ, Safar ME, et al. Aortic and large artery compliance in end-stage renal failure. Kidney Int 1990; 37: 137–42.

22. Gow BS, O'Rourke MF. Comparison of pressure and flow in the ascending aorta of different mammals. Proceedings, Australian Physiol and Pharmacol Soc 1970: 1–68.

23. Avolio AP, O'Rourke MF, Mang K, Bason PT, Gow BS. A comparative study of arterial pulsatile hemodynamics in rabbits and guinea pigs. Am J Physiol 1976; 230: 868–75.

24. London GM, Guerin AP, Pannier BM, Marchais SJ, Metivier F. Body height as a determinant of carotid pulse contour in humans. J Hypertens 1992; 10(Suppl 6): S93–S5.

25. Milnor WR. Aortic wavelength as a determinant of the relation between body size and heart rate in mammals. Am J Physiol 1979; 237: R3–R6.

26. O'Rourke MF. Commentary on aortic wavelength as a determinant of the relationship between heart rate and body size in mammals. Am J Physiol 1981; 240: R393–R5.

27. Kannel WB, Dawber TR, McGee DL. Perspectives on systolic hypertension: The Framingham Study. Circulation 1980; 61: 1179–82.

28. Curb JD, Borhani NO, Entwisle G, et al. Isolated systolic hypertension in 14 communities. Am J Epidemiol 1985; 121: 362–70.

29. SHEP cooperative research group. Prevention of stroke by antihypertensive drug treatment in older persons with isolated systolic hypertension: final results of the systolic hypertension in the elderly program. J Am Med Assoc 1991; 265: 3255–64.

30. Hajdu MA, Heistad DD, Baumbach GL. Effects of antihypertensive treatment on mechanics of cerebral arterioles in rats. Hypertension 1990; 17: 308–16.

31. Baumbach GL, Siems JE, Heistad DD. Effects of local reduction in pressure on distensibility and composition of cerebral arterioles. Circ Res 1991; 68: 338–51.
32. Christensen KL. Reducing pulse pressure in hypertension may normalize small artery structure. Hypertension 1990; 18: 722–7.
33. Darne B, Girerd X, Safar M, Cambien F, Guize L. Pulsatile versus steady component of Blood pressure: A cross-sectional and prospective Analysis of cardiovascular mortality. Hypertension 1989; 13: 392–400.
34. Simon P, Ang KS, Benziane A. Hypertension arterielle systolique isolée chez l'urémique chronique hémodialysé. Arch Mal Coeur 1991; 84: 1205–10.
35. London GM, Fabiani F. Left ventricular dysfunction in end-stage renal disease: echocardiographic insights. In: Parfrey PS, Harnett JD, editors. Cardiac dysfunction in chronic uremia. Boston: Kluwer Academic 1992: 117–37.
36. Lindner A, Charra B, Sherrard DJ, Scribner BH. Accelerated atherosclerosis in prolonged maintenance hemodialysis. N Engl J Med 1974; 290: 697–701.
37. London GM, Guerin AP, Pannier BM, Marchais SJ, Metivier F, Safar ME. Relation of left ventricular mass to arterial wave reflections in chronic uremia. Hypertension 1993; (in press).
38. Hüting J, Kramer W, Schutterle G, Wizemann V. Analysis of left-ventricular changes associated with chronic hemodialysis. A non-invasive follow-up study. Nephron 1988; 49: 284–90.
39. Harnett JD, Parfrey PS, Griffiths SM, Gault MH, Barre P, Guttmann RD. Left ventricular hypertrophy in end-stage renal disease. Nephron 1988; 48: 107–5.
40. Yaginuma T, Avolio AP, O'Rourke M, et al. Effect of glyceryl trinitrate on peripheral arteries alters left ventricular hydraulic load in man. Cardiovasc Res 1986; 20: 153–60.
41. Fitchett D, Simkus G, Genest J, Beaudry J, Marpole D. Reflected pressure waves in the ascending aorta: effect of glyceryl trinitrate. Cardiovasc Res 1988; 22: 494–500.
42. Simkus GJ, Fitchett DH. Radial artery pressure measurements may be a poor guide to the beneficial effects of nitroprusside on left ventricular systolic pressure in congestive heart failure. Am J Cardiol 1990; 66: 323–6.
43. Kelly R, Gibbs H, O'Rourke M, et al. Nitroglycerin has more favourable effects on left ventricular afterload than apparent from measurement of pressure in a peripheral artery. Eur Heart J 1990; 11: 138–44.
44. Guerin AP, Pannier BM, Marchais SJ, Metivier F, Safar ME, London GM. Effects of antihypertensive agents on carotid pulse contour in humans. J of Human Hypertension 1992; 6 (Suppl 2): S37–S40.
45. Fujii M, Yaginuma T, et al. Non invasive detection for wave reflection in the arterial system, by using carotid pulse wave, and its clinical implication. J Coll Angio 1989; 29: 545–51.
46. Ting CT, Chou CY, Chang MS, Wang SP, Chiang BN, Yin FCP. Arterial hemodynamics in human hypertension. Effects of adrenergic blockade. Circulation 1991; 84: 1049–57.

Developments in Cardiovascular Medicine

121. S. Sideman, R. Beyar and A.G. Kleber (eds.): *Cardiac Electrophysiology, Circulation, and Transport.* Proceedings of the 7th Henry Goldberg Workshop (Berne, Switzerland, 1990). 1991   ISBN 0-7923-1145-0
122. D.M. Bers: *Excitation-Contraction Coupling and Cardiac Contractile Force.* 1991
                                                                ISBN 0-7923-1186-8
123. A.-M. Salmasi and A.N. Nicolaides (eds.): *Occult Atherosclerotic Disease.* Diagnosis, Assessment and Management. 1991   ISBN 0-7923-1188-4
124. J.A.E. Spaan: *Coronary Blood Flow.* Mechanics, Distribution, and Control. 1991
                                                                ISBN 0-7923-1210-4
125. R.W. Stout (ed.): *Diabetes and Atherosclerosis.* 1991   ISBN 0-7923-1310-0
126. A.G. Herman (ed.): *Antithrombotics.* Pathophysiological Rationale for Pharmacological Interventions. 1991   ISBN 0-7923-1413-1
127. N.H.J. Pijls: *Maximal Myocardial Perfusion as a Measure of the Functional Significance of Coronary Arteriogram.* From a Pathoanatomic to a Pathophysiologic Interpretation of the Coronary Arteriogram. 1991   ISBN 0-7923-1430-1
128. J.H.C. Reiber and E.E. v.d. Wall (eds.): *Cardiovascular Nuclear Medicine and MRI.* Quantitation and Clinical Applications. 1992   ISBN 0-7923-1467-0
129. E. Andries, P. Brugada and R. Stroobrandt (eds.): *How to Face 'the Faces' of Cardiac Pacing.* 1992   ISBN 0-7923-1528-6
130. M. Nagano, S. Mochizuki and N.S. Dhalla (eds.): *Cardiovascular Disease in Diabetes.* 1992   ISBN 0-7923-1554-5
131. P.W. Serruys, B.H. Strauss and S.B. King III (eds.): *Restenosis after Intervention with New Mechanical Devices.* 1992   ISBN 0-7923-1555-3
132. P.J. Walter (ed.): *Quality of Life after Open Heart Surgery.* 1992
                                                                ISBN 0-7923-1580-4
133. E.E. van der Wall, H. Sochor, A. Righetti and M.G. Niemeyer (eds.): *What's new in Cardiac Imaging?* SPECT, PET and MRI. 1992   ISBN 0-7923-1615-0
134. P. Hanrath, R. Uebis and W. Krebs (eds.): *Cardiovascular Imaging by Ultrasound.* 1992   ISBN 0-7923-1755-6
135. F.H. Messerli (ed.): *Cardiovascular Disease in the Elderly.* 3rd ed. 1992
                                                                ISBN 0-7923-1859-5
136. J. Hess and G.R. Sutherland (eds.): *Congenital Heart Disease in Adolescents and Adults.* 1992   ISBN 0-7923-1862-5
137. J.H.C. Reiber and P.W. Serruys (eds.): *Advances in Quantitative Coronary Arteriography.* 1993   ISBN 0-7923-1863-3
138. A.-M. Salmasi and A.S. Iskandrian (eds.): *Cardiac Output and Regional Flow in Health and Disease.* 1993   ISBN 0-7923-1911-7
139. J.H. Kingma, N.M. van Hemel and K.I. Lie (eds.): *Atrial Fibrillation, a Treatable Disease?* 1992   ISBN 0-7923-2008-5
140. B. Ostadel and N.S. Dhalla (eds.): *Heart Function in Health and Disease.* Proceedings of the Cardiovascular Program (Prague, Czechoslovakia, 1991). 1992
                                                                ISBN 0-7923-2052-2
141. D. Noble and Y.E. Earm (eds.): *Ionic Channels and Effect of Taurine on the Heart.* Proceedings of an International Symposium (Seoul, Korea , 1992). 1993
                                                                ISBN 0-7923-2199-5
142. H.M. Piper and C.J. Preusse (eds.): *Ischemia-reperfusion in Cardiac Surgery.* 1993
                                                                ISBN 0-7923-2241-X
143. J. Roelandt, E.J. Gussenhoven and N. Bom (eds.): *Intravascular Ultrasound.* 1993
                                                                ISBN 0-7923-2301-7
144. M.E. Safar and M.F. O'Rourke (eds.): *The Arterial System in Hypertension.* 1993
                                                                ISBN 0-7923-2343-2
145. P.W. Serruys, D.P. Foley and P.J. de Feyter (eds.): *Quantitative Coronary Angiography in Clinical Practice.* 1993 (in prep.)   ISBN 0-7923-2368-8

Developments in Cardiovascular Medicine

Previous volumes are still available

KLUWER ACADEMIC PUBLISHERS – DORDRECHT / BOSTON / LONDON

The manufacturer's authorised representative in the EU is Springer
Nature Customer Service Centre GmbH, Europaplatz 3, 69115 Heidelberg,
Germany. If you have any concerns regarding our products, please
contact ProductSafety@springernature.com

Printed and bound by CPI Group (UK) Ltd, Croydon, CR0 4YY

29/04/2026

02099460-0006